The WHOLE WOMAN

The WHOLE WOMAN

Take Charge of Your Health
in Every Phase of Your Life

LILA A. WALLIS, M.D., M.A.C.P.
WITH MARIAN BETANCOURT

Illustrated by Hilda R. Muinos

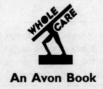

An Avon Book

This book is meant to educate women about their health and suggest ways in which to care for their health. It is also meant to encourage women to enter into a partnership with their physicians and healthcare professionals. What we know about health and how we treat and prevent illness is constantly changing, so it is vital to use this book only as a guide to getting the best healthcare possible, in tandem with a doctor's recommendations and not as a substitute for a doctor's care.

AVON BOOKS, INC.
1350 Avenue of the Americas
New York, New York 10019

Text copyright © 1999 by Lila A. Wallis and Marian Betancourt
Illustrations © 1999 by Hilda R. Muinos
Published by arrangement with the author
ISBN: 0-380-78081-X
www.avonbooks.com/wholecare

Library of Congress Cataloging in Publication Data:

Wallis, Lila A., 1921–
The whole woman : take charge of your health in every phase of your life / Lila A. Wallis with Marian Betancourt ; illustrated by Hilda R. Muinos.
p.   cm.
"An Avon book."
Includes bibliographical references and index.
1. Women—Health and hygiene.   2. Health education of women.
3. Self-care, Health.   I. Betancourt, Marian.   II. Title.
RA778.W2163   1999   99-20885
613'.04244—dc21   CIP

First WholeCare Printing: May 1999

WHOLECARE TRADEMARK REG. U.S. PAT. OFF. AND IN OTHER COUNTRIES,
MARCA REGISTRADA, HECHO EN U.S.A.

Printed in the U.S.A.

QPM   10   9   8   7   6   5   4   3   2   1

Dedicated to my husband, children, grandchildren,
and to the memory of my mother.
—L.A.W.

●   ●   ●   ●

This is for Karen, Mary Ellen, Hilary, and Julia.
—M.B.

Acknowledgments

• • • •

During nearly fifty years of practicing medicine I have had the privilege of caring for thousands of women. And as a professor of medicine at Cornell Medical College, I have had the added advantage of teaching hundreds of medical students and doctors. I have benefited enormously from these experiences, and from my own early education with a long line of distinguished teachers and colleagues. I am but one link in this chain.

The wisdom I have gained over the years as a physician also came from my patients who shared their views with me about their health and the care they were receiving. I am grateful and pleased for this opportunity to share this acquired knowledge, not only with my students and patients but with all women. This book is my expression of thanks to my teachers from both sides: my colleagues and my patients.

—L.A.W.

We are grateful to our editors, Lisa Considine, who acquired the book while at Avon Books, and Ann McKay Thoroman, who then took it over and continued the commitment and hard work in bringing it to fruition. We also want to thank our literary agent, Vicky Bijur, for her continuing commitment to this book.

—L.A.W / M.B.

Contents

• • • •

PHASE II: AGES 20–45
THE ADULT WOMAN

Introduction:
Why Women Are Special

Before I tell you what's in this book, I want to tell you a story about Margaret, who is only one example of how women are put at great risk by the health care system when it fails to understand how women's bodies—and health care needs—are different from men's.

Margaret, at 38, had never experienced a pain like the one that shot into her upper back and shoulder blade when she tried to get out of bed one morning. After a few minutes the pain subsided, but when she tried to get out of bed, it returned. Her husband called their primary care doctor, who told him to take Margaret to the emergency room. When Margaret tried to dress, the pain became more severe and she began perspiring profusely. Her husband called an ambulance, and a neighbor came to stay with their two small children. Covered with an old robe, Margaret was carried on a stretcher to the ambulance. On the way to the ER, the pain went away and she stopped perspiring.

The resident on duty in the ER took an electrocardiogram (EKG) and found nothing abnormal, although he had no previous EKG for comparison. Margaret's blood pressure was a bit high, but her urine and blood tests were normal. A sonogram showed several calcified gallstones, and a gastrointestinal series of tests showed a hiatus hernia. By the time the tests were done, Margaret's pain was gone. She had lost interest in pursing the cause of her pain and was eager to get home to her children.

The resident phoned the family doctor, and after they conferred, Margaret was diagnosed with gallbladder disease and hiatus hernia, rupture of the stomach into the chest through a small opening (hiatus) in the diaphragm. The pain, the doctors decided, could be from either one of those conditions. The resident gave Margaret a pill for her blood pressure and an antacid gel for indigestion. He told her to report to her own doctor in three days. The next day Margaret's pain returned

1

worse than ever. Trying to get out of bed, she collapsed and died. An autopsy revealed extensive coronary artery disease.

While the workup in the ER seemed thorough, the tests only clouded the cause of Margaret's pain, and the correct diagnosis. In women, angina (chest pain) is different than in men. Pain may not be in the chest, but it can shoot up to the back and shoulder. Such pain is often stimulated by exertion, or it can be caused by mental stress. Neither doctor took into consideration Margaret's weight (210 pounds at five-foot-five), her mild diabetes, or her smoking habit (a pack of cigarettes a day), all of which had canceled out most of her biological advantage of being female and being protected from cardiovascular disease by the ovarian hormone, estrogen. Had they taken a thorough medical history from Margaret, her doctors would have learned that her menstrual cycle had been irregular recently, indicating a lowered estrogen level and possible early entry into menopause. Heart disease should not have been ruled out with one single EKG.

Had Margaret been more aware of her own health risks, and how her obesity, cigarette smoking, elevated blood pressure, family history of diabetes, and her irregular periods endangered her cardiac status, she could have alerted the doctor and insisted on having follow-up EKGs, perhaps every twenty-four hours. Such monitoring could have uncovered silent ischemia (poor oxygenation of the cardiac muscle) or arrhythmia (abnormal rhythm indicating malfunctioning of the cardiac conducting system). Had Margaret and her doctors had more insight, they would have ordered a carefully performed stress test under the vigilant supervision of a cardiologist—which would likely have led to a coronary arteriography and a correct diagnosis.

Angioplasty or a bypass surgery would have prevented Margaret's death, and drastic changes in her lifestyle would have stopped or even reversed the coronary disease. Margaret could have grown into a healthy and mature woman and enjoyed watching her children and grandchildren grow up.

I have observed this lack of understanding of the differences in treating men and women firsthand in fifty years of practicing internal medicine, endocrinology, and hematology, in all of which I have achieved board certifications—a unique combination achieved by no other woman or man. The lack-of-understanding bias and what I have learned from my women patients have motivated me to seek ways of changing the education of all doctors on issues of women's health to insure that women get the kind of care they need and deserve.

Like most women physicians, I was educated, trained, and professionally socialized by men; I had male mentors, educators, and supervisors. Despite my good fortune to attend a top-notch medical school (Columbia University College of Physicians and Surgeons) and serve as a resident and fellow in several prestigious training programs at the

New York Hospital–Cornell Medical Center, when I went into practice, I felt unprepared to deal with many of the health needs of my women patients. This amazed me. Why were there so many gaps in my other-- wise ideal education? I enrolled in seminars and workshops, I took courses with other medical specialists—and in so doing I found out how little *anybody* knew about women's health.

At the same time, I was learning from my patients by listening to them, examining them, sharing my knowledge with them, sometimes arguing with them. It was through my patients that I learned what women's health needs actually were.

After caring for thousands of patients, the majority of whom were women, I have learned that women's health is *very different* from men's health. Not only because of different hormones, or because we can bear children, but because during our life span our health does not follow the linear pattern of men's health. Men move along an increasingly high but straight pathway, like a rocket, in all systems. Women go up and down through cycles, more like a boat on a choppy sea.

Because men age along a pretty straight line and the intensity of their health needs parallels their advancing age, the incidence of heart disease, stroke, and most other chronic illnesses grows in men from a low in the twenties to a high in old age. Except for short blips in the late teens and early twenties for death by violence, men's mortality also follows a straight line upward. You might say that as they age men are essentially the same but more so.

Our lives, on the other hand, take a more circuitous route from beginning to end. We go through four major life phases, although there is considerable overlap and individual variation, such as having children at 18 or 42. Hazards to the life and health of a teenage girl are very different from those of a 30-year-old woman, and both are very different from those of a woman in her fifties or eighties. It is precisely because of these transitions from one phase to another that our health care requires special understanding and close cooperation between our doctors and ourselves to make that care effective. At each phase, we face different risks and therefore need different therapeutic strategies.

THE FOUR PHASES OF OUR LIVES

This book deals with these age phases chronologically. Each section covers a different life phase, outlining how you are different from men at this time, and explains conditions that are particularly common to women so that you can become a well-informed partner in your health care. (This book does not elaborate on conditions such as the common cold, or peptic ulcer, which would require similar treatment for either sex.) The primary aim is to help you understand your needs for prevention and make the best possible choices about treatment. The life phases are:

Adolescence: Ages 12 to 20

Adolescence begins with puberty and is a very different experience for girls and boys. As the adolescent girl gropes for a new definition of herself at home, at school, and in society, her health encompasses not only her beginning menstrual cycles and changing body but her nutritional needs, her susceptibility to disease, and a host of new concerns.

The emotional impact of adolescence has a critical effect on health, especially as it leads to eating disorders, unprotected sex, and substance abuse. Adolescence is also a time when a girl's self-esteem often takes a nosedive because of the biological events of puberty as well as the peer pressures. The adolescent must understand her risks for the four health epidemics of the teenage years: AIDS, drug addiction, early pregnancy, and violence.

This section will also inform the adolescent girl (and her parents) about the risks of poor nutrition, eating disorders, the changing nature of illnesses, and the development of good health habits for her inner and outer self. It will advise her on when she needs to get a pelvic exam and what to expect from doctors, including confidentiality.

Adulthood: Ages 20 to 45

Important during this phase is not only the assumption of an autonomous position in family and society, but in the latter part of the twentieth century, it is a balancing act of multiple roles of woman, worker, wife, and mother. Our career and marital decisions dominate our health in this phase. Being at optimum health before planning pregnancy, while pregnant, and after giving birth are outlined in this section. Gynecological concerns and procedures are included.

The stress generated by our multiple roles places us at risk for chronic fatigue syndrome and depression. This is the phase during which we are most vulnerable to immune system disorders such as lupus and rheumatoid arthritis. If poor diet and exercise habits begun in earlier years continue, this can lead to diabetes and other chronic conditions. There is a chapter on one of the worst health hazards of this time, domestic violence.

The Perimenopausal Phase: Ages 45 to 65

Menopause was once considered—by society and therefore by women—as the end of life. If we could no longer give birth, and were considered to have lost our sex appeal, we had no role in the male society except as grandmothers. Very few women understood how the drop of estrogen levels affected their physical and mental health. Men have no abrupt cessation of the testicular function; their blood testosterone declines gradually.

Exactly what happens when estrogen levels drop? You need to know not only what causes the hot flash and other symptoms, but how it affects your cardiovascular system, your bones, your central nervous system. Adjusting to the end of menses carries great emotional impact as well. While the biological clock is ticking, women approaching this phase may have a sense of urgency in making decisions about childbearing, career, future retirement plans, and possibly the care of aging parents.

Health decisions involve whether or not to get hormone replacement therapy for treatment of the menopausal symptoms, as well as preventive and therapeutic management of the newly created risks caused by the estrogen deficiency such as heart disease and osteoporosis. It is important to know how to evaluate your needs vs. the risks, and to know about the alternatives.

The Postmenopausal Phase: Ages 65 and Up

In this phase, your life and health depend on freedom from heart disease, osteoporosis, and cancer. They depend on continued good nutrition and exercise, and a continuation of interest in life and in other people. This period may also include premature bereavement of a spouse or intimate partner because, statistically, we outlive men.

In this period women are also burdened by the domino effect, the accumulation of chronic ailments that require dependence on a longer list of specialists. Many women during this phase suffer from locomotion problems like osteoarthritis and loss of vision or hearing. How to keep all systems going, from the cardiovascular (the risk of hypertension and stroke), to the central nervous, to sexuality, to mental health is the subject of this section. It is your responsibility to yourself to live as well as you can for as long as you can.

This book will help you learn to take charge of your health in the way the medical profession has not taught you up to now: how to recognize health challenges special to each phase and risk factors for common illnesses; how to avoid the specific behaviors that put your health at risk; how to anticipate health hazards that come with each stage of your life, so you can prepare yourself in advance for each phase and thus live a longer, happier life.

Differences in women's health go beyond the reproductive tract and affect every biological system. In addition to making us male or female, our hormones play a complex role in our physical and psychological well-being. Not only are our anatomy and our social roles in the family and community different from men's, so are the way our bodies respond to disease, our emotional reactions to life's adversities, and even how we metabolize certain drugs and chemicals.

• Our cardiovascular system is different from that of men. Estrogen can cause some of our blood vessels to dilate, while the testosterone of men constricts their vessels. Estrogen protects us from heart disease until menopause, when cardiovascular disease becomes our leading cause of death. Heart and blood vessel diseases usually affect us later in life than men, but they are more likely to cause complications and death. Fewer women than men fully recover from a heart attack.

• Our immune system is different from that of men. Our bodies do not reject the "foreign body" that is an unborn baby. A man does not have this immune capability. At the same time we are more at risk for autoimmune disorders (where the body's immune system attacks itself) such as lupus, rheumatoid arthritis, and multiple sclerosis.

• Our gastrointestinal system is different from that of men. Estrogen predisposes us to more gallbladder disease than men. One disease of the liver, *primary biliary cirrhosis,* is almost exclusively a disease of women. And because we have a smaller liver and blood volume, and some of our enzymes are different, we react differently than men to certain medications and drugs such as alcohol. We are more often stricken with irritable bowel syndrome and diverticulitis.

• Our endocrine system is different from that of men. We have more adult-onset diabetes and thyroid disease.

• Our bones and muscles are different from those of men. The cartilage and bones in the pelvis and chest are more flexible to allow for expansion during pregnancy, but we are endowed with a smaller muscle mass because we have less testosterone.

• Our epidermal system is different from that of men. We have thinner skin but a thicker protective layer of fat.

• Our respiratory system is different from that of men. Our lungs have a smaller capacity.

• Our urologic system is different from that of men. Disorders such as cystitis, urinary tract infections, and urinary incontinence are overwhelmingly more common in women.

• Our emotional response system is different from that of men. We more easily succumb to depression, while men are more prone to violence.

Despite the knowledge of all of these important and measurable differences in our internal systems, many studies still document poor health care to women by the existing medical establishment. Women experience this personally on many encounters with physicians. We can see how our health gets lost in the gaps between medical specialties.

We are referred back and forth between gynecologists, internists, family practitioners, and psychologists. A woman seldom receives thorough, comprehensive care as an individual, with attention to all of her organ systems. Such fragmentation is expensive and wasteful. It also generates resentment. A man is not referred to a urologist for a routine digital rectal exam and examination of his genitalia. His primary care physician does that. But a woman's primary care physician is likely to skip such exams. She must go to her gynecologist for a routine pelvic exam and Pap smear.

Because health care has been focused on our reproductive system, the gynecologist has traditionally been the primary care physician for most women. *This means we are not getting comprehensive care for the rest of our body. We are not acknowledging that we are more than our reproductive system.*

At a landmark hearing in the House of Representatives in 1990, Congress learned that the National Institutes of Health (NIH) had not adhered to its own regulations about gender equality in biomedical research. The media, and the public at large, were stunned. The hearings revealed that clinical research studies on illnesses common to both women and men had been conducted *exclusively on men.* For instance, in animal trials, drugs were tested on male rats only! Trials of medications designed for anxiety and depression—conditions much more common in women—were carried out only on males, whether animal or human. The Food and Drug Administration (FDA) now requires that appropriate drugs be tested on women, as well as men, before they get FDA approval. With such gender bias in research, is it any wonder that female bodies and minds have been disregarded in the medical school curriculum? Medical research both shapes and changes medical education, which in turn molds the clinical practice of medicine.

As a result of the 1990 congressional hearing, the NIH created the Office for Research on Women's Health to insure that those seeking grants include female subjects in the trials, that women's health conditions receive equitable funding, and that women be recruited as biomedical investigators. Researchers now need to include equal numbers of women and men subjects in their clinical trials or have a very good excuse as to why a study of women is not germane to their research.

Finally, at the end of the twentieth century, medical education is beginning to include the study of women's health. A number of medical residencies and fellowships for training in women's health have become available to medical school graduates. Several hundred doctors—internists, family practitioners, gynecologists, psychiatrists, surgeons, and other specialists—have taken courses in Advanced Curriculum on Women's Health (ACWH), which I initiated, acting as the chair of the American Medical Women's Association's (AMWA's) Task Force on Women's Health Curriculum. The ACWH is the first medical course dealing with women's health systematically structured along the life phases of the woman.

Since I retired from active practice (I see patients only occasionally on consultation), I have devoted all of my time to trying to correct the inequities in women's health care. In 1979, I developed and directed the Teaching Associates Program, in which nonmedical men and women teach doctors and medical students how to do painless and sensitive genital (breast and pelvic, and male genitorectal) examinations. (This method is outlined fully in the second chapter of this book.)

In 1986, patients contributed funds for the establishment of the Dr. Lila Wallis Distinguished Visiting Professorship in Women's Health at Cornell University Medical College, which allows physicians and biomedical scientists engaged in women's health research and education to come to the university and interact with students, house staff, and faculty, sharing their knowledge and research and sparking more ideas for future research. This is the first such professorship in this country, and I am very proud of it. And in 1997, the American Medical Women's Association's Board of Directors established the annual Dr. Lila Wallis Award in Women's Health, to be given to a person, man or woman, member of AMWA or not, who has demonstrated commitment to and outstanding contribution to improvements in research, education, and practice of women's health.

Recently, I have had the honor of being editor-in-chief of *Textbook of Women's Health,* written with 150 contributors, the first textbook ever for doctors and medical students devoted to women's health.

What do all these developments mean to you? They mean you have more choices and opportunities than ever before to find doctors who are well informed and well trained about your health. In these new special women's health medical training programs, the doctor is learning diagnosis and treatment of women in the appropriate life phase. He or she will have been taught to treat you not as a collection of organs but as a whole human being who is subject to physical, psychosocial, and hormonal environments. In the future, it is my hope that you will not have to see one doctor for a routine pelvic exam and Pap smear and another for colds and headaches. But we have a long way to go before we get there.

The health care system is still fraught with inequities. Why did it take so long for Medicare to finally include coverage for mammograms for older women when we are at such a high risk for breast cancer? Who decided that a mastectomy did not require an overnight stay in the hospital? (It took Congress to change that one!) A man, after all, is permitted to stay in the hospital for as long as five days after a prostatectomy. And why was the insurance industry allowed to decide that a woman and her newborn baby can stay only one day in the hospital? The limit is now two, but that, too, needed to be changed by law.

And you have a role to play, too. Take the time to be better informed about your body, your health, and your health care. Be ready to ask questions of doctors, and challenge the health insurance carriers if need be. These are times when health care must be negotiated. Think of it less as being a "patient" and more as being an active and effective partner with your physicians in managing your health.

The first, introductory, section of this book helps you understand the basics of good health care, how trends have changed over the years, and how to form a good relationship with your doctors and understand how the health care system works. It will help set a foundation for understanding what you need to do—at each stage of life—to maintain your health and take charge of your health care.

The Whole Woman is meant to empower you with knowledge. There's a little history, some anatomy, guides to diagnosis and treatment, and a continuous message that you must be a full partner in your health care.

A New Approach to Managing Your Health

In almost half a century of practicing medicine, I have had many satisfying experiences—the thrill of diagnosing the correct reason for otherwise unexplained symptoms, rescuing patients from overwhelming catastrophes and bringing them back to good health. Of equal satisfaction is the feeling that I have taught a patient something about self-care, that I have engaged her interest and empowered her to be a true partner in the lifelong effort to protect her health.

Many women physicians throughout history have felt the same way. In the nineteenth century, Elizabeth and Emily Blackwell, Marie Zakrzewska, and Mary Putnam Jacobi took very seriously the importance of educating women about their own health. These lonely pioneers in the otherwise male medical world instructed their patients on the dangers of sexually transmitted infections. They taught them personal hygiene. They encouraged them to exercise during their menstrual periods, breaking with the male physicians of the time, who advocated complete bed rest for the "delicate" time of the month.

Elizabeth Blackwell was the first woman to graduate from a "legitimate" American medical school, Geneva Medical College in New York, which is now a part of Syracuse University. Together with her sister, Emily, she started the New York Infirmary for Women and Children to treat thousands of poor immigrant women and children. Today's Beekman Downtown Hospital is the offspring of that infirmary.

The New England Hospital for Women and Children in Boston's South End was established by Marie Zakrzewska in 1902. Zakrzewska, a former head nurse and midwife in a Berlin hospital, came to America and with Emily Blackwell, graduated from the Cleveland Medical College. Marie went on to establish the first medical school for women in New England.

Mary Putnam Jacobi was the first American and the first woman to graduate from the famous Faculté de Medicine in Paris. She returned to New York to practice and teach. Her lectures were so popular there was standing room only. She started the first women's medical society, currently known as Women's Medical Association of New York City, which offers an annual fellowship in her name.

While the male medical establishment overwhelmingly ignored women's health, there have always been a few exceptions. Ironically, one of the best pieces of advice I came across while researching this book is from a twentieth-century male internist, Dr. Thomas Argyros of New York City. He believed a woman should be well educated about her body and health so that "she could become her own doctor and use her physician as a consultant."

CHOOSING YOUR PRINCIPAL PHYSICIAN

Whether you are moving to a new region or you simply want to find a new doctor, it is important for you to establish a relationship with a physician who will become your principal physician. Officially, this person is known as a primary care doctor. I prefer the appellation "principal physician" because this describes the person who will be principally responsible for overseeing all and any of your health needs.

Your choice of an appropriate physician is influenced by the life phase you are in. Adolescent girls, for example, overwhelmingly prefer women doctors because they do not feel as confident talking about sexual or reproductive issues with a man.

If you are planning a family, you might want to consider a gynecologist and obstetrician. On the surface, this may seem logical, but you are limiting your health concerns to your reproductive systems. Where do you go for your flu shot? Many women have doctors who specialize in one area of their health care. An older woman with heart problems, for example, may rely on her cardiologist as her primary caregiver. She might also visit an orthopedic surgeon, and possibly a urologist, but these doctors do not necessarily communicate with each other. It is important to have one physician who oversees your general health and is your principal partner in your health care.

Your best bet is to choose a well-trained internist or family practitioner with special additional training in women's health, or perhaps a gynecologist with special training in primary care. These specialties are defined below. In each case, it is not the gender, age, or even specialty that counts, but the physician's competence, attitude, and training.

How can you be sure that the physician you choose is one of the few who has cared enough for women patients to take and complete courses in women's health care? One way is to ask if the physician is a graduate of AMWA's Advanced Curriculum on Women's Health. Or, while you are sitting in the office waiting for your doctor and looking at all those framed certificates on the walls, see if there is one for completion of the course.

Another way is to ask a crucial question. (I consider this the litmus test.) Does the doctor perform a routine pelvic exam with a Pap smear on every woman seen for the first time or at periodic intervals? If the answer is no, and the doctor routinely refers patients to a gynecologist, that doctor is not a candidate for your principal physician. It is my belief that only 10 to 15 percent of primary care physicians who are internists include the pelvic exam as part of their routine checkup of women. This is mostly because it adds to the time involved in the physical exam and challenges the declining skills of a doctor who does not perform this exam routinely.

I also want to warn women that any specialist, such as a gastroenterologist, who is trying to diagnose abdominal pain must include a pelvic exam as part of the procedure. In women, abdominal pain is often caused by a condition of the reproductive or urinary system, and no accurate diagnosis of abdominal pain can be made without a pelvic examination.

The Internist

Internists are medical doctors who have specialized in the study of internal medicine. They are diagnosticians who treat everything that does not require surgery, and should offer the full range of services we've been describing. Internists often have a subspecialty such as endocrinology, oncology, hematology, cardiology, gastroenterology, and allergy. Some, in fact, limit their practice to the subspecialty.

The Family Physician

The family physician has eclipsed what used to be known as the general practitioner. General practitioners took care of medical, pediatric, surgical, gynecological, and urological problems. In the age of specialization in the middle of the twentieth century, this area of medicine went out of favor, as medical students chose specialties that seemed more interesting and glamorous, in addition to being more lucrative. As our population migrated to cities, forsaking small towns, the numbers of general practitioners diminished. The pendulum swung too far, however, and soon it became obvious that we had plenty of specialists to treat various parts of people, but nobody to treat the whole person anymore.

The pendulum began to come back in the 1980s, and family physicians emerged to oversee family medical problems from children to great-grandparents. Most family physicians have training in internal medicine and pediatrics. They also do gynecology and minor surgery. A few actually deliver babies. With the changes in our medical system and the emergence of managed health care in the 1980s and 1990s, family practice is attracting larger numbers of medical school graduates. Many family practitioners become primary care physicians.

Primary Care (Principal) Physician

This title defines a system for providing managed health care services rather than an area of specialty. Our health care delivery system now works around the principle that one doctor should oversee a person's health. This doctor can be a general internist, a family practitioner, or a specialist such as an endocrinologist or oncologist, but must provide the primary care and make referrals only for specialized care.

This physician is one who can examine you, will give you your annual physical exam, and if anything is wrong, should be able to diagnose it. The primary care physician will refer you to specialists for particular problems out of his or her area of expertise, such as a surgeon, an orthopedist, an endocrinologist, or an oncologist.

The Obstetrician/Gynecologist

The OB/GYN specializes in reproductive medicine and related surgery such as hysterectomy or Cesarean section childbirth. We need the OB/GYN for prenatal care and delivery as well as for surgery of the reproductive tract. Many women see a gynecologist for what they perceive to be primary care: pelvic and breast examinations, periodic Pap smears, and obstetrical care. However, gynecology is a surgical subspecialty and emphasizes, in its training as well as in clinical practice, surgical skills and invasive procedures such as dilatation and curettage (D&C), a scraping off of tissue from the lining of the uterus. Numerous studies have demonstrated that, after tonsillectomy, the hysterectomy and Cesarean section are the most common *unnecessary* procedures performed on American women.

With the recent advancement of women into the residency programs of obstetrics and gynecology, there has been a subtle shift in the orientation of gynecology training programs. A number of educators have attempted to broaden the scope of gynecology training and practice to embrace more primary care problems. These recent changes in orientation foretell a shift in future practice, but they affect only a small proportion of gynecologists practicing now. The overwhelming majority of gynecologists are concerned mainly with diagnostic and therapeutic surgeries of the reproductive system.

In today's managed care plans, a gynecologist is one of the few specialists who does not have to be referred to by your primary care physician.

Women's Health Centers and Clinics

Many women's health centers have sprung up in recent years, but it is important to know the difference between a true women's health center and a glorified gynecology clinic. A true women's health center will have internists on staff as primary care physicians and an internist as the medical director. It will have specialists dedicated to caring for all phases of a woman's life. The Center for Women's Healthcare at the New York Hospital–Cornell Medical Center is one example of a multi-faceted center where women can come for all aspects of health care. The center is organized around internal medicine and primary care, and includes care in orthopedics and sports medicine, infectious disease, obesity, and endocrinology. Gynecologists, obstetricians, psychiatrists, urologists, nutritionists, and other specialists are available for consultations. In some such centers, nurse-practitioners and nurse-midwives also play an important role.

In the mid-1990s some managed care programs were assigning nurse-practitioners with advanced training as primary health caregivers. These nurses handle routine health care such as colds and flu and help patients manage chronic conditions such as diabetes and asthma, but refer patients to specialists when needed. Some work under the supervision of physicians, and some do not. In some states nurse-practitioners are allowed to prescribe medication. There is still a great deal of controversy about this, with many physicians opposing. The other side of the argument is that nurses might provide better routine care than physicians and spend more time with patients.

A health center that is, in fact, a gynecology and obstetrics practice might simply add to the gynecological exam some amenities such as a diagnostic facility for mammography or bone density testing. To distinguish between the two, ask about the medical specialty of the director of the center.

Finding the Doctor Who's Right for You

There are many ways to find a good doctor. They are often referred to by other doctors or by your family members and friends. As Americans become more sophisticated about health care, many patients often do their own research to find qualified physicians. There are many sources of information, from local hospital referral services to medical societies to the World Wide Web.

Hospital Referral Services. These are usually citywide or regional services with an 800 number. You can find the number by calling a hospital or medical center in your city or by looking in the yellow pages under "Hospitals" or "Physician referrals." For example, Thomas Jefferson University Hospital in Philadelphia sponsors a referral service called Jeff Now. This service will provide you with names of several doctors who fit your specifications. Information provided includes the names and addresses of doctors as well as their office hours; where they were educated; their accreditation, licensing, and any board-certified specializations; any limitations on types of patients the doctors will treat; and which medical insurance they accept.

County Medical Societies. These are local branches of the American Medical Association, organizations of physicians in the same geographic area. Medical societies generally give out the names of licensed doctors, usually those newly licensed and looking for patients. At one time this was the best source for finding the type of doctor you needed. However, in some less-enlightened counties, the referral service sometimes fails to give out names of female physicians in various specialties and erroneously states that there are no women in a particular field. If you hear this response, check another source. There are almost equal numbers of women and men graduating from medical schools today.

Medical Schools. Your inquiry for an appropriate physician could be directed to a nearby medical school. Many medical schools maintain a faculty practice clinic and make referrals.

American Medical Women's Association (AMWA). This is a professional association of women physicians whose purpose is to improve the professional and personal lives of women physicians and to further women's health advocacy. Call AMWA in Alexandria, Virginia, at 703-838-0500 for the telephone number of the branch nearest you. Most AMWA local branches have a referral service that will provide you with three names of doctors who, in addition to being competent and well trained, are more likely to have a proper attitude toward women's health needs.

Public Libraries. Most libraries carry reference books you can use to get information about doctors. *American Medical Association Directory of Physicians in the United States* lists each doctor's medical school, year of licensing, specialty, and board certification. *American Board of Medical Specialties (ABMS) Directory of Board Certified Medical Specialists* indicates a physician's certification in particular specialties.

WHAT TO EXPECT—AND NOT EXPECT—FROM YOUR DOCTOR

In all professions there are good and not-so-good practitioners, and doctors are no exception. You might find a doctor who is charming and easy to get along with but who rushes through the exam and does not seem to take seriously your complaints. There might be a doctor who seems cold and distant but who goes over every detail of your diagnosis and health history with you. Such a doctor can inspire trust and confidence even if you do not personally like him or her.

If you sincerely do not feel comfortable with a particular physician, you might not be able to talk freely about your health. You might feel shy about confiding information about your menstrual problems or bowel movements with an arrogant doctor who seems to be patronizing you. Only you and your physician can tell if this will be a positive or negative association.

A survey by the Commonwealth Fund Commission on Women's Health found women more likely than men to be dissatisfied with doctors and twice as likely to report the problem. In a 1993 survey, 25 percent of women reported being "talked down to" and 17 percent were told by their doctors that their complaints were "all in your head." The survey discovered that the majority of doctors failed to counsel women on smoking, substance abuse, nutrition, exercise, and sexually transmitted infection.

However, personalities aside, there are some professional guidelines that any good physician will follow. As a patient, you have the right to expect the following things from your physician.

• Expect your physician to see you reasonably promptly if you are on time for your appointment. If the doctor is detained in the hospital or with an emergency, the nurse or receptionist should let you know and apologize for the delay. However, you should not be forced to wait for hours to see a doctor. This only happens when doctors chronically overbook. (This is quite common.) If you live by a very tight schedule, ask the nurse or receptionist to schedule you for the very first opening in the morning or the very last at the end of the office day. If the doctor still keeps you waiting, consider finding another physician.

• Expect your physician to greet you courteously and respectfully, and to address you by your last name unless you know each other personally on a first-name basis.

• Expect your doctor to listen to your story during the consultation, ask you questions, and listen to your answers, as well as review your filled-out questionnaire.

• Expect her or him to take a thorough personal and family health history from you.

• Expect your doctor to perform a thorough physical examination, including a competent, painless, and sensitive breast and pelvic examination.

• Expect that after your examination your doctor will explain the findings and their significance, whether additional tests are needed to clinch the diagnosis or rule out other possibilities, and present you with the working diagnosis.

• Expect your doctor to suggest preferred and alternate approaches to treatment, clearly giving you *choices* and indicating the chances of success. Such choice might be between a lumpectomy or a mastectomy for a woman with breast cancer.

• Expect your doctor to listen to your opinion and any special reasons for modifying the approach to treatment. Your doctor should respect and accept your decision and cooperate in its execution.

On the other hand, patients sometimes make unreasonable demands on a doctor's time, or they might have unreasonable expectations that the doctor will spend the rest of the day holding their hand if they have serious treatment choices to make.

• Do not expect your doctor to come up with the right diagnosis without your effort to produce a coherent history or to cooperate in the physical exam.

• Do not expect your doctor to make the correct diagnosis without ordering any reasonable, although possibly expensive, tests. As you will discover throughout this book, many conditions are extremely difficult to diagnose except through a process of eliminating all the possibilities. This sometimes requires a good deal of testing; insurance does not always cover all of this testing.

• Do not expect your doctor to lead you to good health without your participation and cooperation in giving up health risks such as smoking or refusing to exercise.

Patient Abuse and Sexual Harassment

Although the vast majority of doctors would never abuse their patients sexually, there are unfortunate exceptions. It is sometimes difficult to decide where patronization becomes abuse. Women have frequently suffered from subtle abuse, such as slightly prolonged or unnecessary touching of any part of the body that is medically not called for, or the use of endearing but fundamentally condescending language. Use of your first name combined with a caressing gesture is one of many borderline abuses. No woman should be an object of open or subtle abuse or rape.

We have all heard reports of psychiatrists having intercourse with a woman patient in order to "rid her of her sexual inhibitions." Also, a gynecologist in Massachusetts had routinely been having intercourse with his patients while they were draped and lying flat and helpless on the table for their pelvic exams. After victimizing several women this way, one finally reported him.

To respond effectively to committed or implied abuse is not easy, especially if you are not feeling well. However, identification of an inappropriate behavior is half the struggle, and effective response favors a prepared mind. A woman who is visiting a doctor because she is ill is less likely to be as assertive as a healthy woman. Report any such behavior to the head of the medical center, the police, or the American Medical Association—or all three.

KEEPING YOUR PERSONAL HEALTH RECORD

A Woman's Personal Health Record (Appendix II), as opposed to her doctor's medical record, represents a serious effort on the part of the woman to keep a careful account of her health. Just as you keep a bank record, or a family stock portfolio, or a car-repair record, your personal health record is a housekeeping device to keep track of your family medical history, your own history, conditions, symptoms, the course of treatment, and results. This is an important source of information for yourself and your doctor. Make a copy and share it with your doctor on your first visit. Update your Health Record after each comprehensive visit to your doctor.

Organizing Your Medical Records

The first thing most people say when you tell them to get copies of all their records is that the doctors won't give them out.

For a long time, most patients believed that they could not have copies of their medical records, that they belonged to the doctor. This is not true; they belong to you. It is important for you to know what is in your medical record and to keep a copy of it over your lifetime. You might have many examinations, consultations, tests, and surgeries, all at various points in your lifetime. It is much easier for you to keep track of them all if you have copies of your records on hand. This way, when you visit another doctor for a consultation, or go for a second opinion, you can simply take your latest reports or records with you.

Doctors do send information to each other when a specialist is called in, but not all doctors and doctors' offices operate with the same degree of speed and efficiency. You might need to request copies of your medical records in writing, and in some cases (depending on the records) you might have to pay a small fee to cover the cost of photocopying.

There might be a time when your family needs to know what you have had done or which doctor was in charge of your case for a particular illness. If the records are at home, it is much easier for everyone to coordinate information.

Medical records include all the written reports made by physicians, correspondence among physicians about your case, laboratory reports, diagnostic films (including mammography films), and even pathology slides with tissue samples. These are kept in pathology laboratories, and if you wanted to get a second pathology opinion, you would be entitled to take the slides with the tissue samples with you.

Whenever one of my patients sees another doctor—say, a dermatologist or an allergist—I ask the patient to hand in to that doctor my prescription blank asking the doctor for diagnosis and treatment. When I get a medical chart on my patient from another physician, I make a point of "deciphering" it and summarizing it for the benefit of my medical chart and the patient's own Health Record. I usually make a copy of all test results for the patient's record. It is a good idea for every patient to ask the doctor to do the same.

MANAGING WITH MANAGED CARE

The health care system is changing daily, and it is impossible to predict what will or will not be covered by a particular medical insurance policy next week or next year. Throughout this book, we will point out instances where it is necessary to ask questions about what is covered by your insurance plan. And it is critical to ask questions, always, because often you will not be told about a treatment option or diagnostic test that might be ideal for you because your insurance will not pay for it and therefore your physician will not voluntarily tell you about it.

State and federal laws are being enacted to make such practices illegal, but it is more important than ever to be informed. Even when a plan does not cover a particular procedure, women have challenged the insurance company and gotten the test or treatment paid for. Never turn down an important test or necessary procedure because of cost alone. If you can afford a particular test—say a colonoscopy, which can cost from $1,000 to $2,000—and it is not covered, talk with your doctor about having it done and paying in installments while you are fighting the system so you can get reimbursed.

Far too many women have no health insurance at all, and most who do are in managed care programs. Because women tend to earn less than men, they have less coverage. Also, women change jobs more frequently because of family concerns and hold more part-time jobs, which often do not include health insurance benefits.

In the managed care system, if you plan ahead and find out what is available, you can make better choices. Before you sign up for any particular plan, investigate the doctors, hospitals, and diagnostic laboratories that are included. Then select the best ones—regardless of their convenience. Many people want to go to a doctor near their homes and often settle for inferior care. If visiting your doctor means an hour's commute to another part of your region, then consider doing that if it means better care.

·· 2 ··

Your First Visit with
a Principal Physician

Being a good partner in your care means, first of all, that you prepare
yourself carefully for your visit with your doctor. Plan what you want
to accomplish and make a list of your key concerns. Have all the information you need with you, so that when the doctor questions you in
detail about your symptoms or complaints you will be able to give very
precise answers. When you are unsure of details, or forget the sequence
of events or symptoms, it is more difficult to correctly diagnose the
condition. Whenever you keep a record, or write things down, you see
patterns, make logical connections between cause and effect, and help
make the diagnosis easier.

If you have been keeping your Woman's Health Record (see Appendix 2), make a copy and bring it with you. The doctor can review it
with you and ask further questions to clarify your problems. Of course,
without this, the taking of your medical history will take longer, even
if you are prepared with the answers.

Plan to bring with you copies of any medical records, such as reports
of past illness or diagnostic test results, that may be relevant to your
current visit. These records will help your new physician develop a
better idea of your health persona during that important first visit. The
doctor might want them for the medical file he or she is building
with you.

Bring a pad and pen so you can take notes. It is easy to forget
information given quickly in a doctor's office, especially if you are feeling anxious about your health or if a great deal of medical jargon is
used in the explanation. By the same token, you are likely to forget to
mention to the doctor some of your concerns that seemed very important
before the visit. This is why taking notes, writing down symptoms, and
bringing lists to the doctor is conducive to receiving better health care.

Think about whether or not you want to bring someone along with you, especially on your first visit to a new physician. Some women bring their spouses or other relatives with them when they believe they have a serious problem to deal with. Often, when two people hear the same diagnosis or information, they can talk it over later and be sure they both understood it the same way. This can be the basis for deciding and writing down additional information you need from the doctor. Patients who do not speak English often bring along someone to act as a translator.

HOW MUCH TIME WILL YOU NEED?

A woman once told me of having to wait for four hours to see her doctor. She learned later that this doctor left his patients waiting while he was picked up in a limousine and taken to a television studio where he appeared on a panel of medical experts. After he returned to his office—four hours later—he offered no apology. Since most of his patients were women, he assumed they had nothing important to do and would not mind waiting. Most doctors are not like this, and an efficiently run medical office should mean you rarely wait more than a few minutes.

When you call to make an appointment with a doctor, ask for an estimate of how long you will be in the doctor's office from the time you arrive until you leave. The first visit with your principal physician, such as an internist, usually takes between forty-five minutes to an hour and a half. This accounts only for the time with the doctor—discussions and examinations—and does not include the time involved in collection of blood and urine specimens or additional procedures such as an electro-cardiogram or X ray.

Women usually require more time per visit with a primary physician than men do because the pelvic exam is time and labor intensive, and because women tend to ask more questions. Still, most doctors allot the same amount of time for all patients, regardless of sex.

The time restriction, while affecting physicians in private practice, will more definitely apply to HMOs and other clinics in which the administration will demand of its doctors greater "productivity." There are various determinants, but in some settings doctors allot only fifteen minutes per patient. Indeed, some doctors rush through an exam as if their cars were double-parked outside. Ask ahead of time how much time your doctor will spend with you.

You need to know from the doctor your diagnosis, the cause of your illness, and the proposed and alternative treatments, as well as future steps for prevention. This type of comprehensive, educational care takes time, and the constraints on some doctors might not allow them to render it.

HOW MUCH WILL YOUR VISIT COST?

When you call for an appointment you need to ask if the doctor accepts your health insurance. Some doctors accept all types, others accept none. There is uneven distribution among doctors who take Medicaid. If you are covered by an HMO, your visit might be entirely covered except for a small copayment. If your insurance includes a deductible that has not yet been fulfilled, you might be asked to pay the cost of the visit before you leave. Most physicians will expect you to pay for the services as the services are rendered, and will expect you to seek reimbursement from your insurance later. There are some who will wait to be paid after you are reimbursed. It is always wise to inquire about this before your visit.

In addition to the office visit, you may be charged for laboratory tests for blood and urine analysis and a Pap smear. The bill for these services will generally come to you later, directly from the laboratory.

If the cost of your visit and the tests is more than you can afford, ask if you can work out a payment plan. Some doctors will do this with their patients. Some will not, but it always pays to ask.

THE CONSULTATION: TELLING YOUR STORY

Before any examination takes place, the doctor should talk with you in his office while you are fully clothed. Some practitioners prefer to have a nurse take patients into an examination room so the patients can change into gowns, and then talk with them before they begin the examination. If you know this to be the case, ask if you can talk first before you disrobe. Without your clothing you are at a disadvantage and might not feel confident talking with the doctor candidly.

If you are shy, or unsure, let the doctor know that. Ask if you can be heard without interruption. This way, the doctor will not interject questions into your recitation and possibly cause you to miss telling him some important details. Also, if there is a symptom you feel awkward or embarrassed about, such as a vaginal discharge you might believe occured because of a particular sexual encounter, tell that one first and get it over with.

According to a study by the American Society of Internal Medicine, 70 to 95 percent of correct diagnoses are made on the basis of what the patient tells the doctor about her health. This is why it is so important to keep track of your symptoms and write things down. You can tell your doctor the story of your present illness, and he or she can ask you further questions and listen carefully to your answers, without having to dig out information that could be vital to your diagnosis. For example, if abdominal pain occurs before or after eating, it could make a difference. Gallbladder pain would most likely occur after eating, while an ulcer might cause pain before a meal and be soothed by milk or other bland food.

Your doctor will ask you about your own and your family's health history, including surgeries, pregnancies, diseases, and allergies, as well as habits such as smoking and drinking, and about any medications you are using. Most doctors now routinely ask about diet and exercise as well. A doctor needs to know if you drink ten cups of coffee a day, or that you eat nothing but fried foods, whether you are a couch potato or work out regularly.

All the planning ahead, and the careful keeping of your health records, such as the Woman's Health Record, will pay off now. You have dates and times, onset of symptoms, but do you know how to describe your symptoms accurately? For example, if your symptoms are bowel related, the doctor needs to know not only how many and how often, but what they look like. What is the color of the stool? Is it black like tar or white as chalk? Does it show blood? And is the blood bright red or dark?

What and When: Chief Complaint and Duration

Chief complaint does not mean that you deplore your having to wait in the doctor's office a long time. In medical jargon it means any specific symptom or "thing" that bothers you or worries you. Doctors have a system for evaluating symptoms, and it begins with the chief complaint. This is the what and when. For example, if you have been running several times a week for years with no problems, but you noticed an irregular heartbeat all last week when you ran, then this would be the chief complaint.

The chronology of symptoms or events is very important. Describe these in chronological order. What happened first? When did it happen next? You may remember the onset of illness in relation to a family event or vacation; while this may be relevant the exact time and day the symptoms started are more important. Even the hour may be important if symptoms are acute. The year may be important if you had the condition in the past. Have the symptoms increased or decreased with the passage of time, or do they occur in cycles? Do they occur in response to a body function such as eating or moving your bowels?

How to Describe Pain

Because everyone's perception of pain, and their tolerance to it, is different (it's also different in men and women), it is important to think about and describe the pain from several angles.

Quality. Is the pain piercing or stabbing like a knife in the heart? Or is it a dull throbbing or ache? Is it constricting, like a vise tightening around your chest?

Degree. Is it mild, moderate, or so severe that you cannot think of anything else?

Duration. How long does it last? How many times does it recur?

Location. Precisely where is it? We need to know more than just that it is in your abdomen. Ask your doctor to show you a simple illustration so that you can point out where the pain is located or use Figure 36 in Appendix II to point to the location of the pain.

Radiation. Does the pain radiate from one site to another? For example, is the left shoulder pain radiating into your left hand? Or is the pain in your right side radiating into your groin?

Change. How does the pain change with time? Does it continue or get worse with time? Or is it intermittent with long or short pauses in between, lasting a second or a few minutes? What makes it worse?

Relief. Does anything relieve the pain, such as taking an aspirin, changing the position of your body, deep breathing, lying down, sleeping, or having a bowel movement? How does the pain affect your sleep or waking hours?

THE COMPREHENSIVE PHYSICAL EXAMINATION

After the consultation, the physician or a nurse should escort you to the examination room so you can change into a gown. When your physician comes in he or she will observe your general state of health and check your vital signs—blood pressure, pulse, and temperature— although some may be taken ahead of time by a nurse or physician's assistant. Your height and weight may be recorded, too.

Checking Vital Signs

Temperature. Confirming that you have a normal temperature of 98.6° F.

Blood Pressure. The force of the blood pumping through your arteries is your blood pressure. Pressure is generated by the action of the heart pumping blood into the arteries and the resistance supplied by the arteries. There are two phases: the heart pumps into the arteries and this is the systolic pressure. When the heart relaxes and the blood comes back from the veins to the heart, the pressure transmitted by the relaxing heart is the diastolic pressure. A normal reading might be 110 over 70. The systolic reading would be higher if the arteries were clogged and the heart had to pump harder to push the blood through the arteries.

The classic technique—which is seldom used by doctors today—is to elevate the arm to empty the veins, place the cuff and pump it up, then have you lower your arm so the doctor can listen to the sounds generated by the blood flowing through the arteries to measure the pressure. Blood pressure should be taken twice, before and after the exam, to account for any possible anxiety about the exam itself.

Pulse. When the doctor holds your wrist, or presses on the carotid artery in your neck, while watching his or her wristwatch, it is to record the number of beats per minute your heart is pumping. This is your heart rate.

Respiratory rate. The doctor simply watches you breathing when you are not speaking.

After checking your vital signs, the exam includes a check of the rest of your body.

Checking All Systems

Eyes, Ears, and Nose. By shining a light into your eyes, the doctor can examine your eyes for any abnormalities such as conjunctivitis or signs of glaucoma. Your retinae (the back of your eyes) are examined with an ophthalmoscope. In the nose, the doctor looks for any redness that could be infection or paleness that could indicate the presence of allergies. He or she checks for polyps or a deviated septum, and palpates the cheeks and forehead for sinus tenderness. Ears are checked for redness, bulging from fluid, wax, or a foreign body.

Mouth and throat. The doctor will use a tongue depressor to push down on your tongue and ask you to "Say aghh!" to check for inflammation, unusual color, or swelling in the throat and mouth. The physician looks at the teeth for oral hygiene or signs of gum disease or herpes blisters. Anemia could be detected by color of the tongue. It may be red or pale or black or brown. The tonsils may show signs of swelling or redness. The lining of the cheek may be examined for salivary stones.

Neck. By palpating both sides of your neck, a doctor can check your thyroid gland and lymph glands for any swelling that could indicate an abnormality or infection. Pulsating or distended blood vessels may also suggest abnormalities.

Breasts. An examination of your breasts is performed while you are sitting up and lying down. Your underarms are palpated to check for possible swelling of the lymph nodes, which catch fluids from the breast, chest, and lungs.

Heart and Lungs. When the doctor holds the stethoscope in various places on the front of your chest, it is to listen for particular sounds in chambers and valves of your heart. For example, if you have a prolapsed mitral valve (MVP), which about 10 to 20 percent of women do, blood backing up through the prolapsed valve will emit a particular sound, a "click" caused by the abnormal opening of the valve. Sometimes murmurs can be heard with high blood pressure.

By pressing the stethoscope against your back as you breathe deeply in and out, the doctor can hear how air enters and leaves your lungs, and note any obstruction. Communication during the exam is difficult for the physician, who must listen with a stethoscope to your heart, lungs, and your blood pressure.

Abdomen. By inspecting and palpating in various spots, your doctor will be able to find any swelling such as a mass, enlarged liver, or obvious intestinal obstruction.

Arms and Legs. Your upper and lower extremities are inspected and palpated and checked for symmetry. Hands are checked for tremors and heat radiation. Legs are checked for any swelling at the ankles, varicose veins, or tenderness at the back of the calf, which could indicate phlebitis. The markings and color of the nail bed are checked for signs of malnutrition and infection.

Reflexes. By tapping your knee with a hammer, we can check your reflexes. An abnormal reflex can indicate a condition of the central nervous system or an underactive or overactive thyroid. The knee reflex consists of a short nerve circuit. The impulse, without going to the brain, goes from the knee to spinal cord to leg and makes it jerk. This is where the term "knee-jerk," as in "knee-jerk reaction," comes from.

Pelvic Exam. A painless, competent, and sensitive examination of your pelvic organs—uterus and ovaries—should be performed with gentle but purposeful skill, with gloved hands and a speculum that has been warmed. A digital—that is, with the doctor's finger—rectal exam should be part of the pelvic exam. A complete description follows later in this chapter.

Blood Tests

A first visit to a doctor is likely to include a routine complete blood count (CBC) to check your red and white blood cell count; your chemistry profile, which includes cholesterol level, electrolytes, calcium, phosphates, thyroid levels, and lipids; and any other indicators your doctor might want to look at. The nurse or physician's assistant will draw blood from your arm or finger. Blood is sent to the laboratory, where it is tested. Be sure to call your doctor the following week if you want to know what this blood test reveals. Most of us want to know what our cholesterol level is, and doctors do not always send these findings to their patients. They just put it in the file unless something abnormal shows up.

Producing a Urine Specimen

Before the physical exam, you might be asked for a urine specimen. Be aware that a urine specimen can sometimes lead to false results if the urine becomes contaminated by any secretion from the vagina. (This is why urine should *not* be collected for testing during menstruation.) When white blood cells, which are normally present in vaginal mucus, are seen in the urine, it can be interpreted as an infection. This can lead to unnecessary treatment or tests. There is a way to prevent this contamination, and we call it a "clean catch." Here is how to do it.

In the privacy of the bathroom, pour warm water over cotton balls. Then, while sitting on the toilet, spread the lips of your vagina with your fingers. With your dominant hand, wash your vulva and the perineum (the area between your vagina and rectum) thoroughly by gently mopping up the area with a wet cotton ball. Wash from the front to the back (from the top of the vulva to the bottom of the rectum) and throw the cotton ball out. Avoid scrubbing the area vigorously as this may contaminate the specimen with red blood cells. Repeat the procedure until the area is scrupulously clean. Now, keeping your vagina lips spread with your fingers, void directly into the cup, holding the cup away from the skin and high up so that no vaginal mucus gets into the cup. Label the cup with your name. Let the nurse know that you have left a clean-catch urine specimen in the bathroom.

THE PAINLESS PELVIC EXAM

Historically, pelvic exams were so unpleasant and hurtful that women avoided them at all costs, even if they had symptoms that needed to be checked. There is no reason for a painful pelvic exam—other than the physician's failure to learn how to make it painless.

Few women know that! They have hated the clinical invasion of their bodies, the sight and cold feel of a steel instrument (the speculum) entering that private space. In addition to the discomfort and pain, women resented the frequently unfeeling, brusque, and condescending attitude of the doctor.

The women's health movement of the 1960s, 1970s, and 1980s exposed the patronizing attitudes of many physicians toward their female patients. The pelvic exam became a symbol of female subjugation and abuse. A call was issued for a more meaningful partnership between the physician and patient regarding her care and the examination of her reproductive organs. This led to an entire literature of resentment, such as the books *Our Bodies, Ourselves, Vaginal Politics, The Doctors' Case Against the Pill*, and articles in journals such as *"The View from the Other End of the Speculum,"* and *"A Funny Thing Happened on the Way to the Orifice."* (I believe the books are still in print.)

The doctor should communicate with you as a partner in your care and let you know what will be happening during each step of the examination. The first pelvic examination for a young woman should include an explanation of the anatomy. Ask if there is a plastic model or detailed illustration available to make the instruction clear. This will give you a better idea of what the doctor is going to do during the examination. Hold the speculum in your hands and ask what part of the instrument actually goes into your vagina.

The doctor should ask you about your sexual experience as well, whether or not you are a virgin, if you have had sex, and whether any part of it was painful and if you used contraceptives. The doctor should ask if you have been performing breast self-exams or if you have noticed any changes in your vulva. This lets you know your doctor considers you a partner in your health care.

The physician's hands and instruments must be warm, and he or she should tell you before touching each part of your body. The caring physician should also offer you some choices about how you wish to proceed by asking you some questions.

• *Do you want to be draped during the exam?* The drape is used to avoid exposing your body and to create a sense of privacy. However, if you want to watch the examination, or see with the aid of a mirror, then you would not have the drape.

• *Would you like to watch?* If you do, ask if your head can be elevated, the drape displaced. A mirror and lamp can be arranged so that you can see your own vulva, vagina, and cervix. This is the beginning of empowerment. It involves you in the process.

• *Are you comfortable on the table?* With your head elevated, you will be able not only to watch but also to relax your abdominal muscles and make it easier for the doctor to feel your ovaries and tubes. The traditional flat table is not as comfortable. You are more in control if you are positioned with your head elevated.

• *Are you able to relax?* It is impossible to be totally relaxed during a pelvic exam, but your physician can teach you some ways to relax your perineal and abdominal muscles. First tighten these muscles, as if you were interrupting urination, and then relax them several times before the instrument or doctor's fingers are inserted. Take deep breaths or a series of panting breaths to relax.

• *Are you comfortable in the foot brackets?* These can be shortened to allow your knees to bend. This helps you bear down when necessary, so the cervix moves closer to the vaginal opening. If you have a condition that made your movements difficult, such as arthritis, you should ask for the foot brackets to be lengthened. If you do not like putting your heel into the cold metal foot bracket, keep your socks and shoes on or ask for foam booties.

Above all, the examination should be gentle. No doctor would consider being brusque or squeezing hard on a man's testicles, so expect the same sensitivity from a physician who is palpating your ovaries and uterus.

What the Pelvic Exam Includes
A doctor performing a pelvic examination is following a certain procedure designed to provide information. There is usually a nurse present during the examination because assistance is sometimes needed. You always need to empty your bladder before a pelvic exam because a full bladder makes it difficult for the physician to feel the internal organs. There are five parts to the exam.

External Genitalia. First, the doctor will examine the vulva, clitoris, labia, and glandular ducts to look for anything out of the ordinary. After examining the external genitalia some doctors may wish to do a "mini pelvic," using one finger to identify the position and direction of the cervix for the speculum insertion.

Speculum Exam. The speculum is an instrument that is inserted into the vagina and pushes the walls of the vagina apart to allow light and other instruments to be inserted and the cervix visualized. The speculum should be warmed first by holding it under warm water. As long as they are cleaned and sterilized after each use they don't need to remain sterile; the vagina is not sterile. Some doctors use disposable plastic specula. These are thicker than the ones made of steel, they make a loud click when they are opened or locked, and might frighten the patient.
A smaller, narrower speculum is used when a girl's hymen is still intact. If insertion is difficult, the doctor might teach the girl how to gently dilate her hymen and come back for the completion of the exam.

Collections of Specimens. These specimens are taken for routine laboratory studies. While the speculum is inserted, the doctor can insert instruments such as cotton-tipped applicators, cervical brushes, and wooden scrapers and take scrapings and specimens of secretions from the cervix and vagina or endometrium for various tests, such as a Pap smear and sexually transmitted infection cultures.

Bimanual Vaginoabdominal Exam. This means the doctor is using both hands, one inside your vagina and one outside your body, pressing on various locations on your abdomen. The uterus, ovaries, and tubes are located, and any abnormalities are detected. The uterine size might alert the doctor to the possibility of pregnancy, an irregular

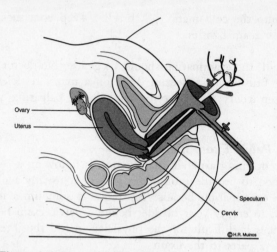

Figure 1. Pelvic examination. Examiner collects secretions and cells from the cervix by using an Ayres' scraper.

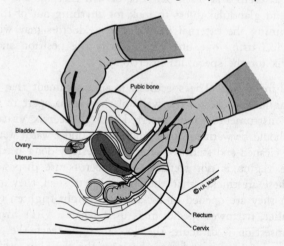

Figure 2. Bimanual pelvic (vagino-abdominal) examination.

uterine outline to the possibility of fibroids. The ovaries and tubes are usually small. Often they are difficult to palpate either because a patient cannot relax her abdominal muscles, or because she is overweight and a layer of fat interferes, or she has intestinal bloating. In that case, a pelvic sonogram would be needed to visualize the ovaries.

Bimanual Rectovaginal Exam. Here the doctor inserts his or her middle finger into the rectum and the index finger into the vagina while pressing with the other hand on the abdomen to recheck the findings of the bimanual vaginoabdominal exam. Ovaries are found in the back of the uterus so they are better palpated on the rectovaginal exam. Standard procedure for this examination is to check any fecal matter on the doctor's glove for blood, which could indicate the presence of ulcerative colitis, a bleeding peptic ulcer, polyps, colorectal cancer, hemorrhoids, or fissures and lacerations from rectal intercourse.

FORMULATION: DIALOGUE WITH THE DOCTOR

Once again, get fully dressed after the examination before you talk with the doctor. One woman told me her doctor discussed his findings with her for ten minutes while she sat naked and vulnerable, having just had a breast exam in the examination room.

Once you are dressed and back in your doctor's office, you will hear what the doctor has to say. I call this step "formulation." This is a summary of what has been found on examination. Your doctor should explain the working—or possible—diagnosis as well as other possibilities, and what additional tests might be needed to confirm the diagnosis. If the working diagnosis is correct, then expect a detailed explanation of recommended treatment.

Now is the time to ask some questions. Don't be embarrassed to ask the doctor to repeat things you missed, to define medical jargon, explain to you the procedures, draw clear pictures for you, or refer to medical diagrams and illustrations.

Listen carefully and take good notes or have your friend or relative take the notes. If medications are prescribed, write down instructions for their use. Ask about side effects and remind your doctor of other drugs you take, including oral contraceptives or hormone therapy, in case there is potential for additional side effects. Find out if a generic drug can be substituted. Some insurance plans will pay only for generic drugs. Some will pay for certain drugs. Often the newest or most expensive drugs are not included.

If the proposed plan of action interferes with your work schedule or other plans, ask the doctor to work out a more convenient timetable, as long as it does not endanger your health.

Find out when results of your blood and urine tests will be available, and ask that a copy be sent to you, or ask if you may call the doctor the next week and ask about the findings. Ask if you should call the doctor with a report of your condition—for better or worse—in a few days or weeks.

Before you go home, make a follow-up appointment if you need one. As soon as you get home, bring your Woman's Health Record up-to-date.

Questions to Ask Your Principal Physician

Here is a list of questions to remind you what you need to know before you leave the doctor's office.

IF MORE TESTS ARE NEEDED

Why do we need those tests?

What will they tell us?

Will they clinch the diagnosis or are they important to monitor the course of illness?

Is there an alternative to the tests or to the treatment?

Are there any side effects to the tests?

How much will the tests cost?

What would happen if you postpone the tests or the treatment?

What would happen if you do not do either?

Are my choices of further tests restricted by my health insurance?

ABOUT THE DIAGNOSIS AND TREATMENT

What is the working diagnosis and the appropriate treatment?

How long will it take for me to get better?

Is the condition likely to get worse or improve on its own?

Will the condition interfere with my functioning at work or at home?

Is there real danger to my health and my life?

Are there any likely complications I must avoid?

What can I do to prevent the recurrence of the problem?

Is the likely treatment painful, uncomfortable, time-consuming?

Are there side effects to the treatment? How will I know what they are if I have unexplained symptoms?

How much will the treatment cost?

Is this the best treatment, or are you restricted from offering other choices because of my health insurance?

ABOUT MEDICATIONS

If the treatment involves oral medication (pills), how often should I take it?

Should it be taken before or after meals, in the morning or evening?

What happens if I forget a pill; do I simply skip it or double up on the next dose?

How will the treatment interfere with any prescription or nonprescription medication I am already taking?

Does it interact with alcohol, coffee, or any other food or drink?

If it is an antibiotic, should I eat yogurt or acidophilus tablets to restore the balance of the flora? (Antibiotics destroy all of the bacteria in the system, including the good ones that we need.)

Can you prescribe the medication under its generic name, which is usually less expensive?

Will my insurance cover it?

CONTINUING THE PARTNERSHIP

Once you find a competent, compassionate, considerate, and thorough physician, take good care of her or him. Even if you see this doctor only for yearly physical checkups, you are building a relationship of trust and mutual respect. Now you have the peace of mind of knowing you have someone to call if you are ill.

Phone Calls to Your Doctor

Some physicians designate regular telephone hours for talking with patients. Others return calls at the end of the day's office hours. Some never return calls, but leave a voice mail message instructing you to call another number in an emergency or go to the hospital emergency room, and call back during the next day's office hours.

If your doctor has a voice mail system or an answering machine, be sure to leave a short, precise message about what you want and why you need to talk with the doctor personally and as soon as possible. Most physicians will get back to you as soon as they can if you truly need them.

Emergencies

If you are a regular patient and have an emergency, a doctor will usually make an attempt to fit you into office hours or see you before other patients. If it is outside of regular hours, he or she may see you in the hospital or in the emergency room. If you are not a regular patient, an emergency is not a good way to introduce yourself to a new principal physician. Most will not take you in an emergency because they have no previous medical records for you. It would be more efficient for you to go to a doctor who knows you or to a hospital emergency room.

The hospital emergency department is set up to take care of the immediate problem only, but the follow-up and rational comprehensive care must be scheduled at another time.

If you know the doctor you want for your principal physician, find out which hospital he or she is affiliated with and go to the emergency room at that hospital. If you let the doctors in the emergency room know that you have not yet had a chance to meet with a particular doctor you have chosen, they will very likely note that on your chart, and the physician will then have access to the emergency physicians' notes.

PHASE I

ADOLESCENT HEALTH

AGES 12–20

••••

INTRODUCTION:
BECOMING A WOMAN

Becoming a woman can be viewed as a blessing or a curse, depending upon the environment in which a girl develops. For example, when 13-year-old Maria awoke one morning to find bloodstains on her sheet, she ran to tell her mother, who gave her a hug and a box of menstrual pads.

"You are a woman now!" Maria's mother said with pride. That evening the entire family, which had come to America from Mexico ten years before, dressed up and went out to dinner to celebrate Maria's coming-of-age. The response is not so positive in all families, however.

In some African cultures a girl's clitoris is cut away and her labia are stitched together so that she will never feel pleasure in the sexual act, and presumably, will not stray from her husband—who may, of course, stray as far as he likes. The mutilation is done by the tribe's elder women, who are not medical practitioners. The ritual frequently results in infection and sometimes even death.

In some orthodox religions, men claimed that blood made women unclean at certain times of the month, and so they were forbidden from participating in many activities. No wonder menstruation has been called "the curse."

How could a girl's self-image be anything but confused and muddled with centuries of contradictions and uncertainties? Girls like Maria are lucky. They live with families who accept coming-of-age—and menstruation—as a natural and good part of life. They see it as a reason for joy.

The sudden depreciation of self-image that occurs in adolescent girls has been described eloquently by Carol Gilligan in her book *In a Different Voice*. As a psychologist she was concerned with the effect on self-esteem that different socialization processes had for girls and boys. She found that around puberty girls lost a lot of their self-assurance and thought less well of themselves than boys did. A girl's self-image hinges on these physical and emotional changes, and it is important for her and her parents to understand them. Self-knowledge builds confidence. The more you know, the better you cope with change and uncertainty.

Adolescence and menopause are the two great transitions in a woman's life, but of the two, adolescence plays a more formative role. It is also a very fragile period in a girl's mental and physical development; it occurs during adolescence, when the preconceived ideas of self, forged in childhood, collide with the cold reality of the adult world.

Adolescence does not happen at once, but in three distinct phases.

THE THREE PHASES OF ADOLESCENCE

Early Adolescence

From ages 12 to 14, the junior high school years are characterized by the struggle between dependence and independence. A girl becomes involved with peer groups, usually other girls, and her rapidly changing body becomes her preoccupation. While the teenager is developing her intellectual capacity, she might have idealistic and nonrealistic vocational goals and difficulty in controlling her impulses. She might have an impulse to run away, to give away the expensive new running shoes she got for her birthday to a homeless person. She might dream of becoming a pop star like Madonna.

Middle Adolescence

From ages 15 through 17, the high school years, the independence vs. dependence struggle may increasingly develop into conflicts with parents who become upset and worried. A girl acquires a new sense of individuality, and her vocational aspirations are less idealistic. She might now think of occupations such as doctor, teacher, or hair stylist. She still feels omnipotent and immortal and is likely to engage in risk-taking behaviors. While parents are worried about sexual behavior and substance abuse, the girl herself, while possibly engaging in sex and substance abuse, is more concerned with her weight and self-image.

Late Adolescence

From ages 18 to 20, developing plans for college or a job lead to more realistic goals. The girl separates herself more from her family, but is likely to better appreciate her parents' values. She is settled into her new body and identity, although still overly concerned about it. Peer group values become less important to her, and she is likely to spend more time with one person and perhaps develop an intimate relationship.

Girls who marry and have children in late adolescence stunt their natural progression from childhood to young adulthood. Early childbearing, before their bodies and minds stop growing, usually results in diminished aspirations. Girls resign themselves to a lower educational level, lower income level, and greater dependency on the male members of the family, usually the husband or boyfriend.

The dangers teens face today are far greater than they were a generation ago, when the big question was whether or not to "go all the way." Today's young woman must be very well informed about the health hazards of sexually transmitted infection, substance abuse, and violence, including rape. The more difficult part of making teenagers aware of these serious challenges is, of course, their age itself. Few teenagers believe or even think about what they do now as meaning anything later in life. They feel they are invincible. They can worry about it all later.

The five challenges to the health of American women—young and old—begin in youth. They are:

- Coping with the physical and emotional changes brought on by puberty, and the achievement of physical fitness

- Eating well to avoid malnutrition, obesity, eating disorders, and future problems like heart disease, osteoporosis, and diabetes

- Drugs and substance abuse

- Violence

- Teen pregnancy

All of these challenges are included in this section of the book, which begins with a chapter to help girls learn just what is changing in their bodies, and why so many aspects of future health depend upon nutrition and fitness during this time of life. The chapter about menstruation should help clear up some of the medical misunderstandings and myths about PMS, cramps, and other related conditions.

Of importance to young women in this phase of life is an understanding of how eating disorders—anorexia, bulimia, and obesity—affect their future. Everything a girl does during this phase of her life affects her health later, and this cannot be overly stressed. And that is why such topics as skin care, exercise and nutrition, and understanding the basics of good health care are introduced here.

The dangers of this period are outlined in chapters on sexual violence, sexually transmitted infection, and contraception, all meant to stress the importance of protection. A chapter on tobacco abuse should help make it clear why the World Health Organization considers the legacy of tobacco—more than any other single disease— as the world's greatest health burden, a burden that will kill more people than anything else by the middle of the next century.

One of the best antidotes for low self-esteem is organized sports, and this is becoming more widespread. Sports and exercise set a girl on a course of life where she feels competent and strong and does better in career choice and social situations. She is also going to be much healthier than the majority of the population.

··3··

Puberty and Menses: Getting to Know Your Changing Body

A girl is not always sure she likes what is happening to her body as her arms and legs elongate and she loses some of her baby fat. Her breasts grow, and sometimes they hurt. I have heard many girls complain their breasts were "in the way" and held them back from physical activities and sports.

Although the arrival of the first menstrual period is the most obvious manifestation of becoming a woman, many physical changes predate this event. There's usually a spurt of growth, and girls get taller. Breasts develop (*thelarche*) and pubic hair appears (*adrenarche*). It takes approximately four to five years for breasts to mature and about four years for the pubic hair. Some girls accept the changes in their bodies while others rebel and are frustrated by them. The period can become "the curse." Loose clothing, or carrying books close to the chest, can hide the burgeoning breasts.

In the last half of the twentieth century, American girls seemed to be developing the characteristics of puberty, such as body hair and breasts, earlier, but the average age for the beginning of menses is still around 12. A study of seventeen girls from ages 3 to 12, reported in the journal *Pediatrics* in 1997, showed the development of breasts and pubic hair began, on average, at the age of eight and as early as seven. African-American girls tend to reach puberty a year before Caucasians, possibly because, on average, black girls are heavier than white girls. Previous research showed that only 1 percent of girls under age 8 have such development. The new study is the first one that looked at girls under the age of 8, and it is the first multiracial study.

Puberty before the age of 8 or 9 used to be known as "precocious puberty," but today may be considered within normal limits. Precocious puberty meant the brain clock could have been set ahead by many still-unexplained factors, perhaps by the girl's weight or the amount of fatty tissue on her body. It can also be caused by an abnormality such as tumors of the adrenal glands or the ovaries. Researchers had no clear-cut explanation for the earlier onset of puberty but suggested one reason is that children are getting heavier. According to the study, girls who matured earlier were larger and heavier than those who did not. There is speculation among researchers that, in addition to improved nutrition, earlier puberty could be due to higher exposure to environmental estrogens in hair products, insecticides, and plastics. This earlier puberty, scientists believe, is a real phenomenon with important clinical, educational, and social implications. Medical guidelines, as well as timing of sex education programs in schools, need to be revised.

Even if a girl is prepared for and supported during her first menses, as Maria was, seeing that first trace of blood can still be a shock. The ease with which a girl had engaged in sports now suddenly gives way to a careful activity planned around physiological events over which she has no control. She thinks she cannot go swimming whenever she wants. She starts to wonder if some of her organs are normal. Are the lips of her vagina too big or too small? Is this discharge normal? Are her breasts too large or too small? Many girls, genetically programmed for large breasts, stoop or hunch and develop posture problems.

Few of us in the older generations received any education about what to expect from our changing bodies from parents or schools or our family doctors. Today, there is more openness about it in families that are educated, but according to a survey of adolescents by the Commonwealth Fund Commission on Women's Health, most teenage girls learn about their changing bodies and emerging sexuality from the mass media or their friends, and unfortunately, much of what they learn is incorrect. However, many girls do realize they lack important information and would like to know more about health, nutrition, exercise, alcohol, and drugs.

Several excellent books about puberty are listed in Appendix 3.

THE GONADOSTAT: SETTING THE BIOLOGICAL CLOCK

Research at the University of California at San Francisco in 1997 suggested that one of the critical initiators of puberty is *leptin*, a chemical already famed for its role in controlling body fat. It is a protein secreted by adipose cells that let the body know it is fat enough and so it should stop eating. When leptin was injected into young female mice, the animals reached sexual maturity earlier than those injected with an inactive solution. This research seems to confirm the long-held belief that puberty is somehow related to body fat, especially in girls.

There is a "critical fat" hypothesis that holds that a girl must reach a certain weight before her brain feels that her body can handle a pregnancy. When that weight is achieved, the hormones are released and puberty begins. The new research sustains this theory that blood levels of leptin must reach a certain level to allow puberty to happen. If the investigators are right, this would explain why chubby girls frequently begin puberty earlier, and very thin or athletic girls begin later.

For a normal *menarche*—the onset of menstruation—to occur, a complicated process must be initiated requiring sequential coordination of hormone secretions coming from various endocrine glands and brain centers. The process is so complex, indeed, that it makes you wonder how the body ever gets it right. And yet in more than 90 percent of girls menarche does occur on time and progresses in a timely fashion.

Menarche hinges on the maturation and synchronicity of the glands and hormones that connect the brain with the ovaries. The brain's hypothalamus produces a hormone we call GnRH, short for *gonadotropin releasing hormone*. This hormone stimulates the pituitary gland to produce its hormone, FSH, or *follicle stimulating hormone*. The FSH stimulates the ovary to produce estrogen. Rising estrogen levels cause a surge of GnRH and FSH along with a surge of another pituitary hormone, LH, or *luteinizing hormone*. The LH triggers ovulation. This connection between the hypothalamus, the pituitary, and the ovary is called the hypothalamic-pituitary-ovarian axis.

What causes the hormonal axis to mature is not known, but the timing is tied in with attaining a sufficient body weight with sufficient fat. If the gonadostat within the hypothalamus believes a girl is ripe, it sends out signals to the pituitary gland, located under the lower surface of the brain, to start producing special hormones to activate the ovary. These pituitary hormones are called *gonadotropins* since they target the gonads (ovaries in the female and testes in the male). Thus, the gonadostat is set and menses begin. The female hypothalamus is imprinted with cyclicity, which drives cyclic alterations in hormone levels, ovulations and menstrual cycles. This is the difference between men and women. There is no such imprint on the male hypothalamus.

There are three kinds of estrogen produced in the ovary: *estradiol*, the most active; *estrone*; and *estriol*. An estrogen precursor is also produced by the adrenal glands but it is negligible during the reproductive years. Estrogen is beneficial to the bones, blood vessels, heart, immune system, brain, eyes, teeth, and probably more that we do not yet completely understand. On the other hand, it is thought to be linked to breast, ovarian, and uterine cancers, autoimmune disorders, asthma, fibroids, migraine headaches, and mood disorders.

CHANGING ANATOMY: THE VIEW FROM OUTSIDE

Your body is developing inside and out. You can see the outside, primarily the development of breasts and pubic hair. First we'll describe what you can easily see. Then what few women bother to look at—the dramatic changes occuring invisibly inside their bodies.

The Developing Breast

Two to four years before the arrival of the first menstrual period the girl's breasts begin to grow (*thelarche*). This is caused by the building up levels of estrogen. The breast gland is composed of branching ducts with a small bubble at their ends, the alveoli.

Sometimes breasts ache while they grow because the skin is stretching and the alveoli are popping open from a previously collapsed state. Breast pain is common in a young girl, especially if she is injured. When I was a teenager, we played a ball game in my school and it was an unwritten rule that the ball should not be thrown at a girl's chest. One of my patients brought her 13-year-old daughter, Tania, to see me after the girl got hit in the breast with a basketball and developed a lump a few days later.

The lump in Tania's breast was caused by the impact of the ball, which might have caused an accumulation of blood under the skin. In other words, she might have had, in addition to the visible outside bruise in her skin, an inside bruise or a blood clot, a hematoma, deeper in her breast. The hematoma could persist for some time. At first it was tender and painful. As the superficial bruise faded, the inner hematoma caused a red discoloration, which later became black and blue and then slightly green. Gradually the color faded and the lump disappeared. Contrary to many people's beliefs, mechanical injury to the breast does not lead to cancer.

A lump in a breast always frightens women, young and old, and this is good reason to learn about your breasts and how they work. At the time of the first menstrual period and thereafter, it is not unusual for a girl to develop lumpiness in her breasts, lumps that wax and wane, grow and disappear in tandem with hormonal changes during the menstrual cycle. The lumpiness and soreness are worst before the period and usually diminish right after the period. This benign condition, called "fibrocystic breasts," is not a disease but a common response of the breasts to changing estrogen levels. Some of the alveoli become distended balloons (cysts) and compress the neighboring tissue, which becomes scarred (fibrous).

A malignant lump is extremely unusual in a young girl Tania's age. An adolescent does not need to examine her breasts for the presence of cancerous lumps (unless there is a family history of breast cancer), but it is when they are young that girls should become familiar with their breasts. The purpose of breast self-examination is to learn about the consistency and lumpiness of your own breasts and to be able to recognize a new lump that has not been there before (Figure 3).

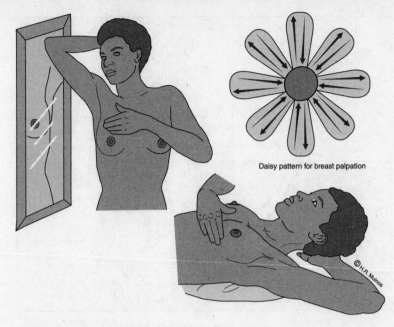

Daisy pattern for breast palpation

Figure 3. Breast self-examination in a daisy pattern. Note two positions.

Vagina: Entrance or Exit?

The vagina is the hollow, partially muscular, somewhat S-shaped canal through which menstrual blood exits, babies exit, and normal intercourse with a man takes place. Contractions of the muscular vagina contribute to the orgasm, a pleasurable sensation experienced with the stimulation of intercourse. In common medical parlance the part of the vagina that marks the exit to the outside world is called *introitus*, or "entrance." Named by male anatomists, our anatomy obviously reflects their own point of view: that the vagina is the way into the woman for sexual intercourse, the pelvic examination, and the pathway of microorganisms carrying sexually transmitted infection.

A female anatomist—and there were never enough of them to make a permanent mark—would have considered the opening of the vagina as an exit, a conduit for menstrual blood to flow out of the body and for babies to come out into the world. In this century of female emancipation I christen the outlet of the vagina *exitus*. And I define *vagina* as "a muscular pouch that leads from the uterus to the outside," not the other way around.

Outside and in front of the vaginal canal are the clitoris, the labia, the urethral meatus, and several small glands. All of this is known collectively as the vulva. The perineum is the area that separates the vagina from the anus (Figure 4). The entire vulva, and especially the clitoris and vagina, are richly enervated so that touch and pressure convey the pleasurable sensations that culminate in orgasm.

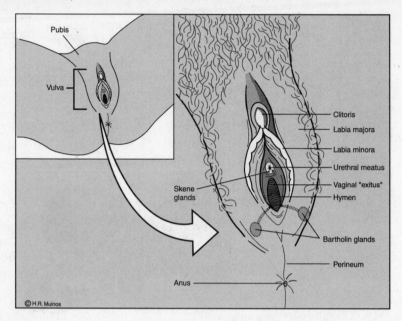

Figure 4. External genitalia.

Hymen

Until a girl has sex or a pelvic examination, the exit of the vagina is usually covered by the hymen, a latexlike membrane that contains some flesh and blood vessels, which is why it bleeds when it is ruptured. As a rule, the hymen does not cover the exit completely. It can be in the shape of a half-moon. Usually it is symmetrical or has one or more pin-sized holes in the center. These variations are normal and have no clinical significance.

One relatively rare (one in 2,000) variation is the hymen that completely covers the vaginal opening; it is called *imperforate hymen.* A small incision needs to be made by a physician before the first intercourse; otherwise it might be painful or even impossible to have intercourse. In some cases, the imperforate hymen prevents menstrual blood from leaving the body and has to be surgically removed. If a woman ages without experiencing sexual intercourse or a pelvic examination, the membrane can become quite tough. I have seen several patients, actually, who had not had intercourse all their lives, with very tough hymens. Three of them were nuns.

Fourchette

The fourchette is between the vagina and the perineum. It resembles a two-pronged fork of flat tissue framed by the inner lips on its sides. It can be stretched gently but it could be injured by forceful entry during intercourse or by careless insertion of the speculum during a pelvic examination, especially in elderly women with shrunken *atrophic* vagina.

Pubis
This is the triangular area bounded on both sides by the inner surfaces of the thighs and above by the lower abdomen, sometimes delineated by a horizontal crease over the lower abdomen. The hair covering the pubis is called the *escutcheon*. In women this triangle of pubic hair is broad at the top and narrows at the bottom, while in men it is the opposite. Their hair generally grows upward from the genitals and narrows near the navel.

Labia
The exit of the vagina is characterized by two pairs of folds, the inner lips (*labia minora*) and the outer lips (*labia majora*). The inner lips are thinner, usually moist and hairless. The outer lips are thicker and frequently covered with hair, especially on their outer sides. These lips are made of the same kind of tissue as the lips on your mouth.

Clitoris
The clitoris is the equivalent of the male penis, a "bump" of variable dimensions where the inner lips come together. It is filled with sensory nerves, and when it is gently stimulated, the woman experiences pleasurable sexual feelings. Like the penis, the clitoris might have a distinct foreskin, or cap, but unlike the penis it is not a conduit for urine. An excessively large clitoris of more than one centimeter (half an inch) might indicate abnormally high levels of male hormones and *virilization*, but this is a rare occurrence due to drugs or tumors of the ovary or adrenal glands.

Urethral Meatus
Situated below the clitoris, this small indentation is the urethral meatus, or the outlet of the urethra, the urinary conduit from the bladder.

Skene Glands
Just behind (or below) the opening of the urethra there are two small openings that drain the area of the vagina and the urethra and might exude pus in case of infection. These are the Skene glands, named after a urologist.

Bartholin Glands
On either side of the posterior end of the labia are the Bartholin glands (also called vulvovaginal glands), which help lubricate the vagina during sexual arousal. You might or might not see the openings for secretions, but you might feel the thickening on either side of the vagina. If these

glands become clogged from secretions and infected, they can become painful and might need to be drained. You might not be able to sit or walk comfortably. A painful swelling, which can become an abscess, appears in the labium, and the skin overlying the gland is pulled tight, becomes swollen, and is painful to the touch. An abscess can also be a sign of a sexually transmitted infection, such as *gonorrhea* or *chlamydia* (see chapter 9).

Treatment for infected Bartholin glands consists of oral or injected antibiotics and hot soaks. Sometimes surgical intervention is necessary to remove and drain the abscess, but that does not always resolve the problem. In the past, gynecologists often prescribed surgery to remove such abscesses. This was unnecessary and often did not resolve the problem as well as hot soaks.

CHANGING ANATOMY: THE VIEW FROM INSIDE

The sexual and reproductive organs fit into the pelvis, which is a cradlelike bone structure shaped somewhat like a catcher's mitt. Because a woman's pelvis must accommodate the growing baby, her pelvis is wider than a man's.

Internal genitalia consist of the uterus, Fallopian tubes, ovaries, and ligaments that keep everything in place in the pelvis. One of the ligaments, the broad ligament, is like a suspended curtain. The other, the uterosacral ligament, stabilizes the position of the uterus. Of these organs, only one part of the uterus—namely, its neck, the cervix—can be viewed on examination.

The Uterus

The muscular uterus (womb) is the size and shape of a small pear in a young girl, and of a somewhat larger pear in a woman who has borne children. It looks like a slightly flattened electric lightbulb, with its narrow part, the neck, directed downward, into the vagina. The neck is the cervix.

The body of the uterus is the *corpus*, and the base—which is actually at the top of the pear, opposite the cervix—is the *fundus*. The position of the fundus varies, and a tilted womb is just a normal variant that can pose some difficulty for the physician who wants to precisely assess its shape. In the nineteenth century, a tilted womb was sometimes blamed for infertility, but this is a myth and today we know there is no direct link between the tilted uterus and an inability to have children.

The wall of the hollow uterus is a powerful muscle called the *myometrium*. The contractions of this muscle are essential for labor and delivery in childbirth. Milder contractions of the myometrium are probably partly responsible for pleasurable sensations during orgasm.

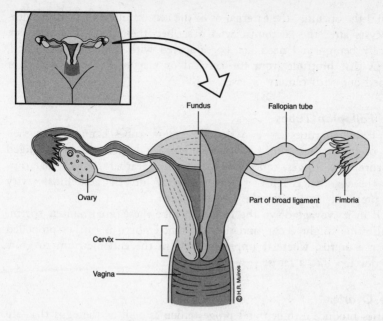

Figure 5. Internal genitalia.

The uterus is hollow to allow expansion for a growing baby. It is lined with a layer of special cells called the *endometrium*. Estrogen makes these cells grow and proliferate, so that the lining becomes lush and thick. Progesterone, the second ovarian hormone, causes microscopic glands to form in the endometrium and begin to secrete mucus and other nutritious material just in case an egg is fertilized and comes to rest on the plush endometrial cradle. Thus, the menstrual cycle is divided into the proliferative (estrogen-controlled) phase and the secretory (primarily progesterone controlled) phase.

The Cervix

The cervix is the open end of the uterus, the exit leading into the vaginal canal. The opening into the vagina, called the *os*, is usually narrowed and protected by smooth muscle. It opens up during the menstrual flow and completely disappears during labor. Its role is to protect the uterus from the influx of foreign and possibly harmful material or bacteria, and to protect the fetus from premature expulsion out of the uterus. There is also another, less prominent narrowing at the upper end of the cervix as it opens into the uterine cavity. This is called the *internal os*. The medical expression "incompetent cervix" means the cervical os (either one) is dilated inappropriately during pregnancy and a miscarriage is imminent.

Cysts are the most common abnormalities of the cervix. They occur around the opening, the external os of the cervix, and are called Nabothian cysts after the anatomist who described them first. The cysts are entirely benign and need not be tampered with. On the other hand, polyps that protrude from the cervical os may need to be excised or burned out with cautery or laser.

The Fallopian Tubes

The Fallopian tubes are two slender, hollow tubes connected to each side of the fundus, the top of the uterus, and that end in a fringed aperture. The fringes, called *fimbriae*, are like feathery fingers that capture the egg that is released from the ovary into the abdominal cavity and propel it down the tube into the uterus.

If in its voyage down the Fallopian tube the egg encounters sperm, fertilization might occur, and the resultant embryo is further propelled into the uterus, where it implants itself in the endometrium to grow and develop into a fetus.

The Ovaries

Ovaries produce estrogen and progesterone as well as the eggs that are released periodically. These are the female gonads. Male gonads are the testes. The ovaries are two solid, bean-shaped organs, about an inch long in a young adult woman, much smaller in the prepubertal girl, and smaller once again in a postmenopausal woman. They are situated outside the fundus on either side below and slightly to the back of the fringes of the tubes. A girl is born with about two million undeveloped eggs in tiny "blebs" in her ovaries. These are called *immature follicles*. After puberty an egg matures each month and ruptures from the surface of the ovary, leaving the remains of the follicle behind.

Lubricating the Passage

Once a girl reaches puberty and her sexual and reproductive organs develop, her genital glands will start to produce secretions. The normal vaginal discharge sometimes concerns girls who first experience it, but the worry is unwarranted unless the discharge is unusual or irritating or has a foul odor. Then it may be a sign of infection or a sexually transmitted infection.

Mucous glands imbedded in the cells covering the cervix and lining the vaginal walls produce small amounts of thin, white or clear, sticky fluid that lubricates the *lumen*, the vaginal passageway. At the time of ovulation, secretion increases and becomes elastic, so that it can be pulled in long threads. The normal vaginal secretion is slightly acid, and this keeps the vagina healthy and resistant to infection.

There is no need to do anything about normal vaginal secretions except to keep yourself clean with regular showers and bathing. There is more information in chapter 9 about sexually transmitted infection and in chapter 16 about conditions of the reproductive system.

MENSTRUATION: MYTH AND REALITY

It seems redundant, in the last decade of the twentieth century, to say that menstruation is a normal, healthy process requiring minimal medical intrusion. Women themselves do not always know what is going on in their bodies. A recent study reported in the *Journal of the American Medical Association* explored the "modern-day menstrual folklore." Forty women of multiethnic backgrounds, aged 17 to 41, were asked for their knowledge about menses. The majority lacked accurate basic knowledge of anatomy. They believed that menstruating women should avoid sexual intercourse, should not swim, should not do any exercise. A few even believed that the menstrual flow created such a suspect aura that women might be attacked by reptiles. A few expressed fear of watering plants lest the plants wither from their contact.

The only "aura" involved with menstruation might be the pheromones, hormonal substances given off in small particles in the perspiration and breath. When inhaled, pheromones can exert a hormonal influence on another person. This might explain why women who live together in a college dorm, summer camp, or military barracks for any period of time begin to have coordinated menstrual cycles. Eventually, they all get their periods around the same time of the month.

Menarche, the beginning of menstrual periods, can normally occur at any age between 10 and 16. The exact age of normal menarche varies, depending on racial or ethnic background, family history, diet, and body type. As already mentioned, because of better nutrition, the age of menarche is getting earlier in modern society. Variations also exist in the duration of the period, the volume of flow, and the degree of discomfort.

All other factors being equal, girls living nearer the equator tend to start menstruating early, while girls in Scandinavian countries tend to start later. An interesting corollary is that late menarche girls tend to be taller (like the Scandinavians) than those who start early. This is because the estrogen causes the growing regions of long bones to close. Thus, premature menarche is associated with shorter stature.

Ovulation

A woman is born with 2 million follicles in her ovaries. These follicles are small blisters within the ovaries, containing the eggs (*ova*). Under influence of hormones, the follicles grow, mature, produce estrogen, and move toward the surface of the ovary. Then one by one for each menstrual cycle they burst out of the surface of the ovary and the egg is released into the abdominal cavity. This is called *ovulation*. The ovary

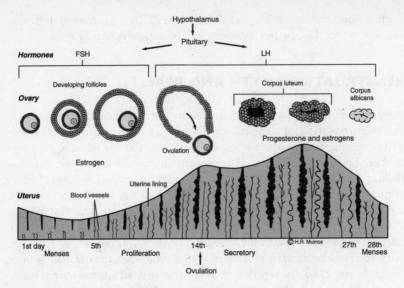

Figure 6. Menstrual cycle.

heals itself after that rupture and forms a yellow body (*corpus luteum*), which produces the second important ovarian hormone, progesterone.

The egg is sucked up from the abdominal cavity by the fringed end of the Fallopian tube to be propelled by the movement (*peristalsis*) of the tube toward the uterus. If the egg, on its voyage through the tube, is fertilized by a sperm, the resultant embryo implants itself in the uterus and in time becomes a fetus. Meanwhile, the uterus is ready for the embryo because estrogen and progesterone have prepared a moist, warm nest for it. Many contraceptives work by interfering with this ovulation process or by interfering with the action of progesterone on the lining of the uterus so that implantation cannot take place.

If the egg fails to be fertilized by sperm it exits out of the uterus. At a signal from the ovary the entire lining of the uterus is sloughed off. This sloughing is accompanied by uterine bleeding, otherwise known as menstruation.

Early Menarche

One mother, anxious over her 9-year-old daughter's early menses, came in to see me. "Look at her; she has the figure of a grown woman. Isn't it too soon? I was almost thirteen when my periods began." Eve, a husky, brown-eyed girl, had obviously undergone her prepubertal growth spurt, and her breasts were developing. She had pubic and underarm hair, but no abnormal hair such as on her face or breasts, which would indicate a hormonal imbalance.

Eve was fine. It was just that her biological clock had been set slightly ahead. I reassured the mother and daughter that this was not abnormal, and predicted short stature for the girl, which was not of concern to them. It turned out that Eve did not grow much taller than she was at the age of nine. Fully grown, she reached only two inches over five feet.

Early menses can also be caused by an underactive thyroid. The thyroid gland is a busybody. Its hormones, thyroxine (T-4) and triiodothyronine (T-3) affect every organ, tissue, and cell in the body. These hormones regulate metabolism and the speed with which the cells burn fuel, consume oxygen, and turn out carbon dioxide. Too little thyroid hormone (hypothyroidism) or too much (hyperthyroidism) can slow down or accelerate menarche.

In some cases, hypothyroidism can cause sexual precocity in girls. Taking thyroid medication will postpone the menarche. It is important to recognize this abnormality in young girls. However, with long-standing severe thyroid deficiency girls might not start menstruating at all, or will start very late. Paradoxically, after menarche has arrived, thyroid deficiency might speed up the menses and increase the bleeding. The interval between the periods becomes shorter and the girl bleeds more profusely and more frequently. Hyperthyroid women, on the other hand, might have shorter, scantier, and less frequent periods.

Premature menarche, or any irregular menses, needs to be investigated by an endocrinologist trained in pediatric and adolescent medicine.

Delayed Menarche

If there is no menstrual period by the age of 15, a girl might be experiencing normal *delayed menarche*. If it does not appear for several years after 16, there could be an abnormality in the chromosomes, ovaries, or adrenal glands.

Delayed menarche is frequently a source of worry to parents, if not the girls themselves. Susan, a thin, pale, 17-year-old, had not yet begun to develop or menstruate, despite her advanced height. A student and athlete, she was always in a rush, with little time to eat. She weighed 88 pounds, having recently lost 12. Her mother brought her to see me despite the girl's protests.

Susan seemed unable to sit still, and her hostility was evident in the knife-plunging glances at me and her mother. Her face had a haunted, depressed look, like those anorexic models in the Calvin Klein clothing ads. Susan's breasts were just beginning to develop but there was no hair yet visible on her pubis. Tests showed very low estrogen in her blood. Her thyroid function was normal. A pelvic sonogram revealed normal ovaries and no abnormal masses.

My working diagnosis was anorexia nervosa, a potentially life-threatening disease needing prompt intervention, both physical and psychiatric (see chapter 10). I told Susan her diagnosis and that if she had not gained a pound or two in a week, she would have to be hospitalized for intravenous feedings. My bluntness and a referral to a psychiatrist worked. Four months later, she had gained 10 pounds, her breasts had enlarged, and pubic hair had appeared. After a few more weeks, her first period arrived.

Once the secondary sexual characteristics have appeared, menarche is not far behind. It is simply a delayed menarche. The reasons for the delay are sometimes difficult to determine.

Irregular Bleeding

In the first two to five years after menarche begins, it is perfectly normal for menstruation to be irregular. It could come every fifteen days or every forty-five days, or any time in between. The norm would be from twenty-eight to thirty-two days from the first day of the last period. It might even stop for months, most commonly in the summer, with a change of environment from the school year. The hypothalamus is a sensitive organ and is subject to stimuli from everywhere in the body and brain, including thoughts and emotions.

In the first few years, ovulation might be sporadic. That brain-to-ovary hormonal axis takes time to mature, and many cycles occur without actual ovulation. Bleeding in a cycle not preceded by ovaluation is not a regular shedding of the endometrium resulting from the interplay of estrogen and progesterone. It is due to fluctuation in the level of estrogen only. With a rise in estrogen level, the endometrial tissue grows actively. With a sudden drop in the estrogen level, the endometrium loses its hormonal support and sheds. This type of estrogen withdrawal bleeding is not a real menstrual period.

Sometimes girls perceive moderate and heavy bleeding as excessive because the pattern is irregular, or they are afraid too much blood means they are hemorrhaging. A lack of familiarity with their normal menstrual flow patterns and a general fear of blood are often the reasons why young women tend to describe moderate and marginal bleeding as excessive.

The absence of bleeding is called amenorrhea; too much bleeding is a condition called *menorrhagia*. Excessive vaginal bleeding at the time of a normal expected period seldom requires medical intervention except when a true hemorrhage occurs with a spontaneous and incomplete miscarriage, vaginal laceration during a sexual assault, masturbation with a foreign object, infections, or certain drugs and medical conditions. If these conditions are ruled out, excessive bleeding is usually treated with a progesterone compound that stops the bleeding. In rare cases where this does not work and heavy bleeding persists, the gynecologist may perform a diagnostic dilatation and curettage (D&C) (see chapter 14).

AMENORRHEA: WHEN MENSES DO NOT COME

Amenorrhea is the absence of menses for longer than three months, although some authorities define it as absence for a year or longer. *Primary amenorrhe*a means your period never came, and *secondary amenorrhea* means it stopped coming.

Both anorexia nervosa and extreme and chronic physical exertion associated with weight loss, such as sometimes occurs in professional athletes and ballet dancers, are examples of amenorrhea that can be secondary or primary when these conditions interfere with the very establishment of normal menstrual function.

In more than half the cases of primary amenorrhea, however, the fault lies with the ovary. It can be either polycystic (filled with many cysts that interfere with the development and function of the egg-containing follicles) or there can be ovarian dysgenesis (see Turner syndrome, below). This means that the ovary never developed properly in the fetal life of the girl. It could be due to chromosomal abnormality or an environmental complication such as particular medications or recreational drug abuse (see chapter 11).

Congenital abnormalities of the adrenal glands can cause primary amenorrhea, but this can be treated with medication. Developmental abnormalities of the uterus and tubes might also be at fault, and can sometimes be corrected with surgery. During fetal development the proper connection between the Fallopian tubes, the uterus, and the vagina might not occur. This, too, however, can be corrected by surgery.

Secondary Amenorrhea
Secondary amenorrhea is more common than primary amenorrhea and usually engenders much less anxiety. This is when normal periods stop. The most common cause is an inadequate estrogen level. In other words, the ovary has suddenly given up production. Sometimes malnutrition can affect the ovary and cause its failure, as in the case of Susan, mentioned earlier. Occasionally, psychological trauma of various degrees, even travel or summer vacation away from home, can cause temporary cessation of menses. A correct diagnosis of secondary amenorrhea frequently requires a consultation with a reproductive endocrinologist in order to consider and rule out ovarian, pituitary, adrenal, and thyroid dysfunction and tumors.

Little Menses
Oligomenorrhea, or little menses, is a markedly diminished menstrual flow and menstrual cycles with intervals of up to three months. This is not uncommon. If it is not due to hyperthyroidism, it's most likely due to excitement, travel, or excessive exercise.

Hidden Menses

Theresa, a 17-year-old who came to my office, had breasts and pubic hair but no periods. However, she did have lower abdominal pain every month. Examination revealed that her hymen covered the entire exit of the vagina so there was no way out for the menstrual blood. This variant of the normal hymen, the imperforate hymen, completely covers and encloses the vaginal exit. Theresa had actually been menstruating, but the blood remained in the vaginal canal, causing pressure and discomfort. This condition is called *cryptomenorrhea*, or hidden menses. A simple procedure by the gynecologist, incision of the hymen and drainage of the fluid, relieved her of pain and allowed her to experience normal menstrual periods.

Turner Syndrome

Normally, a female has two X chromosomes in every cell of her body, which is described as XX. In Turner syndrome, or *ovarian dysgenesis*, a girl possesses only one X chromosome, which is described as XO. The ovaries never develop sufficiently to produce estrogen and certainly not progesterone. Therefore, a girl must receive estrogen and progesterone replacement in order to prevent catastrophic osteoporosis and premature arteriosclerosis. Girls with Turner syndrome also receive growth hormones to prevent very short stature. This syndrome is not very common, but it is the most common chromosomal abnormality in girls. Endocrinologists see quite a bit of this.

Other Causes

When hyperthyroidism, polycystic ovaries, and hypothalamic causes are not the apparent causes of the amenorrhea, a more extensive workup needs to be considered. A scraping from inside a girl's cheek, called a *buccal smear*, and an examination of her blood cells for chromosomes (a *karyotype*), might be needed to rule out such rare conditions as mistaken male gender with superficially female features. This testicular feminization syndrome means the girl is really a boy whose body is insensitive to testosterone so he looks like a girl. A defect of one of the two X chromosomes could also be involved.

MENSTRUAL DISCOMFORTS EXPLAINED

For far too long menstrual cramps were considered psychosomatic. They were a sign of a woman's denial of her sexuality or her need for attention. Ovulatory pain (pain experienced when the ovarian follicle ruptures), or *Mittelschmerz*, is also a real discomfort for 50 percent of women. Premenstrual syndrome acquired a great deal of notoriety. It has been blamed for emotional problems women experience before and around menses and for aberrant and even criminal behavior. It has served as an excuse for not promoting women to higher levels of responsibility in all types of jobs. It has brought discomfort and nuisance to many, perhaps 25 pecent of all women of reproductive age.

Until very recently, women suffered from premenstrual syndrome and menstrual cramps without relief. It was all in our heads, the doctors (men) told us. They were wrong, of course, because research into personality factors and cramps found that women with dysmenorrhea were not significantly different from those who had no cramps.

We know now that the "psychosomatic" theory was wrong. Doctors calling the pain psychogenic did harm to women's self-esteem.

Primary Dysmenorrhea: Menstrual Cramps

There is a sound physiologic basis for cramps—a high level of prostaglandins in the uterus. We do not know why excessive prostaglandins are produced in some women or why cramps are less severe for some women after childbirth.

Prostaglandins are substances made of unsaturated fatty acids that are found in almost all body tissues and fluids. They act like hormones but are not carried by the bloodstream to act on remote organs the way most other hormones do. As the progesterone level drops before menstruation, there is a dramatic increase in the production of prostaglandins in the uterus. These prostaglandins produce an inflammatory reaction and initiate powerful laborlike contractions of the uterus. They also cause constriction of the small arteries of the uterus, cutting down on oxygen supplied to the endometrium.

Cramps are sharp spasmodic pains in the lower abdomen that sometimes radiate to the lower back and thighs. Cramps can also cause nausea, vomiting, diarrhea, headache, irritability, and even fainting. Prostaglandins also lead to contractions of the intestinal tract that speed up the digestive process. It is not unusual to have mild constipation before menses and then mild diarrhea and menstrual cramps during the first three days of flow.

Intrauterine devices (IUD) have also been associated with severe cramps because the device itself stimulates the release of more prostaglandin, probably through an irritative effect. The IUD as a method of contraception is not recommended for most adolescents. (See chapter 8 for more on birth control methods.)

Primary dysmenorrhea usually begins six to twelve months after menarche. Young women who have not borne children are more likely to have severe symptoms. It tends to improve after the first pregnancy. The majority of young women suffer from some degree of dysmenorrhea. A 1970 survey found a 60 percent incidence of dysmenorrhea among 12-to-17-year-old females. In 50 percent of those, dysmenorrhea was described as mild; in 14 percent, it was described as severe.

Bonnie, a 17-year-old who suffered from cramps for a year, complained that when her period came she was done in by the pain. "I cannot go to school or out with my friends. Everybody knows when I get it." At first, Bonnie's pain was tolerable, but it gradually worsened until she had to stay in bed during the first day. The acute pain caused her to double up. At the same time, she had searing headaches and gastrointestinal problems. Tears rolled down her cheeks as she described her symptoms.

Treatment for Cramps

The purpose of medical treatment of menstrual cramps is to decrease the inflammation caused by prostaglandins by using medications that inhibit the production of prostaglandins and thus prevent the spasms. Nonsteroidal anti-inflammatory drugs (NSAIDs) such as ibuprofen can also reduce the menstrual blood flow in some women. Aspirin also possesses anti-inflammatory properties but is not as effective for menstrual cramps as NSAIDs. In some women aspirin can increase blood flow and irritate the stomach.

NSAIDs are relatively safe in the small doses found in over-the-counter preparations. If you start taking them three to five days before your period begins and continue until the end of the second day, they are usually effective. (NSAIDs are also used for other conditions, such as arthritis, and when they are used for long periods of time can cause ulcers and kidney damage.) If cramps do not ease up with NSAIDs, see your doctor to rule out a condition called *endometriosis*, explained in chapter 16.

Despite the availability of safe, effective short-term therapy since the 1980s, dysmenorrhea is still the leading cause of absences among women from school and work. Overall, 14 percent of adolescent girls, including 50 percent of those with severe dysmenorrhea and 17 percent of those with mild dysmenorrhea, reported missing school due to cramps.

Most adolescents with dysmenorrhea never seek help from a doctor (only 14.5 percent did this), and 30 percent of parents were unaware of their daughters' symptoms. The most important reasons for not obtaining relief from cramps? Lack of education or access to informed health care.

Fortunately, Bonnie achieved considerable relief from her menstrual cramps by taking ibuprofen regularly, starting two days before the expected period and continuing for the first three days of the flow.

Commission E (the German equivalent of the Food and Drug Administration) has approved the use of the extract of black cohosh for menstrual cramps. This herbal medication has not, however, been adequately tested in this country.

PREMENSTRUAL SYNDROME (PMS)

PMS is a collection of symptoms occurring in many women regularly for three to seven days before menses and disappearing when their period begins. Women might complain of any combination of physical and emotional symptoms.

Physical symptoms include water retention with bloating and discomfort (aching) of the abdomen and pelvis, constipation, sweet-cravings, swelling of feet and ankles, swollen and tender breasts, aching of the bones and joints, headache, logginess, clumsiness, and loss of balance.

Psychological symptoms are dominated by feelings of unexplained sadness (depression), restlessness, tension, mood swings associated with crying spells, anxiety, poorly controlled outbursts of anger, and difficulty in concentration.

We have several fancy names for PMS—such as *late luteal dysphoric syndrome*, which means there is not enough progesterone present. But we don't know if it is a lack of progesterone or not enough estrogen that causes the symptoms. Is there some imbalance between the two that temporarily inhibits the kidney from excreting water or sodium? This could explain the bloating, but what causes the cravings?

What to Do About PMS
Since we don't know the cause, we cannot yet cure it. But there are ways you can feel better during that crucial time.

First, be sure there is no other possible reason for the discomfort. Ask your doctor to check your thyroid for deficiency. Low thyroid exacerbates the symptoms of PMS, and replacement therapy with thyroid hormone is likely to ease symptoms.

Resist the urge to eat sweets and salty food. It will simply make you more hungry, especially for sweets, and you'll retain more fluid. Complex carbohydrates (starches, grains), on the other hand, might relieve mood-related symptoms by boosting the level of a precursor of the brain chemical *serotonin*, which appears to elevate mood. A recently available over-the-counter powdered supplement called PMS Escape consists of complex carbohydrates, vitamins, and minerals; a trial of this mixture reported a decrease in depression, anger, confusion, and sweets-craving. Your doctor might also recommend consuming more calcium, magnesium, vitamins E and B_6 and eliminating caffeine, nicotine, alcohol, and salt, although there are very few well-conducted trials to document the effectiveness of these measures. You may also find that certain exercises, especially yoga, are helpful.

Most over-the-counter PMS remedies found in the drugstore contain a mild diuretic and a mild sedative. Diuretics help rid the body of water by making it excrete more urine. Be careful of diuretics. The most commonly used diuretics, such as Hydrodiuril (hydrochlorthiazide) and Lasix (furosemide), also cause excessive excretion of potassium. Loss of potassium can create serious side effects such as heart palpitations and, when extreme, a lethal cardiac arrhythmia. A moderately low potassium level in your muscles and in your nerve cells can also cause you to become jumpy, irritable, and restless, and predisposes you to leg cramps. You would need to restore your body's potassium level by eating bananas, orange juice, or other high-potassium foods. If you must use a diuretic, ask your doctor to prescribe a potassium-conserving type, like Aldactone (spironolactone). Certain over-the-counter nonsteroidal anti-inflammatory drugs (NSAIDs) such as ibuprofen might help the headache and body aches of PMS. Recently calcium supplements have been found to help some women with PMS symptoms.

A mild tranquilizer reserved for life's specially trying moments will get you over the stress peak moments, but don't do this without consulting your doctor. In more severe cases of PMS, the doctor might prescribe antidepressants like fluoxetine (Prozac) that are effective in about 75 percent of women.

The options for treating PMS are increasing. Because PMS symptoms wax and wane spontaneously, try dietary changes and exercise first. If medications are prescribed, they should be used for a brief period; even when the drug is stopped the symptoms may never return.

Mark your calendar and anticipate your PMS days. Try to keep your sense of humor about it.

HEALTH CARE FOR A CHANGING BODY

Most young women today are not afraid to inspect their own genitals. The prudery of the past meant women were not supposed to look "down there." Some young girls would even engage in intercourse with many partners—but refuse to look inside their own vaginas because they felt it was immodest! A man cannot help but see his penis and scrotum and watch them develop. But girls can pretend their sexual organs do not exist. They can watch their breasts and pubic hair develop but never explore further.

The Pelvic Self-exam

The best way to examine yourself is in a sitting position, with a hand mirror, a good source of light, and by spreading the lips of the vagina with your fingers. This self-examination is not intended for self-diagnosis but as an aid in observation and collaboration with a trained health professional. You can also do this during a pelvic examination at the doctor's office. Ask for a mirror so you can see what the doctor sees. This will give you a chance to see deeper inside with the help of the speculum and a high-intensity light. Being a partner in your care requires the ability to make and share decisions, which implies knowledge and adequate information.

Personal Hygiene

Your vagina is self-cleaning because of its acidic environment, which protects you from most germs. Douches, especially medicated ones, can irritate the vagina, and clumsy poking can lead to trauma of the hymen in a young girl. A daily bath or shower should be enough to keep you perfectly clean.

In the 1970s, pharmaceutical manufacturers marketed feminine hygiene sprays so heavily that most women were convinced they needed to spray their vaginas or they would not be clean. The sprays ended up clogging the pores and causing glandular abscesses in some women, and so most of them did not stay on the market for long.

In many European countries, a bidet is a standard fixture in all bathrooms, and this is an ideal way to clean yourself each time you urinate or defecate. But without a bidet, and without proper knowledge about how to clean yourself after a bowel movement, the perineum, the area separating your rectum and vagina, is teeming with bacteria, and infection can ascend into the vagina and the urethra.

To prevent the bacteria from getting access to the vagina, always wipe yourself from front to back, never the other way. The best way to cleanse is to wash the area with warm water after each bowel movement. A piece of cotton soaked in warm water is an inexpensive way to insure personal hygiene. Let the warm water run over one or two cotton balls and, while sitting on the toilet, wash your vulva from the front to the back several times, using new cotton balls each time. Gently wash over the clitoris, the inner and outer lips, the grooves between them, the fourchette, and end with the perineum and the anus.

To Douche or Not to Douche

Douching is cleaning inside the vagina, but because our bodies have such an efficient self-cleaning system, this is rarely necessary. The acidic environment of the vagina keeps it clean. In rare instances a douche is needed to flush out medication, semen, or a particularly persistent discharge.

Standard douching equipment consists of a rubber or latex bag and a long tube with a nozzle at the end. A clamp along the tube closes off the water flow. Warm water with a small amount of plain white vinegar, about one teaspoonful per quart of water, is the best cleanser. If you use a commercial solution, be sure to dilute it properly; painful chemical burns of the vagina can occur as a result of a too-strong solution. Check the temperature of the water against the back of your hand to make sure it is not too hot.

Douching is best done in a tub, where you can suspend the bag from a shower rod and lie back. Spread the lips of your vagina with one hand and insert the nozzle about halfway into your vagina with the other. Open the valve of the tube while closing the lips of your vagina around the nozzle. Never use force or pressure. By closing the lips around the nozzle, you increase pressure only slightly while the solution flows in by gravity alone. Alternately, fill the vagina and open the lips and allow water to flow out with any debris and liquid.

It is important that you do not use a syringe and that you do not force water into your vagina under pressure. The pressure of a syringe might be excessive and can force the fluid, along with some infective particles, up into the cervix, especially if the cervix is partly open during or after menses.

Do not douche during your period and soon after giving birth, because the cervix might be open and nonsterile fluid could get into the uterus and cause infection.

Using Menstrual Pads and Tampons

Menstrual pads and tampons have come a long way since those big bulky pads that felt like diapers and made us constantly aware that we had something between our legs. When active women began to protest the discomfort of sanitary napkins, the designs got better, and now we have so many types, styles, and sizes to choose from it is even more confusing. They are not yet perfect, just better.

Tampons, too, have improved since women doctors designed some of them to conform better to the shape of the vagina. But once again, the failure of the establishment to thoroughly test new products for women caused a scandal in the 1970s. Toxic shock syndrome, a fatal infection, was the result of using superabsorbent fibers in tampons (see below).

Always wash your hands before inserting a tampon. Try not to contaminate the tampon after you remove it from the wrapper. Keep in mind the natural curve of your vagina, which is like a reversed S. Exploring with your finger, follow the curve of the vagina and feel the cervix at the very end. The tampon usually rests behind the cervix, in the pouch called the *posterior fornix*.

If your vagina is moist, as it usually is during the menstrual flow, you need not moisten the tip of the tampon for ease of insertion. If the vagina is dry after removing the last tampon, which soaked up all the flow and then some normal secretions, you must be careful not to force the tampon. Moisten the tip with KY jelly or tap water.

Never keep a tampon in too long—that is, not more than a few hours or, at most, overnight. Use a pad with the tampon to protect yourself on heavy flow days, rather than using a super tampon or two super tampons at the same time. On the other hand, do not change the tampons too frequently as that can dry out the vagina excessively. When flow is scant, do not use tampons at all, just the pads designed for light days.

Check your vagina at the end of your period to be sure you have not left a tampon inside. It's easy to forget and find out only days later, when you have foreign body vaginitis! One of my patients, Natalie, could not understand why there was an unpleasant odor and a continuous brown discharge from her vagina, despite her daily shower and careful hygiene. When I extracted a tampon from her vagina that had been lodged there for over ten days, since her last menstrual period, she was horrified. Sometime during the menstrual flow, she inserted a fresh tampon without removing the previous one. The string of the old tampon had wandered up and disappeared from where she could feel it. Natalie frequently used two tampons during the heavier flow days to prevent "accidents."

She was relieved by my discovery of the simple cause, but she was also terribly embarrassed by what she called her own "stupidity." I assured her scores of my patients came in with the very same problem.

Toxic Shock Syndrome (TSS)

Toxic shock syndrome can be caused by a streptococcus bacteria when there is soft tissue infection and bacteria get into the bloodstream. This type affects both sexes equally. Half the cases of toxic shock syndrome are related to menstruation, and the other half are not. The nonmenstrual toxic shock syndrome affects men and children, too, but it targets mostly women. The menstrual TSS usually affects younger women. TSS is a systemic disease characterized by fever, low blood pressure, and a diffuse rash that peels off. Many organs of the body are involved.

Symptoms of TSS include fever, chills, and muscle pain, along with an overall feeling of weakness. Small patches of redness might develop on the skin, and these small circular patches will eventually become thick and peel off. The rash typically involves hands and feet, which also swell, and develops a week or two after onset of the illness. Joint and muscle pain can be severe. A sore throat and a "strawberry" tongue—yellowish speckles on a deep red background—can also develop. Conjunctivitis, abdominal pain, headache, and perhaps even vaginitis might develop.

To diagnose the menstrual type of TSS, cultures of the vagina must be taken to identify the bacteria. Blood tests will find out if the white blood count has shifted; often it does. A variety of tests will be made.

TSS is treated with antibiotics for ten to fourteen days—or longer, if the infection is deep-seated. An aggressive attempt must also be made to bring the blood pressure up to normal levels and keep it there.

··4··

Nutrition and the Adolescent

When I was in grammar school, we learned about the circle of food groups, a chart showing equal pie-shaped wedges of protein, vegetables and fruits, grains and starches, and dairy products. The circle has now become the food "pyramid," a much better visual presentation of the portions of our daily nutritional needs. We should now be "bottom feeders," that is, the largest amounts of food in our daily diet should be grains, vegetables, and fruits—shown in the bottom of the pyramid. Animal products are in the middle, and at the narrow top of the pyramid are tiny amounts of fats and sweets.

Doctors are certainly beginning to take nutrition more seriously today, and any good doctor will question his or her patients about what they eat. We know there are health risks associated with consuming too much fat or sugar, or not enough vital nutrients such as calcium or iron.

Enthralled by fast-food establishments that offer greasy but tasty food in a social "hangout" setting, few teens consider seriously the importance of a balanced diet. The adolescent all too often skips breakfast, has a bag of fries for lunch, and munches cookies when studying or watching TV. And they are not alone. I have even witnessed physicians gathering at a fast-food hamburger place after sitting for three hours in a medical seminar on heart disease!

Poor nutrition can contribute to depression; it can lead to sluggish mental function, poor memory, anemia, impaired ability to fight infection, fainting spells, heart palpitations, and weak bones and teeth, among other complications.

THE OXYGEN-BURNING BODY: VITAMINS AND ANTIOXIDANTS

Our bodies are oxygen-burning machines. We cannot live without oxygen in the air we breathe. By combining with the food we eat, oxygen gives us energy. This "oxidation" process is similar to the burning of fuel by a car engine—it makes the car move. But the car is made of inert materials and the oxidation that makes the car go also builds up layers of rust, grease, and soot. This, of course, can be cleaned off, or, when it is bad enough, the car can be traded in for a new one.

Our bodies, however, are made of organs and cells that are harmed by *too much* oxidation. Proteins, carbohydrates, fats, and DNA are all combustible compounds that drive our human engine. Of these, fats are especially susceptible to oxidation. A stick of butter will go rancid when exposed to air long enough, and the lipids (fats) in our cells can get rancid if they are not protected from atmospheric oxygen and from the byproducts of metabolism, the so-called oxygen free radicals. The free radicals might cause oxidative damage to the body that is now believed to be responsible for aging, cardiovascular disease, cataracts, other degenerative diseases, and even cancer.

Thus, we need antioxidants to prevent this damage. These vital nutrients are like our body's traffic police, chasing down the offensive free radicals to keep our systems going. Antioxidants keep the free radicals in check but do not arrest the entire gang. We need free radicals to defend ourselves from invaders (bacteria, viruses, foreign cells). Our white blood cells utilize free radicals to kill (burn, oxidize) the invaders. The cells lining the intestine utilize free radicals to digest food.

However, like all body systems, a delicate balance must be maintained. We need some free radicals to fight off invaders, but if we have too many free radicals, they will kill off everything in sight, including our DNA. Then serious trouble arises, like cancer. When we do not eat properly, or when we use drugs or alcohol, free radicals can get the upper hand. We need antioxidants to keep our engines clean and prevent free radicals from taking over.

A diet of fruits and vegetables contains a number of antioxidants that help us maintain the body's balance. Vitamin C, Vitamin E, and beta-carotene are the primary antioxidants contained in a vegetarian diet.

• Vitamin C is found in peppers, broccoli, strawberries, kiwi fruit, cabbage, oranges, cantaloupe, grapefruit, asparagus, and onions.

• Vitamin E sources are fat-laden nuts, seeds, and oils; and most experts recommend taking vitamin E in supplements, rather than increasing your fat intake.

• Beta-carotene, the precursor to vitamin A, is found in deep yellow and red fruits and vegetables and in dark green vegetables such as carrots, sweet potatoes, winter squash, spinach, red bell peppers, apricots, cantaloupe, lettuce, broccoli, and Brussels sprouts.

Other possible antioxidants are selenium; zinc; other carotinoids such as lutein, found in tomatoes; and polyphenols, which are found in yellow onions and red grapes.

There is a controversy as to whether supplements work as well as the natural vitamins and antioxidants that are contained in our food. Most supplements are not as safe and do not work as well, probably because there are other ingredients in food that make the antioxidants work better.

IRON-DEFICIENCY ANEMIA

Abby was always tired. She constantly fell asleep while doing her homework and blamed it on the fact that "'there's just so much!'" Her mother complained that she was unable to wake the 15-year-old in the morning and she was always late for school.

When excessive fatigue and sleepiness affect a young woman, the two most likely culprits are hypothyroidism and anemia. Anemia is primarily a female problem, more common in teens when menses begin because many fail to make up for the loss of iron caused by the blood loss. (This also occurs sometimes in menopause when bleeding is irregular.) Fewer than 0.2 percent of men are affected, because their blood has more hemoglobin to begin with because of androgens and they do not lose blood regularly through a period. Iron deficiency is particularly dangerous in pregnancy because it may cause low birth weight and lead to premature births and to abnormalities in the fetus.

Anemia means you do not have enough red blood cells and hemoglobin, a protein that imparts red color to the blood cells and to the cheeks on your face. Iron helps the hemoglobin transport oxygen from the lungs to all tissues of the body. Hemoglobin also transports carbon dioxide (the end product of burning fuels by the tissues) from the tissues to the lungs, where we get rid of carbon dioxide by the simple act of exhaling. It is hemoglobin that allows us to breathe, to exchange carbon dioxide for oxygen. Without iron, the production of hemoglobin stops and the body does not get enough oxygen. With a drop in hemoglobin, you might be easily fatigued, sleepy, even occasionally dizzy. The brain does not function well either.

Iron plays an important role in the functioning of liver and muscles and in the immune mechanisms of fighting infections. It is possible to have a mild iron deficiency without being anemic. With mild iron deficiency, there is enough iron to fulfill the bone marrow needs for hemoglobin production but not enough to cover the other needs.

Anemia can come from lack of other nutrients such as vitamin B_{12}

or folic acid in the diet. Or it can come from the failure of the body to absorb iron because of a chronic infection, rheumatoid arthritis, liver disease, lupus, or cancer.

Our intestinal tract is designed to protect us from too much iron intake, but not from too little. When there is too much, our bodies won't absorb any more iron. Women are protected from iron excess by menstruation. Some researchers attribute the low incidence of heart disease in women before menopause to lower iron levels. Ironically, this protection from too much iron can be the cause of too little.

Abby began menstruating at the age of 12 and has been doing so every twenty-four days for six to seven days each month. When questioned, she told me she used about five pads or tampons each of the first four days, then about four. A quick calculation produces a figure of about forty pads or tampons a month. That is probably double what most young girls require, even taking into account habits of keeping clean and dry and changing the pad or tampon at each urination.

Further questioning revealed that Abby is a vegetarian and eats no meat or fish, both good sources of iron, but she does not balance her diet with iron-rich vegetables or supplements. Abby had an iron deficiency and anemia, most commonly caused in adolescence by loss of menstrual blood and failure to compensate for the loss of iron.

The treatment I prescribed was oral iron supplements with added vitamin C to improve iron absorption. Two months later, Abby bounced into the office, her cheeks pink and her blood count normal.

Natural Sources of Iron
The iron supplement protected Abby from anemia, but she could have prevented her iron deficiency with a balanced diet and more awareness about nutrition. Many foods we eat every day contain iron, so read labels and find those that you like and will give you part of your daily requirement. Vegetarians, like Abby, need to be extra aware and educate themselves about where to find the nutrients they need.

- meat and poultry, especially liver and organ meats
- fish, especially shellfish
- legumes such as lima beans, dried beans and peas, and canned baked beans
- leafy green vegetables in the cabbage family such as kale, collards, and broccoli
- peaches, apricots, raisins, especially dried fruits
- whole-wheat bread, wheat germ
- enriched white bread, pasta, cereals, and rice

CALCIUM DEFICIENCY:
THE BEGINNING OF OSTEOPOROSIS

Osteoporosis begins in childhood. The effects of calcium malnutrition in early life are delayed but deadly. It is the adolescent girl who is likely to avoid milk and quench her thirst with sodas and other soft drinks, containing phosphates, which turn any calcium they do ingest into calcium phosphate. This is what some rocks are made of. It is not easily absorbed and is excreted and wasted in the stool.

Calcium is essential for the proper development of strong bones and teeth. It is also involved in normal blood clotting and in normal muscle and nerve function. The bony skeleton is not an inert rock. It is a living organ the parts of which keep resorbing (melting) and rebuilding all the time. The movements of the body, especially weight-bearing exercises, stress the appropriate bones and stimulate rebuilding.

It is in adolescence and in the twenties that a woman's skeleton can reach its peak mass and density—provided an ample supply of calcium is available. At about 35, bone growth plateaus until a slow bone loss begins and accelerates at menopause with loss of estrogen. According to the National Institutes of Health, the *elemental calcium* needs of women are:

- 1,200 milligrams per day for a teenage girl.

- 800 milligrams per day from age 25 till menopause.

- 2,000 milligrams a day in pregnancy to accommodate the growth of the fetal skeleton.

- 1,500 milligrams in menopause and later to overcome bone loss and to compensate for the decreased absorption of calcium in the intestine of the aging. A woman on estrogen treatment would require only 1,200 milligrams.

The guidelines were revised in 1997 by the Institutes of Medicine, a branch of the National Academy of Sciences. Their research indicates that the teenage girl should be taking 1,300 rather than 1,200 milligrams, the adult should take 1,000 rather than 800, but in menopause a woman needs 1,200 rather than 1,500 milligrams. This research indicated that no additional calcium was required during pregnancy—or in menopause, whether a woman was or was not taking estrogen replacement. This is not without controversy, however: Most scientists agree that 1,200 milligrams is enough if the woman takes estrogen, but insist at least 1,500 milligrams of elemental calcium is needed by the menopausal woman.

Ask your doctor for the latest guidelines, because they might change again as more research is done. At any rate, the average adult gets only about 500 to 700 milligrams in a normal diet, so it would appear that everyone should increase their intake of calcium. In order to ingest 1,000 milligrams a day, you would need three to four servings of calcium-rich food—that number of glasses of skim milk, for example. A glass of skim milk contains about 300 milligrams of calcium. So does calcium-fortified orange juice. Eight ounces of lowfat yogurt contains 415 milligrams of calcium. One ounce of Swiss cheese has 270 milligrams. Three ounces of salmon (with bones) has 180 milligrams. One cup of cooked broccoli has 130 milligrams.

In addition to helping build bones and perhaps decreasing the symptoms of PMS, life-long ample calcium intake has recently been found to lower the risk of developing high blood pressure and colon cancer.

Using Calcium Effectively

The term "elemental calcium" is important to understand. Calcium does not exist on earth as a pure element and is combined with other elements to form a compound, such as calcium phosphate, calcium carbonate, or calcium citrate. The word *elemental* signifies actual calcium amount in the supplement.

How the calcium is compounded is also important.

Calcium carbonate contains about 40 percent calcium, is easily absorbed, and is relatively cheap. It is the constituent of Caltrate, Tums, Os-Cal, and many oyster-shell-derived calcium preparations. Most women tolerate calcium carbonate very well, but some develop constipation and bloating.

Calcium citrate, an excellent source of calcium, is also absorbed in the gastrointestinal tract. Calcium citrate is less likely to cause constipation or bloating but is more expensive than calcium carbonate.

Calcium phosphate is insoluble in the human stomach and is not absorbed. One way to determine if a coated calcium pill, or other questionable compound, will resist digestion is to give it the vinegar test. Drop the tablet into a glass containing six ounces of vinegar and stir every few minutes. The pill that does not dissolve completely within thirty minutes will probably not do so in your stomach either.

Calcium and iron are chemically similar elements—both are metals. They share the same absorption mechanism in the gut, and each interferes with the absorption of the other. Most frequently it is the calcium that interferes with the absorption of iron.

Taking calcium with a meal improves the absorption of calcium but can interfere with the absorption of iron, so if you take iron supplements and calcium, take them at different times. For example, do not take your iron supplement with a glass of milk.

Various "health food" calcium preparations contain added magnesium, advertised as improving the absorption of calcium. Nothing could be farther from the truth. Magnesium belongs to the same family of minerals as calcium and competes with calcium for the shared absorption mechanism in the intestine. In various experiments it was shown to actually impede the absorption of calcium.

Natural Sources of Calcium

Of all food, milk, in its various forms, is the major source of calcium in our diet. Three eight-ounce glasses of milk contain as much calcium as seven cups of broccoli. Milk is often fortified with vitamin D, which facilitates the absorption of calcium in the intestine. Sardines and salmon are also good sources of calcium as long as you chew and swallow the tiny bones along with the fish flesh. Fruit juices fortified with calcium are good sources.

Foods that contain significant calcium are:

- milk (skim milk is even richer in calcium than whole milk), buttermilk

- yogurt

- cheeses

- sardines and salmon

- tofu made with calcium salts

- kidney beans

- nuts and seeds

- dried figs

- broccoli

- many dark leafy, green vegetables

Spinach also contains a significant amount of calcium, but that calcium is bound to oxalic acid, which makes it unavailable for absorption. While we need plenty of fiber in our diets, it is important to be aware that foods high in fiber decrease the absorption of calcium. Proteins, like soft drinks, produce phosphate (an acid), which before being excreted in the urine binds with calcium. Thus, an excessive amount of protein in the diet (such as large amounts of meat every day) drains the body's calcium.

While protein is essential to the body's structure, growth, and function, it is the important ingredient of all our cells—most of us (unless we live on very low calorie "starvation" diets) don't need to worry that we eat too little protein. The average American consumes about 100 grams of protein a day. A 125 lb. woman needs only about 45 grams of protein a day. Over time, eating too much protein increases the workload of the liver and kidneys and boosts the risk of osteoporotic fracture at a later age. In addition, foods that consist of animal protein also contain fat, which is associated with high risks of heart disease and cancer.

Lactose Intolerance

Some people cannot tolerate milk, and if they drink it they get cramps and diarrhea. This is most frequently due to lactose intolerance, caused by a deficiency of a natural enzyme in the body known as lactase, which helps the body absorb milk products. The unabsorbed lactose lingers in the intestinal tract; gets fermented by the ever-present bacteria; and causes gas, fullness, and diarrhea.

Lactose is a double sugar. It is composed of glucose and galactose, two sugars connected to each other with a strong bond. Before this double sugar can be absorbed through the intestine it must be cleaved in half by an enzyme called lactase. When cleaved, the two separate sugars can be easily absorbed. Lactase is an enzyme present in all infants. Without it, the baby would not be able to digest its mother's milk. But the enzyme disappears after the age of two, or even later in life in many people. Lactose deficiency can be complete or partial, and it is more common in Asians and Mediterranean people than it is in others.

Some women with this condition can tolerate small amounts of milk or ice cream on occasion. There is also a product called Lactaid that contains the enzyme lactase. You can take Lactaid in the form of caplets or add a drop to milk. In yogurt, bacteria partially digest the lactose, so yogurt may be a good substitute for milk in lactase-deficient people (see also Chapter 26, under Irritable Bowel Syndrome).

·· 5 ··

Fitness and Self-esteem

The 1996 Olympic games in Atlanta and the recent sellout crowds attending women's college, and now professional, basketball games made it obvious that women's team sports were here to stay. Since the 1972 amendment to the Constitution guaranteeing equal opportunity for girls in sports at school, the participation of women in athletics has risen dramatically from less than half a million before 1972 to more than 2 million in 1997.

The President's Council on Physical Fitness and Sports reported in 1997 that female high school athletes tended to get better grades. They were also less likely to drop out of school than girls who were not athletic. They will also be more likely to go to college and will develop fewer chronic health problems such as heart disease, high cholesterol, and disbetes. The report also indicated that girls who participate in sports are more mentally fit and have developed social skills more easily than less active girls. The Women's Sports Foundation did a survey in 1989 that showed higher grades, more college entry, and less emotional disorders like depression.

In other words, the beauty of sports is that *they increase self-esteem at an age when girls traditionally lose self-esteem.* Physical competence creates a sense of self-mastery and strength. A girl can make a decision from a position of strength, something boys learned long ago and carry with them throughout their lives. Whether you are short or tall, black or white, if you excel in sports, you are accepted by all.

In the past, exercise for adolescent girls was restricted to gym class or jumping up and down as a cheerleader for the boys' sports teams who were getting a real physical workout. How many girls were turned on by gym class, with its regimen of calisthenics or aerobics, which had no apparent goal or focus? Not to mention those awful gym suits! In the spirit of adolescent rebellion, they looked for any excuse not to participate. Girls grew up to be sedentary women. However, beating the other team, or winning a school championship, or getting an athletic scholarship to a good college would interest a girl enough to make physical fitness a big part of her life today.

Despite the progress, the efforts of educational institutions to enforce participation in physical fitness classes are only moderately successful. According to a 1997 Commonwealth–Fund supported Louis Harris poll, although girls overwhelmingly indicated that they knew exercise was important to health, by high school years only two thirds of girls (67 percent), compared with 80 percent of boys, were exercising three times a week or more. Fifteen percent of older girls said they exercised less than once or twice a week or more, double the rate of older boys (8 percent). Not surprisingly, self-confidence and self-esteem declined sharply in high school for girls (14 percent of older girls and 9 percent of younger girls registered low self-confidence), while self-confidence improved with age among boys.

Upon graduation from high schools and colleges, many women settle down into an existence characterized by a domestic or domestic-and-job pattern, a pattern that does not include regular, self-motivated recreational exercise. Women with access to health clubs might continue to be active, but for the majority of women who are poor, or get pregnant early, exercise is not part of their lifestyle. Physical fitness (or unfitness) patterns that have become established during the young adult life cycle tend to persist, unfortunately, to be further modified downward in postmenopause. The short-term "toxicity" of physical inactivity in women is obesity and depreciation of self-esteem.

I have found it extremely difficult to motivate women to perform regular exercise throughout the year no matter how old they are. I have heard all the excuses, from inclement weather (which should not interfere with an indoor program), to painful knees (usually due to overweight, as a result of a sedentary lifestyle), to boredom (all that repetitive movement), to lack of time (even among retired people).

At the brink of the twenty-first century, Americans are still a sedentary people. The grandsons and granddaughters of pioneers have turned flabby. A 1998 study reported in the *Journal of the American Medical Association* assessed the role of television watching and inactivity in childhood obesity. Eighty-five percent of boys but only 74 percent of girls reported three or more periods of vigorous physical activity each week. In that study the number of hours of television watching correlated with obesity even more directly than did physical activity. Children who watched four or more hours of television a day had the highest body mass index.

With the universality of the car and the airplane as the preferred vehicles of transportation; with urban, suburban, and even rural life being replete with effort- and time-saving devices; with television becoming the major source of information and entertainment, we have become physically unchallenged but mentally stressed, and this has afflicted women with a multitude of chronic diseases.

BUILDING A HABIT OF EXERCISE

Being physically active is not only good for your body, it makes you feel good about yourself. You feel strong and in control. You can achieve physical goals that are as important as the mental achievement of winning a science scholarship.

Physical activity is associated with numerous health benefits: lower incidences of cardiovascular disease, diabetes, osteoporosis, and osteoarthritis. In addition, exercise causes the brain to release substances that elevate our mood. These substances, called *endorphins,* have a well-documented, beneficial effect on a person's sense of well-being while decreasing depression and anxiety.

A 1997 study by the Federal Centers for Disease Control and Prevention together with state health departments revealed that people living in Colorado are the thinnest in the country. Only 19.9 percent of Coloradans are overweight, compared with nearly a third nationwide. Fitness experts in Colorado said the leanness of residents was because of the abundance of outdoor activity. People move to Colorado because they want to participate in those activities.

A safe and effective physical fitness program is essential for all age groups. Eat well, wear the proper clothing, do some warm-up stretches before you begin. One trend I have noticed recently is that once women commit themselves to an exercise program, or to working out every day, they feel bad when something interferes with this program. The body is unconsciously responding, just as if it were having a withdrawal symptom from a drug. Then you know that exercise will always need to be part of your life.

How Much Exercise Do You Need?

The sedentary lifestyle is a serious public health problem, and a number of institutions have engaged in setting guidelines on what constitutes an effective exercise program. In 1985, the American College of Sports Medicine endorsed vigorous endurance (aerobic) exercise for at least twenty minutes three times a week. The definition of a "vigorous endurance exercise" is a level that results in a heart rate equal to 60 to 90 percent of the maximal rate. If you wish to be precise calculate your heart rate by counting the beats in a 10-second interval and multiplying by 6. Maximum heart rate is roughly determined by subtracting your age from 200.

For a sedentary person to reduce her health risks exercising two or three times a week for 15–30 minutes at 40–60 percent of maximal heart rate may be sufficient. If the goal is to achieve physical (cardio-respiratory) fitness you must work out at least four times a week at 70 to 90 percent of your maximal heart rate. At this level the exercise makes you sweat but should not exceed what you consider somewhat hard or make it impossible to carry on a normal conversation.

In 1995, the Centers for Disease Control and Prevention and the American College of Sports Medicine came up with recommendations that are much less stringent and should be no insurmountable obstacle for any age group. These guidelines consist of thirty minutes of moder-ately intense physical activity on most, and preferably all, days of the week.

The more relaxed guidelines by the exercise and health authorities has been interpreted by many physicians and their patients as the target requirement for physical fitness, the target above which no new advan-tages accrue. If that is "enough" for an average person, they reason, then perhaps there is no reason to exercise more.

In reality, this concept is wrong. There is definitely an added advan-tage to the more intensive regimen. It induces cardiorespiratory fitness, which correlates with longer life expectancy and, to a certain degree, predicts survival. Indeed, a study of 17,000 Harvard male graduates (naturally, no long-term studies on women yet) revealed that those who lived the longest had been expending energy at a rate equivalent to running at six miles per hour for about six hours a week. The study found, surprisingly, that in terms of longevity, moderate exercise had no benefits over a sedentary lifestyle. In other words, if cardiovascular health and survival are the purposes of your exercise, you can obtain it only by exercising to the fullest capacity (1985 guidelines). The halfway effort does not insure half of the benefit.

A study of women runners gave evidence that with the increasing numbers of miles run there was a corresponding higher level of the good cholesterol in the blood. On the other hand, elderly women were studied with the intent to outline the effect of exercise on bone. The relaxed guidelines were found to prevent bone loss, thus increasing bone density and slowing the onset of osteoporosis. Obviously, the prescrip-tion varies with age and with the choice of the goal. Younger women who wish to improve their cardiopulmonary fitness and live longer need the intense regimen, working up sweat with at least twenty minutes of aerobic exercise three times a week.

If the goal of your exercise program is to lose weight, you need to work out at least five times a week for 45–60 minutes at 45 to 60 percent of your maximal heart rate.

The Physiology of Exercise

We have three kinds of muscles: smooth, striated, and cardiac. Striated muscles are the large voluntary muscles that move our arms and legs, the neck, and the torso. They are called striated because under the microscope they are composed of alternating stripes that consist of layers of two chemical components of the muscle, components that convey the ability to contract and relax.

Smooth muscles are small involuntary muscles found in the walls of the stomach and intestine, in the uterus, in the walls of the Fallopian tubes, and in the walls of arteries. Under the microscope they do not have stripes.

The heart muscle, the *myocardium,* is an involuntary muscle that responds to its own pacemaker. The myocardium is striated under the microscope, but it is not under our voluntary control, although some people have been able to control it through biofeedback.

Our muscles are made to work, and they do this by contracting (shortening) or relaxing (lengthening). When our muscles work through movement or exercise, they need an oxygen supply for complete burning of the fuel. If our muscles work through weight lifting or other intense exercise that does not allow enough air exchange to provide oxygen for complete burning of the fuel, lactic acid accumulates in the muscles. This hurts and can cause pain and spasm.

Frequently, our bodies have more aches after the first ski trip of the winter, and muscle spasms and aches are not uncommon after the first exercise of the season; but gradually they acclimate. In the shoulders and hips, and, to a lesser extent, all over the body, there are trigger points that set off pain through the muscle chain if we overexert. Acupressure, or "shiatzu" massage, employs pressure on trigger points to relieve the spasm and pain. Rarely, exercise can trigger an asthmatic attack in predisposed individuals.

Energy is stored and used by the body in three ways. Ingested fats are broken down in the gut into triglycerides (fatty acids and glycerin), then are absorbed and reassembled by the liver to be stored as fat within the fat cells.

Proteins are broken down in the intestine into aminoacids that are then are absorbed and processed by the liver to become parts of the structure of the body and contribute to its growth.

Carbohydrates are broken down into simple sugar units such as glucose, fructose, and galactose, then are absorbed and stored in the liver and muscles as glycogen. Glycogen is the most used, most quickly accessible form of energy reserve. It provides the energy by being broken down by various liver and muscle enzymes into glucose-glycogen. It can deliver some energy while being broken down even if oxygen is not available. This is the nonoxidative cycle, in which glycogen gets broken down into lactic acid. Then, if oxygen is available, the lactic acid is further broken down (oxidized) to carbon dioxide and water, yielding much more energy in the process. Oxygen is needed for complete burning.

If, however, oxygen is not available—for instance, during very strenuous exercise, when you cannot catch your breath fast enough—the energy-producing process ends at the lactic acid. It is the accumulation of lactic acid that can be irritating to the muscles and can throw them into a painful spasm. Some people will get a spasm of the chest muscles if they exercise strenuously and cannot catch their breath. When exercise is extreme, we run out of fuel, and so our existing tissue breaks down.

When menses stop in athletic women, it is not exercise that causes the cessation. It is because there is no more fuel to care for the system. Stored fat is used up. The reproductive tract shuts down if the energy reserve is not large enough to insure reproduction. Failure to menstruate is not caused by athletics but by weight loss, for when you gain muscle, you lose fat.

THE ATHLETIC TRIAD: A DANGEROUS TRIANGLE

The "athletic triad" is the combination of excessive athletic activity, weight loss, and menstrual abnormalities. With continued excessive exercise and excessive weight loss, the estrogen level drops, causing menstruation to stop and leading to bone loss. Young ballet dancers and other athletes often get what we call march fractures in the feet and ignore them until pain becomes insufferable. These are hairline fractures that usually cannot be detected without an X ray and are sometimes missed by X rays. The healthy physiologic limit that should be imposed on the vigorous exercising of young women should be absence of side effects. Young women who exercise excessively might experience several side effects.

Intense physical activity leads to injuries of the musculoskeletal system. Thirty-five to 65 percent of runners are injured per year; the risk of injury increases with the total distance run per week. The critical level varies from one individual to another. Exercise that leads to injury is too much exercise.

The pleasant mood associated with physical activity is a great benefit, but a dangerous point is reached when an athlete's "high" makes her disregard physical discomfort and drives her to increasing amounts of exercise. Watch out for these feelings and behavior.

All in all, the dangerous athletic triad occurs in only a small fraction of young girls, while the malignant "pentad" of physical inactivity/overeating/obesity/accelerated chronic illness/premature death affects millions of people in our country—between a third and a half of the female population. Physical inactivity and obesity constitute a far more serious public health problem than the athletic triad, and this is discussed in more detail in the chapter on eating disorders.

CALORIES BURNED WHILE EXERCISING

If you do any of the following exercises for one hour, you will burn calories. This table, from the National Institutes of Health, is based on an average 150-pound person (as usual, there is no difference shown for men or women). If you weigh less than 150 pounds, you will burn fewer calories than what is listed in the table and if you weigh more than 150 pounds you will burn more calories.

ACTIVITY	CALORIES PER HOUR
Walking at 2 miles an hour	240
Walking at 4½ miles an hour	440
Running in place	650
Running at 10 miles an hour	1,280
Jogging at 5½ miles an hour	740
Jogging at 7 miles an hour	920
Bicycling at 6 miles an hour	240
Bicycling at 12 miles an hour	410
Jumping rope	750
Swimming 25 yards a minute	275
Swimming 50 yards a minute	500
Tennis singles	400
Cross-country skiing	700

Fitness Effectiveness Rating

The following exercises are grouped according to their physical fitness benefits including cardiopulmonary, endurance, strength, and flexibility.

EXCELLENT

Racquetball

Soccer

Running combined with upper body workout

Swimming

Karate

Modern dance

Aerobic dance

Gymnastics

Mountain climbing

GOOD

Volleyball

Basketball

Field hockey

Badminton

Tennis singles

Ballet

AVERAGE
Running

Bicycling

Sailing small boats

Horseback riding

Folk dancing

Square dancing

Water skiing

Tennis doubles

Softball

FAIR
Brisk walking

Canoeing and kayaking

Rowing

Backpacking

Golf (walking)

Yoga

Weight lifting

POOR
Walking slowly

Sailing large boats

Bowling

Golf (with cart)

·· 6 ··

Protecting the Outer Self

To an adolescent girl, appearance is of great concern, especially because her hormones are wreaking havoc with her complexion. Many teenage girls are overly self-conscious about their looks, and their self-esteem plunges with the appearance of each new "zit." In addition, the skin, our largest body organ, is often abused at this age with toxic cosmetics, and body piercing and tattoos with less-than-sterile instruments. Yet by far the leading health risk to our skin is cancer. Few adolescents realize that getting a great tan—even a salon tan—can put them in grave danger.

THE ARCHITECTURE OF THE SKIN

Our skin is beautifully designed. It is tough where it needs to be tough, such as on the bottoms of our feet, and delicate where it needs to be sensitive and flexible, as it is on our eyelids. We have three layers of skin: the *epidermis* (top layer); the *dermis* (middle layer); and the underlying *subcutaneous layer,* which is connected to the layers of fat, muscle, and bones.

The epidermis, the top layer, is itself made of four layers. The outer layer is made of dead cells of protein called *keratin.* Just under that is a *granular* layer that moves the keratin cells to the surface. Next is the layer of *squamous* cells that produce keratin and also transport water. Blisters begin here. The innermost, *basal* layer is where the squamous cells are produced. It is here also that the *melanocytes* are produced. These are the cells that produce the pigment, or *melanin,* that determines skin color. The skin cancer known as malignant melanoma originates from these cells. Differences in skin color result from the inherited

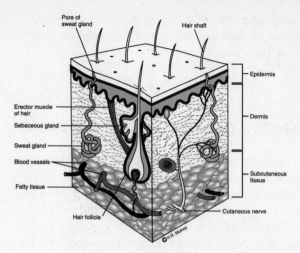

Figure 7. Structure of the skin.

programming of the cells and the amount and concentration of melanin the cells produce.

The dermis is the middle layer of skin, composed of thick fibers of collagen, a tough protein produced by spindle-shaped cells called *fibroblasts*. This layer also contains the *elastic* fibers, with a substance called *elastin*. The collagen and elastic fibers give skin its strength and flexibility. Over the years, the number of fibroblasts and the thickness of collagen and elastin diminish, and this is what we see on the outside as loss of firmness in the skin.

The dermis is also crisscrossed by nerves, blood vessels, and lymphatics. It is here that you feel water retention in your body during PMS or pregnancy. The dermis swells up and your skin feels tight. The dermis also contains the follicles that generate hairs, and sebaceous glands that generate oil (the *sebum*). When these glands are overactive, you have oily skin; if they're underactive, you have dry skin.

The subcutaneous layer consists mostly of fatty cells, although blood and lymph vessels and nerves run through it as well. This layer serves as a heat insulator and shock absorber. Women generally have more fat layer than men. This is where our two types of sweat glands are located: the *eccrine* and the *apocrine*. These glands act as our thermostat. When we are hot, they produce and pump salt with water and other chemicals to the surface of the skin to cool us. As much as a gallon of sweat a day can be produced during times of heat or emotional stress. Most of it evaporates quickly; the rest is perceived as perspiration. The apocrine glands are in the armpits, in the ear canals (where they form ear wax), around the genitals, and in the nipples of the breast. These glands become active during adolescence and are influenced by sex hormones, especially the male hormone testosterone. The apocrine glands respond to emotion rather than heat, and are responsible for the production of body odor.

SKIN CANCER: THE DAMAGE BEGINS EARLY

A single blistering sunburn in childhood (or adolescence) can double the risk of skin cancer. Melanoma is the leading cancer in Caucasian women between the ages of 25 and 29. More than half a million Americans get skin cancer every year, 90 percent of the cases caused by overexposure to the sun and sun lamps. It is the most common cancer and accounts for more cancer than all other types combined. This is a cumulative cancer, that is, the longer you expose yourself to the damaging rays of the sun, the more at risk you become. Few of us realize how fast the sun's damage is done.

Anyone can get skin cancer, but those at highest risk are fair-skinned people with blue eyes, who burn and freckle easily. Naturally, there is more skin cancer in parts of the world where people are most exposed to the sun. Fair-haired women in Norway are not as likely to get skin cancer as women in Florida. Moderate risk is associated with light or dark skin and hair, people who tan easily but who can burn if they stay in the sun too long. The risk is lowest for dark-skinned people with brown or black eyes.

The most common skin cancer is the *basal cell carcinoma*. As we said earlier, the basal cell is in the bottom of the top layer of skin, the epidermis. This carcinoma grows slowly and remains in one place. It does not spread to other parts of the body unless it is left untreated. Then it can invade nearby tissue and bone. It looks like a pearly white pimple, usually with a well-defined border.

The *squamous cell carcinoma* begins in the squamous cells of the epidermis which invade down into the dermis and can spread to other parts of the body unless detected early. Like basal cell cancer, this type is also found mainly on the head, face, and hands, areas that are exposed to sun.

Malignant melanoma is the most deadly type of skin cancer and has a high risk of spreading. It causes most skin cancer deaths. It begins as a growth in the melanocytes, or pigment cells of the skin.

Prevention and early detection, as with most illnesses, are the best treatment. Your family physician should examine you from head to foot periodically to be sure there are no signs of cancer. It is your responsibility to check your body periodically and show any suspicious mole or lesion to your doctor.

Protecting Your Skin from Too Much Sun

Most of the damage to the skin caused by the sun is already done by the time you are 20. The melanin in skin absorbs ultraviolet (UV) rays. If you tan easily, you probably have more melanin than someone who burns. The UV rays are converted to harmless infrared rays, and the tanning is the body's way of defending itself against the harmful rays of the sun.

UVA rays do not cause burning like the UVB rays, but they are not harmless. UVA rays penetrate deeper into the skin than UVB. They also cause premature aging and, it is believed, some cancers. These are the rays—the stealth rays—used by tanning parlors, so there is no safe tanning indoors, either. UVA also causes collagen to unravel after only a few minutes of exposure.

The first rule of good skin care is to protect it from the sun. You begin life with soft, unlined skin, but if you allow the sun's UV rays to penetrate your skin for years and years, it will become wrinkled and leathery long before its time, and you will be at greater risk for skin cancer. If you do not believe this, just compare your facial skin with the skin on the inside of your thighs, for example.

The sun is strongest at high noon and is proportionally weaker before or after that hour. However, people who burn easily can get a sunburn on an overcast day, or early in the morning, so there is a need to use common sense. Keep in mind that the sun reflects off light surfaces, so if you are skiing on a bright sunny day, all that white powder is going to send even more ultraviolet rays to your exposed face.

Sunscreens. The FDA has not yet rated sunscreens, but it is thought that we need at least a sun-protection factor (SPF) of 15 or higher for protection from sun. If you are very fair, 25 to 30 SPF would be better. Zinc oxide, a white paste that is often seen on people's noses at the beach, will block both UVA and UVB rays because it is not absorbed by the skin. It also comes in a finely milled form that is transparent.

Another sunscreen is para-amino-benzoacetic acid (PABA). It needs to be applied before venturing outdoors, especially during the noon hours and in the lower latitudes (Florida, the Caribbean). Cover all exposed areas. According to recent (1998), not yet confirmed research, sunscreens only protect you from sunburn, not from the risk of skin cancer. Avoidance of sun exposure seems to be the only sure way to avoid skin cancer.

Sunglasses. Sunglasses are not only a fashion statement. They should protect your eyes. And the younger you are, the more important that protection is. Damage to your eyes from the sun can cause macular degeneration or cataracts later in life.

Most sunglasses claim to block UV rays by 99 percent, but this claim can be misleading. Most of the sunglasses available will block 99 percent of the UVB rays but might block only 60 percent of UVA light, which, eye doctors warn, can contribute to many eye problems. For full protection, sunglasses should block 99 to 100 percent of both UVA and UVB rays, and 75 to 90 percent of visible light. Look for glasses that have a seal of approval from the American Optometry Association.

BEST FACE FORWARD: HORMONES AND ADOLESCENT ACNE

Because our skin is sensitive, it is the arena for a variety of problems such as acne, dandruff, warts, psoriasis, dermatitis, Herpes infection, and athlete's foot. Many skin conditions develop in adolescence because of hormonal changes, and some earlier conditions from childhood might disappear in adolescence—probably for the same reason.

Acne is not the exclusive domain of adolescents, but that is where we find it most often, even though it is quite common in women in their twenties and even older. It is usually on the lower part of the face (and neck) in older women. In adolescence, it can appear on your face, neck, chest, and back. It can be an occasional blemish—or zit—or a continual outbreak of red bumps.

In puberty, the sebaceous glands become activated in response to the male hormones (androgens), which women also produce in small amounts in the adrenal glands and ovaries. The rate of production varies over the menstrual cycle. In some women, acne flares up during or right before menses. Severe acne is more common in boys than girls.

When the hair follicle and the product of sebaceous glands of the dermis (the middle layer of skin) become sticky from glandular secretions, they form plugs. If the cells adhere near the surface of the pore, then you will have blackheads or whiteheads—open comedones or closed comedones. But deeper blockage is what creates the inflamed postules or the cystic nodules of acne.

Once the plug has formed, sebum from the gland builds up, forming a pimple. If you stretch the follicle or if the pimple is squeezed, the contents spill out into the surrounding skin, causing more tender, deep red pimples to form, and sometimes causing permanent scarring. Consider your face an open wound that does not heal if you pick at it. Instead, wash your face several times during the day with special soaps created to combat acne. While you're at it, wash your hands frequently—and especially before you touch your face.

A young woman patient, Hilda, seemed unable to get rid of the acne that had plagued her for two years. She had tried the over-the-

through infected blood or semen. Hepatitis C is transmitted through the blood and is the cause of more deaths than the other two combined.

The infection is usually traced to contaminated blood supplies, needles used by drug addicts, or sexual intercourse. Those not infected this way are suspected of becoming contaminated through the unsterile and unhygienic procedures used to take care of the needles of a tattoo or body piercing parlor, and through contaminated manicure instruments.

A fad that is coming back in popularity in the end of the twentieth century is skin tattooing. Once the domain of hard-core sailors or Hell's Angels, the tattoo is now considered body art, and tattoo parlors are often operated by art school graduates or dropouts. Women, more than men, are getting tattoos on their legs, shoulders, and breasts—even their faces. Together with the increase in body piercing, tattooing has been cited as an adjunct of self-mutilation, also on the increase among adolescents, mostly girls.

These colorful images are made with chemical dyes that are injected into the top layer of the skin with needles. Tiny holes are punched in the surface of the skin. A dye flows through the needle—made of iron oxide, silver, or carbon pigment. You could be allergic to the tattoo dyes, which could cause localized tissue swelling and crusting around the site. Local antibiotic ointment is used to treat such infections.

Decorative tattooing involves health risks such as hepatitis and HIV transmission, which can occur if the artist doesn't use disposable needles and good sterilization practices. No cases of AIDS have been linked to tattoo parlors, according to the Centers for Disease Control and Prevention, but the risk still exists. In most cities and states, tattoo parlors are not regulated or licensed, and a tattoo artist needs no credentials.

According to the Institute of Dermatologic Laser Surgery in Washington, at least 10 million people have at least one tattoo. More than half wish they did not. Tattoos can be removed with laser treatments, although treatment can also make the tattoo darker instead of lighter, and it could permanently burn away eyelashes when it is used to remove tattooed eyeliner. It may take eight to nine laser treatments, at $1,000 a treatment, to remove a tattoo. This surgery fragments the tattoo pigments, and the body's immune system removes them. It can take six to eight weeks between treatments to let the site heal before another treatment—not a pleasant prospect.

HAIR: PROTECTION AND BEAUTY

Our bodies are covered with hair, but most of it is too light to be seen. The only places hair grows densely are on the head, the pubis, underarms, and legs (and on the faces of men). Our hair protects us from the sun and external trauma. Each live hair follicle is rooted in the subcutaneous skin layer, under the dermis. We have these hair follicles all over our bodies, except on our lips, the palms of our hands, and the soles of our feet. Right next to the hair follicles, and connected by tiny ducts, are the sebaceous glands, which produce sebum.

In medical terms, dandruff is called *seborrhea*. It is actually a very common inflammation of the scalp that causes the stubborn, itchy dandruff. In severe states, it can also cause seborrheic dermatitis: red, scaly patches at the sides of your nose, behind your ears, and on your face and eyebrows. A reddening and scaling of the eyelids and sometimes a mild conjunctivitis come with it. The cause of seborrheic dermatitis is unknown, but the common garden variety is simply dandruff, which flakes off the scalp and drops onto the shoulders. Over-the-counter shampoos are available to control the flaking and itching. Severe cases require a doctor's intervention.

We shed our hair the same way we shed our dead skin cells. New hair pushes the old away. It is shed and regrows about a half an inch a month. Our hair gradually thins out as we age, but young women can lose hair, too, for other reasons. After childbirth there can be a temporary loss of hair, which is probably caused by the changing hormonal balance. Women who stop using the pill sometimes experience hair loss. Crash diets, stress, and other conditions can also affect your hair growth cycle. We have all heard stories of women's hair falling out or turning gray overnight because of an emotional shock. PMS can also give you a bad hair day, but this eventually passes. Severe hair loss, as sometimes happens with chemotherapy, is called *alopecia*.

Like the skin, our hair can be dry, normal, or oily, depending on what our sebaceous glands produce. There are so many different types of shampoos, conditioners, styling gels, and sprays that our hair might feel the effects of substance abuse. If you wash your hair frequently— and gently—these substances will not damage your hair. But over-processing your hair with dyes and perms can have a lasting and cumulative effect and leave you with parched, unmanageable hair. Dyeing is the more damaging of these processes. If you perm your hair as well as dye, leaving it stripped of its natural sebum, your hair will suffer for it.

Body Hair

Women often feel embarrassed if they have excessive hair growth on their arms and legs, or on their upper lips or cheeks. The cause can be genetic or racial, or it can be caused by a slight excess of androgen production, but not enough to be a serious condition. Excess hair in a female is known as *hirsutism*. (This is not the same as *virilism*, which is associated with a deepening voice and enlargement of the clitoris, and could be caused by a tumor of the adrenals or ovaries, or a reaction to medications.)

Most women simply remove unwanted hair with tweezers or depilatories, or by shaving their legs or underarms. *Shaving* is generally safe, but many women consider it uneffective because it leaves a stubble. Hydrogen peroxide can be used to bleach hair on the arms or legs to make it less conspicuous, but always do a patch test first to be sure you are not allergic to the chemical.

Waxing can be done by a trained cosmetician in a salon. When hot wax is applied to the area, then peeled away quickly, the hair is pulled out. This can be painful, because many hairs are yanked out at once. But this technique is effective because the hair takes longer to grow back. Depilatories can dissolve hair protein and leave your skin smooth and hairless. But they can also irritate the skin, so always test them first.

For permanent removal of hair, *electrolysis* is the only effective method. Using a fine needle inserted into the hair follicle, an electrical charge can be delivered into the hair bulb and render it dormant forever after. Theoretically, no more hair will grow from that follicle, but within a month or two some hair will regrow. We don't know why. Perhaps not all of the follicle was or could be removed. Perhaps a new follicle has formed nearby. Still, you are ahead on the number. This is an expensive treatment and must be done slowly over a period of time by a trained technician. It can also damage the tissue around the follicle and cause scarring.

··7··

Health Care and Maintenance of an Adolescent

A mother once berated me loudly in my office waiting room when I refused to tell her what I had discussed with her teenage daughter during an examination.

"What do you mean, that's confidential? How dare you keep my daughter's secrets from me? I am legally responsible for her and I am the one who is paying the bill! I have never heard such a thing!" She continued this tirade in front of my waiting patients until I finally left the room and retreated behind the closed door of my office.

The physician attending to an adolescent is treating at least two people, the child and the parent (three if both parents are involved). The doctor must respect the wishes of both the patient and the parent, but is always bound to protect the patient's confidentiality. The parent, obviously, wants to be involved and should be, if only to provide the history of the family's health and concerns about their child's health. Parents should not, however, expect to be present during the physical examination or while the doctor and patient are talking about the problem—unless the patient herself wishes it.

Despite their feelings of invulnerability, adolescent girls need more frequent health care than adolescent boys. The most common reasons for their visits to doctors are menstrual concerns and results of early experiences with sex, genital infections, sexually transmitted infections, pregnancy, and contraceptive needs.

However, the hormonal changes that send us into puberty set us up for a new wave of conditions, such as eating disorders, depression, and experimentation with risky behaviors (for example, smoking, drugs, sex, and driving fast without seat belts). There is also increased risk of violence, including date rape and incest. The combination of physical and emotional effects of puberty makes girls vulnerable to certain ailments, such as headaches and stomachaches, that are common disorders during adolescence.

Health care of the adolescent girl is complex and requires mastering of medical, psychiatric, and gynecological skills on the part of the principal physician. There is also a medical specialty called adolescent pediatrics. Physicians well suited to care for an adolescent include:

- an internist trained in taking care of adolescents.

- a specially trained family physician.

- a specially trained gynecologist.

- adolescent pediatricians (pediatricians with special interest in the care of adolescents or pediatricians who specialize in the management of adolescents).

- a psychiatrist specially trained in adolescent care.

There has been an increasing number of clinics for women and teens, and a large number of female doctors are entering the field of adolescent medicine.

The Adolescent Health Center at Mount Sinai Hospital in New York City is one of the nation's largest. All seven staff doctors are women. Typical of the trend today toward a holistic approach to adolescent health care, there is a great emphasis on prevention, education, and primary care, as well as the issues of pregnancy, STIs, school problems, and depression. A biopsychological approach is a must in adolescent medicine.

One of the most iron-clad rules of adolescent health care centers is confidentiality. They must guarantee their patients that they will not tell their parents. The only time such a rule can be broken is if a patient is suicidal, and even then the physicians attempt to mediate between the patient and her family.

Understandably, teenagers are often reluctant to communicate any of their concerns when accompanied to the doctor's office by a parent. They might not want to talk about a condition caused by sexual activity, for example. They might not trust the doctor, even alone in the examining room, to keep this information from the parent. And they are often justified in this fear. Insensitive doctors often betray their confidences to parents.

Martha, 17, told me she was fine, yet her mother brought her to me because the girl's behavior had dramatically changed. Her mother was anxious because Martha was about to go away to college, with all the potential dangers that would pose. The mother had no idea if her daughter was withdrawn because she was anxious about the changes facing her or whether she had a fight with her best friend.

On the first visit I explained to both mother and daughter that I would ask many questions that both might want to answer, even if the answers were different. All the information obtained at the visit, however, would be confidential, between the patient and me, and would not be revealed to anyone unless I was expressly instructed to do so by the patient. This is essential for a valid diagnosis and treatment.

In the examination room, I told Martha I was pledged to confidence and asked her, once more, to tell me what was bothering her, hoping to penetrate the wall of indifference. As it turned out, Martha was concerned about having a pelvic exam done, and asked if it would hurt. All of her friends told her it would hurt. A lot. I explained the exam to Martha and told her that it would not hurt, although it might be uncomfortable. I swallowed my frustration at the failure of some physicians to learn the technique of a painless pelvic examination.

THE IMPORTANCE OF A PELVIC EXAMINATION IN ADOLESCENCE

A competent and painless pelvic exam is not only a woman's basic right, it is also a duty of every physician and every health professional who cares for women patients.

The other side of the coin is your own responsibility to do your part. Not only should you practice breast self-examination, you should also try to overcome any prudery or squeamishness that prevents you from becoming comfortable and familiar with your own body in health so you can detect disease.

Feminist activists, including women physicians, developed a new way for teaching medical students, residents, and practicing physicians how to do a competent yet sensitive and painless breast and pelvic exam (refer to chapter 2).

By the time they are 17, most girls have had some sexual experience. If Martha was one of the few who had not, I would have had to make a decision on how to proceed with the pelvic examination. I might have to use a special pediatric-sized speculum to prevent stretching her hymen. A small narrow speculum, however, makes it difficult to see clearly the cervix and the walls of the vagina.

"Have you been sexually active?" I asked her. Her voice registered alarm.

"You won't tell my mom? She would be so upset!" I assured her that what she and I discussed in that room was only between the two of us.

"Just once. An older boy. I shouldn't have let him. And now I have had itching and mucus coming out of my vagina ever since!" The examination revealed a yeast infection.

Back in my consultation office, Martha's mother rose to the occasion and asked me to prescribe birth control. "My baby is going to college. I want her to be protected against sexually transmitted infections and against pregnancy." Martha's eyes opened wide, and her face broke into a grin.

There are many reasons why a teenage girl should have pelvic exams. If she is sexually active, she should have one every six months to test for sexually transmitted infections (STIs), and a Pap smear once a year. In an adolescent girl, an additional pelvic exam is called for whenever there is abnormal vaginal discharge or bleeding, unexplained lower abdominal pain, severe cramps, or pain on intercourse. When there is evidence of sexual abuse, rape, or a pelvic mass, an exam is a must.

THE FRAGILE EMOTIONS

Adolescence can be a period of almost overwhelming stress. The biological changes that are occurring, combined with psychosocial sexual maturation, are a volatile brew. About 40 percent of adolescents cope well with the developmental process, and another 40 percent alternate with smooth and rocky periods of adjustment. But at least 20 percent suffer severe turmoil and stress alternating with periods of adjustment.

Emotional turmoil comes with the physical and hormonal changes of adolescence as well as the struggle for identity. Withdrawal, defiance, eating disorders, substance abuse, depression, and suicide are not uncommon in adolescence. How a young woman responds to the chaos of adolescence depends upon her family, her genetic disposition, and her environment. If she grew up in a dysfunctional home, or is the victim of rape or incest, her adolescent behavior is likely to be deviant. A large percentage of children from such homes run away during the teen years and end up living on the streets.

The adolescent is likely to experiment with a variety of extremes: prolonged sunbathing, excessive dieting, or fast driving. Peer pressure can sometimes result in blind obedience to fads in clothing, music, and vocabulary. This needs to be taken seriously.

CLINICAL DEPRESSION

One confused mother brought her 15-year-old daughter to see me. Lucy had always been a quiet child, but now her sullen and uncommunicative behavior alarmed her parents.

"Lucy is quiet most of the time, but explodes over disagreements with her brother, fights him for every little thing. She is angry with me for even reminding her to wear a hat when it's cold. Her anger persists for several hours, even days. When she is in her angry mood she slams the door of her room, barricades it with chairs so I cannot enter." Lucy's mother, Rebecca, told me her daughter now found boring everything she used to enjoy. Lucy had not lost or gained noticeable weight, but according to her mother she gorged on chocolates and junk food rather than eat a meal, then complained of stomachaches and diarrhea.

When Lucy came in for a checkup, she answered my questions in monosyllables. When I asked her about school, she told me she did not care about her grades and that she was not good at anything anyway. "Perhaps I am better off dead," she said.

This statement triggered an alarm bell. Lucy had been depressed for several months. Her dramatic mood shifts, complaints of fatigue and insomnia, her decline in academic performance and putting herself down, all spoke of severe depression.

I asked Lucy if she felt sad and helpless all the time, but as if sensing I was onto something, she said no. When I asked her if she really meant it about "being better off dead," she said, "Of course not," as if her previous utterance had been a joke. But her dark eyes were not smiling, and she was looking away.

I told her mother of my concern and asked if Lucy had ever tried to end her life. Her mother, shocked at the questions, said, "No, of course not. My daughter wouldn't do that!" Nevertheless, I suggested that she call an adolescent psychiatrist about treating her daughter's depression. When I called the next day, Rebecca told me her daughter was feeling better now that I had found nothing physically wrong.

"She no longer says she is better off dead. And she's being much more congenial—she even gave away her favorite CD to her brother," Rebecca said. Now the alarm bells were ringing louder than ever. Lucy's good-hearted gift to her brother could have been an indication that she had resolved to do away with herself!

"Please watch her." I reminded Rebecca that her daughter was in a deep depression and should see Dr. S, a psychiatrist, right away. Rebecca promised to call as soon as she could for the consultation. "After my relatives visit next week," she said. Thus, Rebecca was concerned initially, but when she faced a serious challenge about her daughter's problem, she went into denial.

It is not unusual for even sophisticated, educated families to go into denial when the possibility of mental illness is mentioned. The stigma of seeing a psychiatrist is still strong. Besides, there is also some territoriality. Rebecca might have resented my coming up with a psychiatric diagnosis. This undermined her assurance that she knew her daughter well, better than anyone else. She would have preferred for me to find a physical reason for Lucy's behavior, such as anemia or something wrong with her glands. In retrospect, Rebecca would have been more amenable to reason if I had ordered an expensive high-tech workup including an MRI or CT scan of the head to rule out organic disease. With a negative workup at hand she would have been more convinced to seek psychiatric help.

I let a few days pass by and called again. No answer! Then, a week later, the psychiatrist called to tell me Lucy had taken a whole bottle of her mother's tranquilizers. Fortunately, the dose was mild, and after a harrowing night in the emergency room, Lucy survived. It took months of intensive psychotherapy to restore Lucy's emotional health.

Lucy is only one example—and a lucky one, at that. The physical and emotional changes of adolescence can precipitate depression, which, left untreated, can escalate into suicide, given the adolescent's propensity for dramatic and high-risk behavior, and the tendency to overreact.

The symptoms that could indicate the existence of serious depression in the young are:

- dramatic mood shifts

- chronic fatigue

- prolonged periods of insomnia or sleeping

- lack of energy

- multiple physical complaints such as headache, stomachache, and fatigue

- hypersensitivity to any adverse event

- exaggerated self-criticism, or an arrogance that masks a sense of worthlessness

- inability to find satisfaction

- decline in academic performance

- loss of interest in activities once enjoyed

Depression in the young should never be taken lightly. Just because emotions are high and low, and part of the transition, does not mean the depression is not real. When adolescent depression is not addressed, the result can be suicide. Lucy's mother was refusing to let herself believe her daughter would do such a thing.

Many suicidal adolescents have a history of problems from childhood that escalate in the teen years. The adolescent witnesses or initiates dissolution of any remaining meaningful relationships while internalizing depression and justifying suicide to herself.

Some adolescents give no warning of their intent to commit suicide, but that is rare. Frequently there are signs that should forewarn family and health professionals. One sign is the sudden elation she feels once she has decided on a plan to end her life. (This is why people are often so shocked when someone takes his or her life—things often seem to be going well right before someone commits suicide.) She might start giving away possessions and taking steps to terminate important relationships. The warning signs of depression mentioned earlier are the same ones that can signal suicide if they are ignored.

There has been an alarming increase in suicide among adolescents—both boys and girls—in the latter part of the twentieth century. According to the Commonwealth Fund American–sponsored Louis Harris survey published in November 1997, one in four girls exhibited depressive symptoms and one in ten of all girls registered depression.

Rates were almost twice as high among girls than boys. Symptoms include crying often, thinking about or planning suicide, feeling as though nothing will work out, feeling sad most of the time, hating oneself, feeling alone, not having any fun, not feeling loved, and not feeling as good as others.

Black girls were least likely to exhibit depressive symptoms (17 percent), Hispanic and Asian American girls had the highest rates of depressive symptoms (27 and 30 percent, respectively), and white girls were at mid-range, at 22 percent. Alarmingly, high rates of suicidal thoughts were reported. Overall, 29 percent said, "I think about killing myself but I would not do it." Three percent responded positively to the statement "I want to kill myself."

We don't know all the reasons behind the increase in depression and suicide among adolescents, but many sociologists blame the change in the quality of family life, changes in competitive pressures for success, violence in our society, availability of guns, and the increased use of alcohol and drugs.

A Way Out of No Way: Treatment of Depression

The use of antidepressive drugs for young people has soared recently even though no studies of their use on the young have ever been done. We have no way of knowing the long-term effects of these drugs on the developing brain. In 1996, more than half a million children and adolescents in this country were taking Prozac and similar drugs for depression. Prescriptions for Prozac for young people from 13 to 18 years of age increased nearly 50 percent that year. Critics say that perhaps we are medicating teenagers simply for being teenagers, while others believe that depressed teenagers need all the help they can get.

Until only recently, it was assumed that children and teenagers could not suffer from depression. Now it is estimated that about 5 percent of American children are clinically depressed. The teen suicide rate now equals that of adults.

Lucy's treatment with antidepressants did not begin until she had a comprehensive physical examination, and it was accompanied by long-term psychotherapy.

OBSESSIVE-COMPULSIVE DISORDERS

Eating disorders, such as anorexia and bulimia, are considered obsessive-compulsive disorders and are common to adolescent women. (For more on these nutritional disorders, see chapter 10.) Self-mutilation, or "cutting," which involves making a row of slashes into the flesh of an arm with a razor blade, is also in this category. Women far outnumber men in this behavior, and there is a great deal of speculation as to why, including the possibility that women more often turn their anger inward. Women are influenced by cultural conflicts and by concerns about their bodies—being too fat, or having breasts that are too large or too small. The same antagonisms that prompt a girl to binge and purge, or starve herself, prompt such mutilation.

Self-injury appears to be part of a growing trend among young girls that encompasses the surge in body piercing and tattooing (see chapter 6), and even branding with a hot iron in some cases. With an estimated 2 million teens engaging in "cutting," and millions more getting pierced and tattooed, health officials are calling it "the addiction of the '90s."

Self-injury begins in the early teens but, if untreated, continues into adulthood. The only large-scale survey ever taken of self-injurers revealed they are also likely to participate in other compulsive behaviors like bulimia or alcoholism. The study was done of 240 female subjects in 1989. The study found the self-injurers to be highly functional, educated, and generally white. The disorder works like any other addiction, needing to be done more and more often in order to receive the satisfaction.

How to Find Medical Help

The American Psychiatric Association should have a referral service for psychiatrists who specialize in treating children and adolescents. Call them at (202) 336-5500.

The American Medical Women's Association includes many psychiatrists. Call your local branch for a referral. The national telephone number is (703) 838-0500.

··8··

A Primer on Contraception

On a hill overlooking my family's farm in upstate New York is an old cemetery. A typical group of gravestones includes one for a patriarch surrounded by several graves of women who died young in childbirth after having married the patriarch. They are joined by the smaller graves of infants who did not survive into childhood.

Throughout the centuries, cultural and religious biases, as well as the patriarchal society, kept women from contraceptive protection. Women were at the mercy of their husbands and the Church, while men simply continued to marry and impregnate new wives.

Nevertheless, women tried to prevent pregnancy. Primitive women knew the herbs that had contraceptive power, and these were the forerunners of chemical and hormonal contraception. The elder women, knowledgeable in these unctions, were eagerly consulted by younger women but were considered witches by men. In ancient Egypt, women placed halves of fruit into their vaginas to cover the cervix in a way similar to today's diaphragms and cervical caps. Others used a vaginal suppository made of crocodile dung to prevent conception. Another method was placing pebbles into the uterus. The pebble acted like an intrauterine device to prevent conception, but it failed to prevent infection. Hippocrates recommended violent exercises to cause abortion. The fact that women continued to use these dangerous methods is testament to their exhaustive struggle against pregnancy and illnesses that culminated in premature aging and death.

The simplest form of contraception, namely withdrawal before ejaculation, the so-called *coitus interruptus*, is referred to in Genesis, the first chapter of the Bible's Old Testament, which describes the actions of Onan, the son of Judah, who spilled his semen, not wishing to impregnate his brother's widow. As was the custom of the day, if a man died without leaving any children, his brother was obliged to then impregnate the man's wife so that any sons would be considered heirs of the dead man. Onan—perhaps we should consider him the first hero of contraception—rebelled at this practice and refused to get his sister-in-law pregnant.

Egyptian and Chinese art shows characters wearing penile sheaths, the forerunners of condoms. The Italian physician and anatomist Gabriello Fallopio is said to have suggested treated linen sheaths as protection from syphilis as early as 1560. Fallopio also was the first to describe the Fallopian tubes, thus the name.

Birth control to protect women was never practiced even though men had long before learned how to protect themselves with condoms from venereal diseases. Medical professionals refrained from prescribing contraception even though they knew how. Dr. Albert Arbuthnot was barred from practicing medicine in England in 1885 for his willingness to provide a safe and effective contraceptive service to his patients.

Margaret Sanger, an American nurse who became a pioneer in providing women with birth control early in the twentieth century, was blocked at every turn by local and federal authorities from sending information about contraception in the mail. Sanger saw many women die in childbirth and from botched illegal abortions. She fought the authorities and was jailed several times, but managed to found Planned Parenthood.

It was not until the 1930s that a variety of barrier devices for contraception, including diaphragms, came into general use. The 1960s brought the development of oral contraceptives, spermicides, and intra-uterine devices. It was in this decade that women's health became a political movement in the United States. In the 1970s and 1980s, doctors became involved in dispensing contraceptive services in an attempt to reduce the growth of the world population.

We have made some progress in the area of contraception, but not enough. While the world acknowledges that sex will not go away if we close our eyes, it has yet to confront it with effective education in children. Safe sex today means not only protection from pregnancy but protection from sexually transmitted infection (STI). The pill would probably give the best contraceptive control and some protection against common STIs, but no protection from AIDS. The male condom protects the male and gives relative protection to the female. But for protection from AIDS, the female condom probably comes closest.

TEEN PREGNANCY IN AMERICA: AN EPIDEMIC

Among industrialized nations we have the highest rate of teenage childbirth. American women under age 20 have double the pregnancy rate of women of the same age in Canada, and almost ten times the rate of similar women in the Netherlands. The fertility rate is increasing most rapidly in girls under 14. Every third birth to an African American female and every fifth birth to a Caucasian female are the result of teenage pregnancy, most often to an unmarried girl.

In 1980, there were 25 pregnancies for every 1,000 15-year-old girls, compared with 5 in England and Sweden and 2 in the Netherlands. American 19-year-olds have 150 pregnancies per 1,000, compared with 85 in England, 60 in Sweden, and 25 in the Netherlands. Teen pregnancy is so rare in Japan that a rate cannot be calculated.

Federal surveys in the 1990s indicate that while sexual activity among teenagers is down for the first time in three decades, and more teens are using contraceptives, we still lack an effective national effort to reduce the teenage pregnancy rate. Nationwide there are 112 pregnancies for every 1,000 young women between 15 and 19. This results in 61 births, 36 abortions, and 15 miscarriages. The birth and abortion rates have declined somewhat in recent years, and a survey by the Department of Health and Human Services indicates the trend may continue.

In 1995, 50 percent of 15- to 19-year-old women engaged in sexual activity whereas five years before the rate was 55 percent. The National Campaign to Prevent Teen Pregnancy began in 1996 with the goal of reducing the number of pregnancies per 1,000 women in that age group to 75 by the year 2005. In the past the mixed messages about sex have hindered national efforts, especially in school programs.

The Failures of Contraception

Unintended pregnancies represent more than half the total pregnancies in the United States. Most of the pregnancies of women under 25 are unintended, even with availability of highly effective contraceptives. Contraceptive failure rates differ with the age of the user, with adolescents way ahead. There is no biological reason for this, so the problem lies in lack of counseling. Users of contraception account for almost half the abortions in America, so contraception is not being used properly and is not effective.

Not only have American girls had higher numbers of teenage pregnancy, they've also had more abortions than their counterparts in other Western countries. There were 60 abortions per 1,000 among 19-year-olds in the United States and only 8 per 1,000 19-year-old Dutch girls. In other Western countries, the percentage of girls engaging in sexual intercourse is about the same or higher than that of American teenagers. The rates in Sweden are considerably higher (80 percent). Sweden, however, has systematically provided adolescents with education and access to contraception for many years. In contrast, both education and access to contraception are lacking here. Americans still operate on the naive premise that if we do not tell children about sex they will not find out.

More than half the American teens who are sexually active receive no counseling. Approximately 28 percent seek such advice in the first six months of sexual activity, while in the Netherlands more than 90 percent do so. No adolescent in Holland is more than a bicycle ride away from a teenage counseling center that can answer questions about health matters including sexuality and contraception.

Lacking adequate knowledge about her sexuality, and having little self-esteem, the rebellious adolescent girl often resists using birth control. "Oh, it won't happen to me. Just this once!" An older girl who is engaged in a stable romantic relationship, educated about her own body, and looking forward to a future educational goal or job is more likely to be successful in preventing pregnancy.

Parents, too, sometimes fuel the resistance. Many wear blinders about their children's sexual activities. Denial is easier than confronting their daughter and teaching her how to protect herself. When one mother brought her 17-year-old in for birth control pills I guessed (correctly) that she was a couple of years too late.

Ironically, there are many television commercials for early pregnancy testing kits, but none for condoms (with one or two exceptions for public service commercials about safe sex).

Contraception in an adolescent is complicated by a number of factors. Foremost is her own ambivalence about seeking advice from the family doctor. She might be afraid that the family doctor, who also treats her mother, father, and brothers, will tell her parents about the nature of her visit. Some teens are unable to pay for medical care and hesitate to use their parents' health insurance for personal concerns. (Refer to chapter 7 about adolescent health care.)

Many physicians, too, particularly pediatricians, are ambivalent about advising their teenage patients about contraception, assuming the girls will go to gynecologists for such advice. One survey showed that almost half of pediatricians either did not wish to see adolescents in their practice or stated that their own knowledge of adolescent medicine and especially of suitable birth control methods, was inadequate.

Some physicians erroneously assume that it is illegal today to distribute contraceptive advice for minors without the consent of parents, and so they often refuse to do so. It is best for all concerned when at least one parent is aware of and approves contraception for a daughter, but there is no legal or moral requirement for the doctor to notify a parent without the consent of the girl. And there is every reason to provide the contraceptive to the girl if she wants it.

Pregnancy can be prevented by placing a physical barrier between the sperm and the fertile egg or by manipulating the female hormonal process to prevent ovulation or to make the uterus unsuitable for an embryo. These are reversible methods. Permanent or irreversible contraception includes having the tubes tied or removing the ovaries and uterus.

There is no such thing as the perfect contraceptive, one that is right for every woman. You must balance the positive and negative effects. The choice of birth control should be a joint decision by you and your physician after a thorough examination and consideration of your age, previous contraceptive history, medical history, allergies, and lifestyle.

The ideal contraceptive for teens would be one that is easy to use, inexpensive, and completely protective against pregnancy and sexually transmitted infections. It should also be reversible, that is, it should not interfere with fertility when she wants a child later. The ideal contraceptive should be unobtrusive and applied at a time separate from the sexual act.

No contraceptive can fit this entire bill, but oral contraceptives and condoms come closest. Oral contraceptives are currently the most popular, effective, and logical birth control for the majority of sexually active teenagers in a monogamous relationship. Condoms, when properly used, are effective against disease. Both the pill and the condoms, however, require motivation and planning on the part of the girl. The best protection against pregnancy and disease is using both.

Other than the rhythm method, barrier contraceptives have the highest rate of failure: male condoms, 12 percent; diaphragms, 18 percent; other barrier methods, 21 percent.

Contraception with hormonal manipulation has lower failure rates. Only 3 percent fail with the pill. IUDs and implants, used by only a fraction of the population, also have low failure rates. In Sweden, for example, about 30 percent of all women who use reversible methods use a copper T IUD, which has low failure rate. In this country, fewer than 2 percent of women use the IUD. Injectable hormonal contraceptives are approved in ninety countries and are used by approximately 15 million women. Here, they have only recently been approved by the Food and Drug Administration.

THE PILL: LIBERATION OR HEALTH HAZARD?

By manipulating the levels of estrogen and progesterone during the month, the oral contraceptive works on several different levels. At the pituitary/ovarian level, it prevents the egg from growing and ovulating. At the endometrial level, it causes thinning of the uterine lining, making it a less hospitable environment for implantation of an embryo. At the cervical level, it causes the cervical mucus to become thicker, so the sperm cannot penetrate.

When the pill appeared in the 1960s it signaled liberation for women, who could now take a pill every day and no longer worry about getting pregnant. But it lost its magical aura when serious side effects were soon discovered. The first oral contraceptives (Enovid, in the 1960s) contained large amounts of estrogen and were associated with major side effects, such as *thrombophlebitis*, a condition in which the veins become inflamed, fill up with clots, and throw bits of clots into the circulation, resulting in embolism to the lung. These are rare, especially in young women, now that the estrogen dose in the modern pills has been greatly reduced. However, women 35 and older who smoke are still in danger of embolism and cardiovascular complications.

The progestin component of the pill also carries some side effects, primarily lowering the good cholesterol, high-density lipoprotein (HDL), and raising the bad cholesterol, low-density lipoprotein (LDL). HDL is protective against heart disease and strokes, and the reduction of this when on the pill should be taken seriously and discussed with your physician. This concern is especially valid for older women, who are more at risk for these conditions.

Once you stop taking the pill, there will be a month or three before your periods return. The pill does not inhibit skeletal growth in adolescents, nor does not it inhibit future fertility unless you are in menopause. There is no evidence that the pill brings on menopause sooner.

Among the myths that persist about the pill is that it causes cancer. Oral contraceptives, in fact, actually lower the risk of ovarian and endometrial cancer. They also lower the risk of ectopic pregnancy and pelvic inflammatory disease (PID).

There are 17.5 million American women using the pill now, and 80 percent of all women will have used it at some time.

Benefits and Risks of the Pill

Oral contraception is ideal for adolescents because all of the health risk associated with the pill—cardiovascular problems or pulmonary embolism—are associated with older women. In the world literature there is only a single adolescent death related to the pill, a 17-year-old girl in Sweden who died in 1968 from a thrombotic stroke preceded by a long history of headaches. In adolescents the pills are helpful in preventing menstrual cramps, ameliorating the premenstrual syndrome, lowering the flare-ups of acne, and decreasing the risk of benign breast disease. There is less buildup of the uterine lining, and it is shed every month.

Women who take the pill for ten years or longer can cut their risk for ovarian cancer, one of the most deadly, by 80 percent, according to a study reported in the January 1995 issue of the *Journal of the American Medical Society* (JAMA). There is also a 50 percent decrease in risk of both endometrial cancer and PID, and 90 percent reduction of the risk of ectopic pregnancy. Taking the pill for any period of time in your reproductive years lowers the risk of these cancers.

The association of breast cancer and oral contraceptives is still controversial. Use of the pill dropped drastically in the 1980s after reports linked it to breast cancer. Most American investigators, in more than fourteen studies, report no increase or only a slight increase in women under 45 after prolonged use of the old-type high-dose pills. European studies indicate a slightly increased risk, which might be due to the old-type, high-dose pills.

Most of the data on the relation between the newer low-dose pills and breast cancer do not indicate increased risk, but longer follow-up is needed. This should not be confused with the long-term studies of estrogen use in menopausal women. There, we know there is a slight risk.

Some studies indicate that a small group of women destined to develop breast cancer at an early age might develop it earlier if they have taken oral contraceptives for many years. However, it could be the tumors are already there to grow and the pill only accelerates the growth. Or it could be due to early detection because women on the pill are getting regular checkups. In late 1996, an analysis of fifty-four studies involving more than 150,000 women in twenty-five countries found no long-term risk for breast cancer among oral contraceptive users.

The only known cancer association with the pill is a rare type of tumor at the base of the brain or in the liver, but this association is very tenuous at best and apparently is the result of very-high-dose pills.

The risk of cervical cancer remains unsettled. While some studies indicate an increased risk—1.2 to 1.8 times greater—for women who used the pill for ten years, the studies failed to eliminate confounding factors such as smoking, early age sexual activity, high-frequency sexual intercourse, and infection with herpes and other viruses, as well as exposure to multiple partners. All of these are known to be associated with the increased risk of cervical cancer. So there is no way to know if the risk is associated with the pill.

Side Effects of the Pill

Life-threatening complications are extremely rare, but some women experience headaches, breakthrough bleeding, weight gain, nausea, and depression. Some of these can be cured by changing the dosage and type of pill. However, pills should be discontinued if you develop hypertension, increased frequency and intensity of headaches, unexplained chest or lower abdominal pain, or milky discharge from the nipple. (Estrogen makes the glandular components of the breast proliferate, and progestin makes them secrete milk.)

Whenever cyclic oral contraceptives or estrogen replacement is used, vaginal bleeding might occur at the end of the cycle once you stop taking the pill. This is called withdrawal bleeding and is a counterpart of normal menstrual bleeding. If vaginal bleeding occurs at any other time of the cycle while you are on the pill, it is called breakthrough bleeding. The significance of breakthrough bleeding is that it draws attention to an abnormal process in the reproductive tract, although in most cases it only indicates an imbalance between various hormones. Persistent and prolonged breakthrough bleeding might call for a D&C (see chapter 16, under Common Treatment Procedures) or other investigation into the cause.

A woman who smokes, drinks, or uses drugs should not take oral contraceptives. Also, if you take medications that affect the metabolism—such as anti-epilepsy drugs, antibiotics, sedatives, anti-migraines, and antacids—the level of effectiveness of the oral contraceptive could be compromised.

A young woman with acne might require a pill with more estrogen. Acne is caused by the male hormone, so giving estrogen restores the normal estrogen/testosterone ratio. However, the increased estrogen could lead to proliferation of endometrial cells, which is why excess estrogen might cause endometrial cancer.

Migraine headaches can get worse on the pills that contain estrogen, so mini pills with progestin only would be better. Similarly, if you are a nursing mother, a pill containing estrogen could stop the milk secretion. Here, too, a mini pill would give you the protection you need.

HOW TO USE ORAL CONTRACEPTIVES

There are several types and combinations of oral contraceptives. Some are a fixed dose, and some are multiphasic. Some pills are taken for only twenty-one days, and others every day of the month. Different colors represent the particular stage in the monthly cycle.

Multiphasic pills contain one of the newer lipid-friendly progestins (norgestimate or desogestrel) and are a good choice for adolescents because they contain lower doses of both hormones, cause less change in blood lipids, and are easy to take. They induce regular menseslike bleeding. Multiphasic pills were introduced in 1984 with small doses of progestin and estrogen that vary according to the phase of the monthly cycle.

The tablets vary the amounts of estrogen and progestin to simulate the normal menstrual cycle. The cycle is sometimes divided into two phases, one for the first half of the cycle (ten or eleven days) with estrogen only, the second for the remaining half with estrogen and progestin. These are biphasic pills. The triphasic cycle, on the other hand, is divided by the weeks, so that each week you are taking increasing amounts of progestin. For the last week of the month the manufacturer usually provides inert pills. These pills do nothing but make it easier to keep count. Originally devised so that there would be less in between bleeding or spotting, the biphasic and triphasic pills do not live up to this expectation, and many physicians no longer prescribe them. They are more expensive than the fixed-dose type pill.

Mini pills are made only of progestin, and the primary action is to render the uterus inhospitable to the embryo and thicken the cervical mucus so sperm cannot get near the egg. Mini pills are somewhat less effective than the pills containing both estrogen and progestin. Under ideal circumstances, when taken as prescribed, mini pills are 99.5 percent effective, while combination pills are 99.9 percent effective.

In fixed-dose preparations, each pill contains the same dose of estrogen and progestin. The pills are taken once a day for twenty-one days. During the following seven days of the cycle you take a placebo or no pill at all. Many physicians believe the fixed-dose pills are less confusing than the multiphasic pills, taken only on certain days. The fixed-dose pill is identified by dose and color such as pink or green.

Oral contraceptives, more than any other birth control program, depend on full commitment to the daily pill. The most common failure of oral contraceptives is forgetting to take the pill. If you are meant to take a pill every morning and you forget, then take it anytime during the day. Just do not skip it.

Emergency Contraception

Women's advocacy groups finally convinced the FDA to publish the correct "morning after" dosage of birth control pills, so information on how to do this will appear with all brands on the market. Regular contraceptive pills taken in a quadruple amount (two pills twice over twelve hours) within forty-eight hours, but preferably twenty-four hours, of exposure will act as emergency contraception. According to the FDA, this regimen works 75 percent of the time by preventing the egg from implanting itself on the uterus. It is estimated that up to 2.3 million unintended pregnancies could be prevented every year by this strategy. It is important to understand the correct dosage because some types of oral contraceptives include placebo pills, which have no potency at all and would, therefore, be useless as emergency contraception.

Late in 1998, the FDA approved an emergency contraception kit, Previn, which is available with a prescription from your doctor or a licensed health care provider. The kit works before the pregnancy begins and should not be confused with RU486, the abortion pill (see below). The kit includes an information book, a pregnancy test, and four birth control pills of progestin (0.25 mg levonorgestrel) and estrogen (0.05 mg ethinyl estradiol). The side effects of such emergency contraception usually include nausea and vomiting but sometimes an anti-nausea medication from your doctor can help.

If you believe you are at risk for pregnancy because of unprotected sex and need a prescription or information, call the hot line: 1-888-

NOT 2 LATE (66825283) and you will be referred to providers in your area. There is also a website at *http://opr.princeton.edu/ec/*.

Mifepristone (RU-486)

Mifepristone (RU-486) was approved for use in this country after many years of popularity in Europe. This is the first antiprogestin to be a major breakthrough in reproductive medicine. It has generated great interest in its various medical uses and its potential to produce abortion.

Along with prostaglandin, RU-486 is now used for induction of abortion, but it can also be used to prevent pregnancy. As this book is written, the details are not all worked out about how to use it safely as a contraceptive, perhaps using smaller doses.

Antiprogestins, like excessive amounts of estrogen, prevent pregnancy by preventing the egg from implanting in the uterus. Studies report that if this drug is used here it could prevent up to 2.3 million unintended pregnancies each year. One million of those pregnancies now end in abortion.

HORMONAL INJECTIONS AND IMPLANTS

Hormonal contraceptives can also be taken in forms other than pills. Progestin can be injected into the muscle of the arm, implanted under the skin of the forearm, or imbedded with an IUD (Progestasert).

Depoprovera (depomedroxyprogesterone acetate)

Injected intramuscularly every three months, Depoprovera is a highly effective method of contraception. It suppresses ovulation, makes the endometrium inhospitable for implantation of the embryo, and causes cervical mucus to thicken. The average dose of Depoprovera is 150 milligrams. Small women may need less, and larger women more. There is also an ethnic variation in the dose. For reasons not well understood, for example, Thai women need a smaller dose than Mexican women.

Disruption of the normal menstrual cycle occurs in the majority of users. Irregular bleeding, heavy bleeding, or very light spotting occurs during the first year of use. After a year, menstruation stops altogether. It will return when the injections stop. Almost 20 percent of women who started on Depoprovera discontinue it because of these irregularities.

Some, but not all, women develop headache, gain weight, or have acne flare-ups. Studies done on beagles showed an early tendency to breast tumors. Subsequent studies by the World Health Organization (WHO) provide evidence of no increased risk of cancer of the endometrium, ovary, cervix, and liver with Depoprovera. They also found no

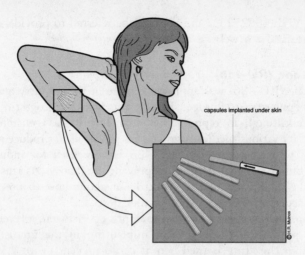

Figure 8. Norplant capsules are implanted under the skin.

harmful effects on the function of kidneys, thyroid, and lipids (fats) in the blood.

Long-term use of Depoprovera reduces menstrual blood loss and decreases the risk of pelvic inflammatory disease (PID), yeast infections, and endometrial cancer. However, there is an unpredictable delay in the return of fertility.

The Norplant System

Developed by the Population Council, Norplant requires implanting six silicone capsules under the skin in the arm, a procedure that takes about five minutes. The capsules release small amounts of progestin into the blood circulation and provide contraception for five years. A heavy woman would require additional capsules. Both insertion and removal require local anesthesia. In some women the surgical procedure of removing the implant might cause scarring; an overgrown scar is a *keloid*.

There is also a Norplant 2 system with three-year duration. No estrogen is used in this system, so the side effects related to estrogen are not a risk. Norplant is very effective—with only a 1 percent pregnancy rate in five-year users. Adolescents can successfully use Norplant, although anyone wanting children at an early age should avoid this method of birth control.

Implants have gotten bad press because of the years-long litigation over silicone breast implants. There are negative feelings about having something put inside the body, and only 1 percent of women in this country use Norplant. Unlike the breast implants, however, which were in use before they were approved by the FDA, the Norplant was approved by the FDA in 1991.

Common problems associated with the implants, such as bleeding,

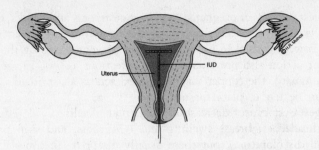

Figure 9. T-shaped intrauterine device (IUD) in place.

weight gain, and depression, are caused by the progestin. There have also been complaints that the removal of the implants can cause pain and scarring.

An international study of over 16,000 women for five years by the World Health Organization revealed that Norplant caused no more problems than the pill or IUD and was 99.77 percent effective in birth control.

THE INTRAUTERINE DEVICE (IUD)

The IUD is more like a barrier contraceptive, but because it is now used with hormonal manipulation, we discuss it here. These are metal loops or rings with strings attached that are implanted by a physician into the uterus, beyond the cervical os. Copper is used for many IUDs because the metal itself has some effect on the environment of the uterus to prevent implantation of the embryo. A string (tail) remains in the vagina, and the physician should explain how to feel for the string in the vagina to make sure that the IUD has not been dislodged or lost in the uterine cavity. IUDs must only be removed by the doctor.

In the past, the IUD was associated with a high risk of pelvic infection. The hanging threads needed to yank the IUD out of the uterus provided an avenue for bacteria, especially yeast infections and gonorrhea, to infect the uterus and tubes. When they are used in a young woman who has not had children, IUDs are sometimes expelled by the uterus, cause perforation of the uterine wall, or result in toxic complications. Because of many class action lawsuits, most of the IUDs were removed from the market in the 1980s. The only two currently available are the newly developed Progestasert, and the Paraguard T380. Both are T-shaped. There is no evidence to suggest that the IUDs now in use cause infection or predispose women to precancerous conditions of the cervix, uterus, or ovary. However, any preexisting cervical infection should be treated before insertion of either Progestasert or the copper-containing IUD.

Progestasert is impregnated with progesterone and works the way mini pills work to alter the endometrial environment so an embryo cannot grow, and thickening the mucus to prevent access by the sperm. The latter action also prevents access of infectious agents. In the copper IUD, Paraguard, the copper that is released acts as an antioxidant. Paraguard can be left in place for ten years.

Progestasert causes decrease of menstrual bleeding. Side effects can include headaches, breast swelling and tenderness, and skin problems (acne and discoloration), but these usually disappear in time. Excessive bleeding could result from incorrect placement within the wall of the uterus. Also, if normal periods return, it is possible the IUD was expelled.

Once the Progestasert is removed, normal fertility is immediately restored. While younger women benefit more from the pill, more mature young adults can enjoy the advantages of less bleeding, fewer menstrual cramps, and protection against STIs offered with Progestasert. In general, these are not used for adolescent girls unless they cannot use other methods.

FUTURE HORMONAL CONTRACEPTIVES

The cervical vaginal ring (CVR) is made of soft, pliable plastic and is slightly smaller than a diaphragm. It contains a combination of estrogen and progestin and can be inserted into the vagina on day five of the menstrual cycle and left in place for three weeks. Then it can be removed to allow for bleeding. The ring can be removed for up to three hours for intercourse, but it does not have to be.

Not yet approved by the Food and Drug Administration as of late 1998, CVRs have been tested in the Netherlands, Brazil, and the Dominican Republic, where women reportedly liked them. The rings have many advantages. One size fits all. It is effective and easy to insert. It is inserted once a month and its use is independent of sexual activity. You need not remember to take daily pills. The ring does not cause nausea; it provides a uniform blood level of the hormones. The ring is extremely easy to remove, and normal fertility will return immediately. Once the ring is approved for general use in this country, it will be an ideal contraceptive for sexually active women, including adolescents.

Vaccines for fertility control are being developed and tested in many countries. They are directed against various hormones and components of the sperm, but they are not ready for wide use.

Skin patches (transdermal devices) are hormonal contraceptives delivered through the skin. While a great deal of research is in progress, nothing is available yet.

GnRH analogs and antagonists are synthetics of the natural hormones that inhibit ovarian function (see chapter 16, under Treatment of Fibroids and Endometriosis). They are expensive and not easily adaptable to adolescent use.

BARRIER CONTRACEPTIVES: MALE AND FEMALE CONDOMS

When those early Egyptian women put halves of fruit rinds into their vaginas to cover the cervix, they were creating a barrier contraceptive. Barriers for a woman are diaphragms, cervical caps, vaginal sponges, and spermicidal inserts—or the female condom. For a man, the barrier is the condom. Such devices block the sperm from meeting the egg during intercourse. None are effective, however, if they are not used properly.

The Male Condom
The condom is the world's oldest contraceptive device. It is inexpensive and easily available in drugstores, vending machines, teen clinics, some school health offices, and family planning clinics. Most condoms in the United States are made of latex, which is impenetrable to viruses. Those made of young lamb intestine do not protect from transmission of viral diseases. They are thinner and improve the pleasurable sensation, especially for the man.

In the days when boys used to carry condoms in their wallets, the shape of the ring showed and was considered a status symbol, a sign of virility. The wallet, and the equally popular glove compartment of the car, were the worst possible places to carry condoms because the heat weakened the latex and the condom would tear or leak during intercourse.

Today girls often buy and keep the condoms because they are so easily accessible in drugstores. There is no longer a need to face the embarrassment of asking the druggist for them. They are well displayed in most drugstore shelves, and there are shops in some malls devoted exclusively to condoms. You can be in control by keeping a supply handy. Some high schools have programs that teach contraception and distribute condoms to students, but this is not universal, and it is still extremely controversial. Parents forced some schools to abandon such programs or limit them to individual counseling with pictures and a video.

Condoms protect from most STIs, but they are not foolproof against AIDS for women. And there is a 20 percent failure rate because they are improperly used.

••••

HOW TO USE A MALE CONDOM EFFECTIVELY

(Adapted from How to Use a Condom, by the Family Planning Council, Southeastern Pennsylvania.)

1. Check the expiration date on the package. If it has passed, the condom might not be safe.
2. Do not keep condoms in a warm place, such as the glove compartment of a car, or in a wallet.
3. Place the condom on the tip of the penis while you keep holding the tip of the condom. Hold the tip of the condom and squeeze out some air so as to leave space for the ejaculate.
4. Unroll the condom on the erect penis all the way down to the hair so that semen will not spill out once the penis relaxes.
5. Put the condom on before allowing entry into your vagina.
6. If you need a lubricant use KY jelly or a contraceptive gel, but not Vaseline or other oil-soluble substances.
7. After ejaculation, make sure that the condom is still on and is pulled out while the penis is still hard. When it relaxes, the condom will become loose and semen can spill out.
8. Use a condom only once and discard it. Use a new condom every time you have sex.

••••

The Female Condom

The female condom is the newest contraceptive device and probably comes closest to protecting you from pregnancy as well as AIDS. It was developed in England and tested in Europe before becoming available here. It's like a diaphragm combined with a male condom. This condom is a soft plastic sheath with an inner ring spanned with a membrane that is placed like a diaphragm between the pubic bone and behind the cervix, thus fitting over the cervix, and an outer rubber rim that is placed outside the vulva. The outer rim provides a protective entrance to the vagina. The rings are connected by a soft tunnellike membrane (sheath) that fits the walls of the vagina.

The female condom is probably more protective than the diaphragm,

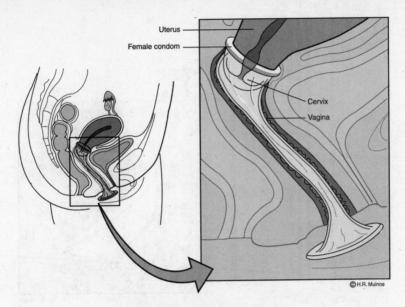

Figure 10. Female condom in place.

although it is more complicated to insert. It is also expensive, and like the male condom it should not be reused. A spermicide is applied to the surface of the inner membrane (the one that goes against the cervix, then the ring is squeezed and inserted into the vagina like a diaphragm; the rest of the sheath is pulled inside the body. More testing is under way on this particular barrier method.

These are now available in the United States directly through the manufacturers or by asking your doctor to order them for you.

The Diaphragm

The diaphragm is a latex dome mounted on a circular metal spring. When properly inserted into the vagina, the dome covers the cervix and the rim fits snugly behind the pubic bone. The metal spring is flexible, allowing the diaphragm to assume a flat oval shape. (A stiffer "All-Flex" rim and stiffer-still "Arcing" spring are also available. Stiffer rings conform to the anatomy better and are less likely to become dislodged. They might be more irritative, however.) When used with a spermicide a diaphragm is 94 percent effective in preventing pregnancy.

The diaphragm comes in various sizes and requires fitting by a trained practitioner. You also need to be carefully trained in how to put it in and take it out, since it does require some manual skill. The doctor should demonstrate the insertion on a plastic model, paying special attention to the direction in which to push the diaphragm. Once fitted, practice putting it in and removing it while in the office, so the doctor can help you.

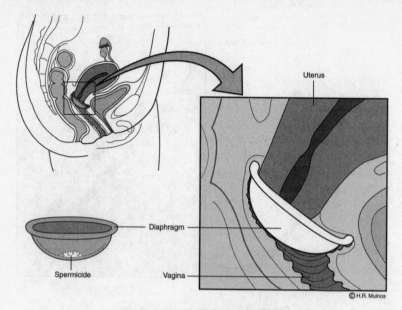

Figure 11. Diaphragm in place.

The diaphragm offers some protection against gonorrhea and cervical cancer but not against HIV.

Inserting a Diaphragm. This should be done well before intercourse begins, so you need to plan ahead for this method to be effective. Before you insert the diaphragm, hold it up to a light to be sure there are no pinholes or tears in it. Then, put one foot on a low stool or chair and bend your knee. With your opposite hand, separate the lips of the vagina. Insert your finger first to ascertain the direction of the cervix. With your hand, squeeze the diaphragm ring to a narrow oval shape and insert it into the vagina toward your lower back. Once the diaphragm is in place, release the pressure on the spring. The diaphragm will then assume a semihorizontal position in the vagina. Insert your finger deeper to make sure that the cervix is covered by the membrane of the diaphragm.

Normally, a properly inserted diaphragm will not cause discomfort. If it does, it is probably not inserted properly. A common error is placing it too high so that its inner rim presses against the cervix rather than resting behind it. Not only is such placement uncomfortable, it also takes away protection by exposing the cervix to semen.

Removing a Diaphragm. Wait for six to eight hours after intercourse before taking the diaphragm out so all the sperm lingering in the vaginal canal are dead.

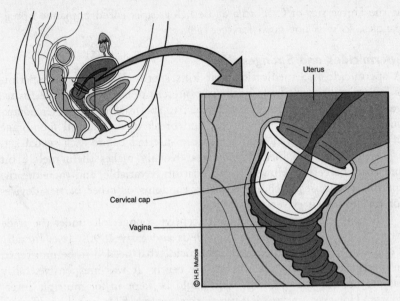

Figure 12. Cervical cap in place.

Caring for a Diaphragm. Wash the diaphragm with lukewarm water and mild soap and let it dry in the air before putting it back into its case. Each time you clean it, hold it up to the light and check the latex for any pinholes or tears.

Cervical Caps

Cervical caps are widely used in England but are not as common in this country because the risk of pregnancy is high. The cap is a small rubber dome-shaped cup smaller than a diaphragm that fits tightly across the cervix like a thimble, preventing semen from entering. Spermicidal gel is placed inside the cap before insertion. The gel provides a snug seal around the cap and additional protection.

Caps come in several sizes and need careful fitting by a well-trained practitioner. After the fitting you need to observe your cervix with a mirror to learn how to insert and remove the cap yourself. Because it is difficult, you need to be committed to learning this technique. The cap cannot be kept inside your body for more than twenty-four to forty-eight hours.

It can also be displaced during intercourse, and it might be associated with an unpleasant vaginal odor. Occasionally it can alter the Pap smear by irritating the cells of the cervix, although there is no real harm done. It is less protective than the diaphragm. Even with a spermicide, the failure rate is 17 pregnancies out of 100 at the end of one year, and 38 out of 100 after two years. Half of a student group studied at the University of California at Berkeley experienced unplanned pregnancies, so it is not good for teenagers.

Spermicides and Sponges

A spermicide is a medication that kills sperm. Vaginal insert spermicides are widely available without a prescription. They include foams, gels, creams, and suppositories. The active spermicides are either nonoxynol-9 or octoxynol-9, which coat and break down the cell membrane of sperm cells. Vaginal inserts must be inserted before each sexual act.

Spermicides are messy. Body heat usually makes them melt a bit and coat the cervix. However, this coating is variable, and therefore the spermicides must be combined with condoms or other barrier devices for maximum effectiveness.

A nonprescription vaginal contraceptive sponge sold under the trade name Today was available in the 1980s and early 1990s. It is literally a cup-shaped sponge filled with spermicide that needed to be moistened in water and properly placed over the cervix. It was inexpensive, fairly easy to use "at the moment," and could be kept in for multiple intercourse. However, it was less protective against STIs and less effective for contraception. Rare cases of toxic shock syndrome were associated with the sponge. Some women complained of vaginal dryness and discomfort. For all these reasons, production discontinued in 1995.

NATURAL FAMILY PLANNING

When you are not using anything "artificial," such as a pill or a condom, but schedule sexual intercourse around your natural menstrual cycle, abstaining when you are ovulating, you are practicing the *rhythm method* of birth control. This is the only method of contraception condoned by the Catholic Church, although in recent years, it is believed, a significant number of Catholics have begun to use other methods of birth control. If a woman is determined to use this method, she must take her temperature every day and keep a chart. She will mark the days when her menstrual flow starts and stops, and note the variations in temperature. (When you are ovulating, your temperature goes up.) Many women keep such a chart when they want to become pregnant.

The failure rate with this method is extremely high. You are at risk of getting pregnant for some time before and after the egg is released, and there is no way of knowing exactly when that is. This method can be used only by women with perfect menstrual cycles and a high level of education about their bodies, and this does not generally include adolescents.

The other natural method is known as *coitus interruptus*, which means the man pulls his penis out of the vagina before releasing his ejaculate.

This is even more risky because a few energetic sperm may precede the ejaculate out of the penis.

It is critical for women to understand how contraception works and to decide what is the best method for them to use depending upon their sexual activity. In the age of safe sex, many more young women are taking this seriously, but there is still a long way to go in convincing the adolescent girl that pregnancy is better when it is planned and that, unless she is in a monogamous relationship with a trusted partner, she needs to use the best possible contraceptive methods to protect herself not only from pregnancy but from sexually transmitted infection.

A recent example of this need was widely publicized in late 1997, when police arrested a 20-year-old man who was responsible for transmitting his HIV infection—which he knew he had—to at least forty high school girls and possibly hundreds of other women.

QUESTIONS TO ASK ABOUT CONTRACEPTIVES

How does it work?

- Will it protect me against STIs and AIDS?

- Will I be in control of it?

- How long will I be protected?

- What are the side effects?

- What are the risks of forgetting to use it or not using it?

- What are the instructions for effective use?

- Will it interfere with my sexual pleasure?

- What does it cost?

- How long will the device last?

- Does medical insurance cover the cost of any possible side effects?

··9··

What to Know About Sexually Transmitted Infections

Few people realize that one in every five people in America gets a sexually transmitted infection (STI)—also known as sexually transmitted disease (STD)—by the time he or she is 21. It is critically important to understand the nature and causes of STIs because often there are no symptoms until the disease is in an advanced stage, when it can cause sterility or death. By the age of 14, 6 percent of girls and 18 percent of boys are sexually active. By the time they are 18, 50 percent of girls have had intercourse, and as you read in the previous chapter, most of them are less than diligent about contraception.

I will never forget Angela's face when I had to tell her she had AIDS. Angela, a slim, vivacious brunette, had had a long-term relationship with a boyfriend at a Midwestern college. She was not promiscuous, and as far as she knew, her boyfriend was not either. She trusted him, but just before graduation the relationship cooled and ended after Don began to date other women. Angela moved to New York. Now 22, she had an exciting job at a top fashion house and an apartment with two other girls in the booming Chelsea section of Manhattan. She was looking forward to finding a new boyfriend.

Angela came to me for a physical checkup soon after she moved to New York. When her human immunodeficiency virus (HIV) test came back positive, the shock would almost not register in those deep blue eyes. How could this be? Acquired immunodeficiency syndrome (AIDS) was for homosexuals and drug addicts, Angela thought. But in fact, in the late 1990s, heterosexual women were the fastest-growing demographic group to be infected with the deadly virus, which came to this continent in the 1980s. Alarmingly, the number of teenagers contracting the infection *doubles* every year.

Having multiple sexual partners carries high risk for contracting AIDS. Female monogamy, however, is not a sufficient protection for women who are threatened by their partners' previous or ongoing high-risk behaviors. Angela had had only one sexual relationship, but her college boyfriend had not. He probably had other partners, one or more of whom might have carried the virus. Men who are bisexual or visit prostitutes can bring the infection home to their female partners. Men away from home for long periods, such as migrant workers or prisoners, often practice homosexuality while women are unavailable to them.

All sexually transmitted infections can wreak havoc with young lives. In the past, syphilis and gonorrhea were the ailments people knew the most about, and it was assumed these were conquered with penicillin. These diseases are making a comeback, along with a host of new microorganisms commonly recognized as the cause of most STIs. Chlamydia, the most prevalent bacterial STI, as well as gonorrhea (both are described below), cause pelvic inflammatory disease (PID), infection of the Fallopian tubes and pelvic structures, and ultimately sterility. Certain types of human papilloma virus (HPV) are implicated in cervical cancer. If a woman with an STI gets pregnant, the baby is also at risk of contracting the disease.

Most STIs are caused by bacteria or viruses. Bacteria are microorganisms with cell walls and can exist and even multiply independently, the way they can in the soil. A virus is much smaller than a bacterium and can survive only within the cell of the host, where it produces more of the viral particles.

HIV AND AIDS IN YOUNG WOMEN

Over 13,000 new female adult and adolescent cases of AIDS were reported in this country in just one year (1994). It is estimated that a total of 200,000 American women were infected by the year 1996. Perhaps most disturbingly, a study by the National Cancer Institute found that *25 percent of newly infected AIDS patients were under age 22.*

Because AIDS hit the homosexual community so hard in the 1990s, women, except for prostitutes, were thought to be at little risk. Women suffering from AIDS were not considered so much as victims but as vehicles for the virus to men and to their unborn children. This is ironic since the transmission is much more "effective" from a man to a woman than vice versa. This disproportion is probably related to a greater volume of exchanged body fluids from male to female and density of the viral particles in the fluids. Seminal fluid contains many more infectious particles than female cervical and vaginal secretions.

Little is known about the risks of HIV transmission among gay women. Salivary secretions contain very low amounts of the HIV virus (less than one infectious particle per milliliter), and no verified case of oral transmission has been reported. The greatest danger for lesbian women has been the transmission from infected donor semen in women who want to become pregnant and from bisexual women who continue to have intercourse with their infected male partners.

Most women become infected with AIDS through heterosexual contact with men who are either bisexual or use intravenous drugs. In women under age 25, heterosexual contact is responsible for 50 percent of transmission and intravenous drug use accounts for 19 percent. Thirty-one percent is attributed to all other pathways (for example, by blood transfusion and unknown causes). Genital sores from herpes (described below) and other conditions that cause ulcerations of the genitals make it easy for HIV to get into the body. Herpes sores can carry high levels of HIV particles, which makes it easy for the person to acquire and transmit the virus during sexual contact. Syphilis and other STIs besides herpes also seem to be linked to HIV, and we believe it is partly because people who have frequent unprotected sex are at highest risk. The other reason is that any ulceration exposes a person to more "effective" transmission.

Except for a handful of cases of unexplained longevity, untreated AIDS has been uniformly fatal within three to four years. With proper treatment, most people with AIDS can live ten or more years. There are differences among individuals in response to treatment and survival time. The AIDS virus kills the most effective immune-responsive cell of the body, the so-called T-helper cell. The weakened immune defense predisposes persons to opportunistic infections such as special forms of pneumonia, various strains of tuberculosis, and intestinal afflictions that cause diarrhea. Women share with men most of the manifestations of AIDS, except for *Kaposi's sarcoma,* a malignant cancer that causes bluish black patches on the skin and in other organs. Kaposi's sarcoma is rare in women with AIDS. But women may have, in addition, other manifestations of AIDS, such as vaginal infections and particularly invasive cancers of the cervix.

Problems with Diagnosis

Because AIDS is rarely suspected in women, it is often left undiagnosed for long periods. Before Angela came to me, she had visited three other doctors (gynecologists), all of whom diagnosed her vaginal discharge and itching as a persistent yeast infection. The first gynecologist prescribed vaginal suppositories. After two weeks, when Angela was no better and called the doctor, he prescribed a new medication over the phone. The second medication did not work either, and Angela went to a new doctor referred to her by a friend. The seconds doctor confirmed the original diagnosis and gave her another medication. The discharge and itching continued, and by now Angela also felt weak and sick. She lay awake at night sweaty and confused, then forced herself to go to work in the morning, but she was unable to concentrate. A co-worker suggested that Angela's yeast infection might respond to cutting back on products made with yeast, such as bread. When this failed, Angela went to a third gynecologist, who confirmed the diagnosis of the first two.

Because her condition was interfering with her work, Angela went to her boss and asked for some time off. The boss, a patient of mine, listened to Angela's story and told her she had been seeing the wrong doctors.

"You should not have been seeing gynecologists but an internist."

"Aren't vaginal conditions part of what the gynecologists should know about?" Angela protested. My patient explained that a localized symptom could signify a systemic condition, an illness located elsewhere or all over the body. "An internist is a diagnostician who can tie all of this together," she told Angela.

"Not another doctor, please!" But Angela was desperate. She appeared in my office looking gaunt. Her skin was hot, and she had a low-grade fever. She admitted she did not own a thermometer so had not checked her temperature. Angela's malaise, nocturnal sweating, and fatigue could be explained by her fever. But why did she have the fever? The dry cough? Her racing heart was probably caused by infection. I discovered a number of enlarged lymph nodes in her neck and armpits. Blood tests revealed anemia and a low white blood cell count. A pelvic exam confirmed the vaginal yeast infection, but some other infection was making it worse. It could be in her lungs or lymph nodes. She needed to be in the hospital for more tests and to monitor her symptoms. I also needed to ask her permission to let us check her blood for AIDS.

The sad fact is that in women HIV coexists with other vaginal infections and STIs. All too frequently, only those are diagnosed and the physician does not look any further.

Treatment of HIV

Although there is yet no cure for AIDS (as of late 1998), treatment is improving and, with earlier diagnosis, can prolong a useful life. Angela was started on AZT, a drug also known as zidovudine, which interferes with the multiplication of the virus. It is a "false" building block of the viral nucleic acid. Once it gets in, it blocks the machinery of synthesizing more viral particles. Unfortunately, the virus usually develops resistance. AIDS is now being treated with a combination of drugs, including the new protease inhibitors, which block an important step in releasing viral particles from an infected cell to infect other new cells. The mechanisms of action of these drugs are diverse, and resistance and side effects are slower to develop.

Angela's pneumonia was due to pneumocystis, a microorganism commonly associated with HIV infection. She was treated with antibiotics and her fever went away. The yeast infection was kept under control with a combination of vaginal and oral therapy. Angela has done pretty well on her medical therapy and psychological counseling that helps her cope with knowing she will not live long enough to fulfill many of her dreams. Because Angela had a high-stress job, she had to eventually give it up, but many people are able to continue working while they are being treated for AIDS.

HERPES SIMPLEX: THE FOREVER VIRUS

Herpes has been with us for centuries. Once you have contracted it, you have it, period. Forever. There is no permanent cure, only periods of remission and flare-up. Treatment does not wipe it out, but merely controls its symptoms. Fortunately, in most people, the herpes infection is controlled and not life-threatening.

The two most common Herpes simplex viruses are Type I, *Herpes labialis,* which affects the face, the mouth, and other parts of the body. A cold sore on the lip often causes worry that the other herpes is present, Type II, *Herpes genitalis,* which appears on the genitals. Ninety percent of all genital herpes infections are caused by the Type II virus. A doctor usually cannot tell if a cold sore on the lip or nose is Type I or Type II, except with sophisticated research tools not widely available. Most commonly, it is the less serious Type I, but even this type can be transmitted to the genitals through oral sex.

Genital herpes is among the most frequent sexually transmitted infections (STIs). About 25 million people in the United States are infected with this virus, with an estimated 2 to 3 million new cases every year. This is about 16 percent of the population over age 15. The majority of primary infections occur between the ages of 15 and 35.

A recent study by researchers at the University of Washington has shown for the first time what had long been suspected, that people infected with the virus that causes AIDS can transmit the virus through genital herpes sores. Since the first AIDS cases were diagnosed, physicians noticed the link between herpes and AIDS, as well as other STIs. Approximately two thirds of those with AIDS also carry the genital herpes virus. Both the herpes virus and the human papilloma virus (HPV) have been suspected of causing cervical cancer, but this association is stronger for the papilloma virus.

Herpes is transmitted by sexual intercourse or passionate kissing. It produces painful and/or itching blisters anywhere on the vulva, vagina, cervix, and anus. In the male, the penis is usually involved, and sometimes so is the scrotum. Approximately 16 percent of women suffering from Herpes Type II infection develop the blisters on areas other than the genitalia: fingers, groin, buttocks, thighs, and eyes. A severe, widespread disease rarely develops, but death may occur in a woman whose immune system is compromised.

The first—primary—outbreak of Herpes Type II tends to be the most dramatic, with flulike symptoms, low-grade fever, muscle pains, nausea, swelling of the lymph glands in the groin, and very severe and painful sores for three to six weeks. These blisters could last from four to twenty days. Burning, itching discomfort on urination and exquisite pain and tenderness of the vulva make intercourse unbearable.

Eventually the blisters rupture and a clear fluid drains out. The remaining ulcerations then heal spontaneously with no scarring unless they become infected with other bacteria. Lesions recur periodically for reasons we do not yet understand. They have been known to reappear after a fever, another infection, psychological stress, menses, and even friction. Subsequent attacks are never as ferocious or involve as much territory as the primary episode. After one or two episodes, weeks, months, or years might elapse before another attack. Some patients suffer from frequent, although short-lived, recurrences. Scratching the lesions decapitates the blisters sooner and will bring on more pain by leaving many shallow, tender herpetic ulcers, and can cause secondary bacterial infection.

The appearance of the blisters is so characteristic that most doctors can make the diagnosis by inspection. If in doubt, definitive diagnosis is made by testing scrapings of the lesions. A viral culture is usually not necessary but can be helpful when the diagnosis is unclear.

Before planning pregnancy, tell your doctor if you have suffered from herpes. The baby's immune system is immature and herpes may cause *encephalitis* (brain infection). This is very rare, but you eliminate any risk at all with prevention, and if your doctor is aware of your history.

Treatment for Herpes Types I and II

Zovirax capsules are used as oral treatment, and the medication is also used in a topical ointment to relieve itching and burning. These capsules must be taken 5 times a day because the drug is short-acting. For women with recurrent herpes infections, prophylactic treatment with Zovirax is sometimes given indefinitely. While very effective, this treatment is quite expensive when given over a long period of time. Zovirax, like all medications, may cause side effects: nausea, vomiting, headache, diarrhea, dizziness, and fatigue. Fortunately, these side effects are rare with short-term treatment.

In addition to Zovirax a new drug famciclovir has been recently introduced for suppression of recurrent genital herpes. More potent than Zovirax, it is longer acting and needs to be taken only twice or three times a day.

Prompted by some of my patients' experiences, I have successfully prescribed the amino acid lysine hydrochloride twice a day for prevention of recurrent genital herpes.

To alleviate the discomfort of genital herpes and to help prevent serious problems, try these remedies:

• Sit in a tub of warm water (sitz bath) three to five times a day for fifteen minutes each time.

• Dry your genital area with a blow dryer instead of a towel. A herpetic lesion might be so tender that even touching it with a towel can be painful. Also, a warm moist towel might cause self-inoculation in other parts of the body.

• Wear 100 percent cotton underwear that prevents accumulation of moisture, which may predispose you to the rupture of the herpes blisters.

• Avoid tight-fitting jeans and pants.

• Wear panty hose with cotton inserts in the crotch.

• Eat well and get enough sleep. Being run-down makes you more vulnerable to infection.

• Avoid sexual contact during the entire time that lesions are present.

• Use of condoms and spermicides will help prevent the spread of herpes.

HUMAN PAPILLOMA VIRUS (HPV): A RISING PROBLEM

The appearance of a genital wart on the lower vaginal area is a sign of human papilloma virus (HPV), the cause of one of the most common sexually transmitted genital viral infections in the nation, and its prevalence is on the rise. The wart frequently is painless or only slightly tender and appears to be nothing more than a nuisance. However, some HPV strains are strongly associated with cervical cancer. HPV is quite common, especially among promiscuous teens, although the carcinogenic effect might appear much later.

The HPV genital wart (*condyloma accuminatum*) is a sharp outgrowth like a Christmas tree and is acquired through sexual contact. On the male it appears on the scrotum. The presence of other sexually transmitted infection produces a favorable environment for growth of the genital warts, which also flourish during pregnancy. We do not know why.

Condyloma accuminatum can cause itching and excessive vaginal discharge that might be foul smelling.

Other strains of HPV show up as flat warts that might appear within the vagina and on the cervix, and a woman might not even be aware of them. Sometimes a Pap smear will alert the doctor because of minor abnormalities. It is the flat HPV rather than the protruding genital wart that is more associated with the risk of subsequent cervical cancer.

Treatment for HPV

The genital wart can be removed or destroyed by applying a cauterizing chemical, or with electrical cautery, or with ice. Larger lesions are best removed surgically in the doctor's office.

Fluorouracil (5-FU) eradicates the lesions, too, but causes redness, and might cause blistering and superficial ulcerations. Alpha interferon injections into the wart have also been successful, but flulike side effects frequently accompany that treatment.

Like herpes, HPV tends to recur and might need repeated treatment. Genital warts grow rapidly during pregnancy, and cesarean delivery might be preferred to avoid transmission of the infection to the baby.

CHLAMYDIA: THE LEADING CAUSE OF INFERTILITY

Chlamydia is the most prevalent bacterial STI in the world, with 4 million cases a year in the United States alone. It is the leading cause of infertility in women.

Chlamydia can affect anyone—women, men, and newborn babies. It might cause only a slight discharge before it ascends to the upper genital tract, where it can lead to infertility if it is not treated. Infections might produce no symptoms or signs. Seventy-five percent of infected women and 25 percent of infected men are asymptomatic, but even unrecognized infections can cause serious complications.

Chlamydia trachomatis is a very small bacterium that lives inside of cells. The first tissue it attacks is the inner canal of the cervix (the endocervix), which connects the vagina to the uterine cavity and the Fallopian tubes. In addition to sterility, it can cause ectopic pregnancy, endometriosis, and pelvic pain. It can cause respiratory and eye infections in babies of infected mothers.

Chlamydial infections plague the health of many women. Because symptoms are often mild or absent in men (urinary frequency and discomfort), few men ever seek treatment unless they develop a serious complication or after their female partners have been diagnosed. Males, therefore, are major carriers of chlamydial infection and are sources of reinfection in women.

Chlamydia trachomatis can be identified in the secretions of the infected endocervix and in the urine of infected men through a special tissue culture medium (expensive) and with a recently perfected polymerase chain reaction (PCR) test that uses a DNA probe to identify the microbe. Less expensive tests include an immune assay of the blood and a direct antigen detection system using a monoclonal antibody.

Unfortunately, at present testing for chlamydia is not part of a regular visit to the urologist for males. Using a newer ligase chain reaction (LCR) test on the urine, chlamydia infection was found in 54 percent of males attending an adolescent clinic and school-based clinics, and those in a juvenile detention facility in Seattle, Washington; the prevalence of this infection increased with age. Among the female participants in those populations, chlamydia infection was found in 8.6 percent. This new LCR test, performed on urine, might, in the future, simplify the diagnosis and recovery of large populations of all susceptible individuals, including male adolescents who engage in multiple-partner sex.

Treatment for Chlamydia

Many physicians believe that chlamydia testing should be a part of routine screening of any sexually active woman, even if there is no discharge, so that early treatment can be instituted before she winds up with a tubal infection and infertility. Other physicians feel that screening for chlamydia should be limited to at-risk populations, such as women who come to STI clinics, abortion clinics, juvenile detention centers, family planning clinics, and teen health clinics.

It is extremely important that both partners be treated simultaneously for chlamydia and other infections. Treatment is a seven-day course of antibiotics, which might have to be repeated if the infection is resistant. Intravenous antibiotics might be required if there is an abscess in the tubes or ovaries. Treatment should be started as early as possible before damage is done.

A 1998 Swedish study correlated the dropping rates of ectopic pregnancies (abnormal pregnancies occurring outside the uterus) with a decline in genital chlamydial infections in Uppsala county. A public health program of screening for chlamydia, treatment and contact tracing has been aggressively and consistently carried out there since 1985.

TRICHOMONIASIS: STRAWBERRY CERVIX

Trichomonas vaginitis, or trichomoniasis, is one of the most common STIs, and you can get it through infected hot baths, warm pools, shared towels, and underwear. This bacterium is able to survive up to twenty-four hours on a wet towel, six hours on a dry surface, and as long as four days in a cool place, such as a bench.

Typical symptoms are a profuse—watery or foamy—greenish yellow puslike discharge with a disagreeable odor. Vaginal itching and burning might keep you awake at night. The vulva, vagina, and cervix are fiery red and covered with copious discharge. Friable spots might be present in the vagina and cervix, which might bleed easily on intercourse or on examination with the speculum. Physicians sometimes refer to this as the "strawberry cervix." About 15 percent of affected women have no symptoms.

It is imperative that the male partner be treated because he is likely to harbor the bacteria in his urethral glands and can reinfect a woman. The parasites can hide in a woman's Skene glands, too (see chapter 3, page 41). Using a condom or abstaining from intercourse for the duration of treatment will help you avoid passing the infection back and forth.

Treatment for Trichomoniasis

Flagyl (metronidazole) tablets remain the most effective treatment for *Trichomonas vaginitis*. Flagyl is an antibiotic that is also used for infections that beleaguer AIDS sufferers. Flagyl is taken as a one-day intensive high-dose treatment, or over a period of seven days, which is somewhat more effective (90 percent cure).

Tablets and suppositories are also available and should be inserted high in the vagina. Local therapy with sulfa cream might help while you wait for the medication to do its work. If you are unable to ingest Flagyl, your doctor might perform several insufflations. This is a procedure of blowing powder into the vagina with a bulb containing medications every two to four days.

The side effects of Flagyl can include a disagreeable, metallic taste in the mouth and nausea. Occasionally, Flagyl causes a decrease in the white blood cell count, but this returns to normal once the medication is stopped. A form of colitis can be associated with large doses of Flagyl and prolonged treatment.

You cannot drink alcohol when you are taking Flagyl without very unpleasant side effects like violent nausea, vomiting, and chest pain. These symptoms are called "antabuselike" effects because antabuse is a medication used for conditioning alcoholics to refrain from drinking. Flagyl is not recommended for pregnant women.

Oral ampicillin is also frequently used, yet is somewhat less effective than Flagyl.

Trichomoniasis thrives with other bacteria, so it is important to observe rigorous personal hygiene once diagnosed. A daily douche with diluted vinegar or with Vagisec solution can remove the discharge and decrease the collection of infected material. (See the section about douching on page 61.)

GARDNERELLA VAGINITIS

Gardnerella vaginitis is also known as bacterial vaginosis. It is common among young women, possibly because they are likely to have more sexual partners than older women. It is not well understood how one gets bacterial vaginosis, or why it is also called Gardnerella vaginitis, because there is no "itis," which means inflammation. It is believed, but not proven, that the transmission is sexual, and treatment is recommended for both the female and male partner. However, it is not clear that treatment of the male partner prevents a recurrence in the woman.

This condition does not always show redness or irritation, but does cause a copious, malodorous discharge resembling a thin flour paste that adheres to the vaginal wall. Bacterial vaginosis changes the vaginal flora. The most characteristic sign is the fishlike odor when the physician adds a drop of potassium hydroxide to a drop of the discharge. The resulting strong fishy odor constitutes a positive, so-called whiff test.

Bacterial vaginosis is often asymptomatic and might clear up by itself. In a pregnant woman, however, it can cause complications.

Treatment for Gardnerella Vaginitis

Like trichomoniasis, Gardnerella vaginitis can be treated with a one-day or seven-day course of Flagyl, which is also available as an intravaginal cream and gel. Other treatments include vaginal suppositories and creams, and sulfa drugs, as well as broad-spectrum antibiotics. This disease has a tendency to recur no matter what treatment is received.

GONORRHEA

Gonorrhea is caused by the gonococcus, bacteria in the epithelial cells, the mucous membranes. Ejaculate from a man with gonorrhea can spread through a woman's entire genital tract. It tends to ascend through the cervix and the tubes and cause infection of these organs. It can cause pelvic inflammatory disease (PID), abscesses in the tubes and ovaries, chronic abdominal pain and fever, and finally acute peritonitis, a serious and frequently fatal infection of the abdominal lining. Mortality used to be 100 percent. Even now, despite available antibiotics, when sepsis (blood poisoning) occurs, mortality is very high.

Gonorrhea might also affect the skin, causing infectious blisters anywhere in the body and abscesses on practically any organ. If it gets into the joints, it causes painful arthritis.

By the time the initial stage of gonorrhea is apparent, it is usually too late to stop the irreversible consequences, which include infertility. Every sexually active woman, and especially one with any discharge, should be tested for gonorrhea at every routine pelvic exam.

Although the vast majority of cases are sexually transmitted, any contact with the gonorrheal pus can transmit the disease. Dr. Elizabeth Blackwell, the first American-educated female doctor, lost sight in her left eye when interning at a Paris hospital. A drop of discharge from the patient fell from a sore onto Blackwell's unprotected eye, thus ending her long-cherished hope of becoming a surgeon. Babies are also susceptible to eye infection as they pass through the infected mother's birth canal.

Treatment for Gonorrhea

Most uncomplicated gonorrheal infections of the lower genital tract (vulva, vagina, cervix, urethra) are eradicated with a single shot of penicillin, ampicillin, or intravenous ceftriaxone. For penicillin-resistant infections, another group of antibiotics, the quinolones, are used—unless the woman is pregnant.

Anyone having treatment for gonorrhea should be treated for chlamydia as well because the two frequently coexist. Both these infections, if in the upper reproductive tract, can cause the tubes to become deformed and closed off, leading to infertility. If this happens, plastic surgery to open the tubes might be needed to restore fertility.

SYPHILIS

Like gonorrhea, syphilis is caused by bacteria that attack mucous membranes. Syphilis spreads to the rest of the body through the bloodstream, while gonorrhea spreads through adjacent tissues and only rarely enters the bloodstream. Both enter through mucous membranes but each targets a different set of tissues and organs.

Syphilis is transmitted through intimate kissing or sexual intercourse. An untreated syphilis infection follows three stages. First, a lesion—the primary lesion—appears on the lip if acquired by kissing, or on the vulva. This lesion is called a chancre. It has a hard base and usually heals within three to eight weeks, with or without treatment.

If it is not treated, however, the secondary phase of syphilis develops as a result of the spread via the bloodstream. This includes a low-grade fever, headache, sore throat, and enlargement of the lymph nodes. A rash appears on the palms of the hands and the soles of the feet, as well as over the genital areas and on other mucous membranes such as the mouth, lips, and nose. Within twelve weeks, the lesions of the secondary stage resolve and, if left untreated, are followed by a latent stage.

About 40 percent of patients in the latent stage of syphilis develop tertiary syphilis, which affects the blood vessels—especially the aorta—and the brain. If a pregnant woman is not treated, she might suffer preterm delivery or a stillbirth. If her baby is born alive, it will develop congenital syphilis. Mortality is high, and the baby might have many congenital anomalies.

Diagnosis and Treatment of Syphilis

Syphilis is diagnosed in the primary stage by examining scrapings of the chancre under the microscope and with a blood test in the subsequent stages.

The treatment of choice for syphilis is penicillin. If the patient is allergic to penicillin a desensitization procedure is performed prior to therapy or one of the newer cephalosporins is used.

PROTECTING YOURSELF FROM STIs

If you are in a monogamous relationship, both you and your partner should be tested for preexisting STIs and HIV before you begin having sex. If you are both clean, and neither of you has unprotected sex with others, then you should be safe. Nevertheless, you are vulnerable. It is important that you go to the doctor or clinic together to do this, so that a competent health care professional or physician can guide you about any positive findings or about STIs in general.

Because it is impossible to be absolutely protected from STIs, be alert to any changes in your body. Do regular self-inspections of your pelvic area. Get tested for STIs twice a year, and if you have any suspicion there could be something wrong, go to your doctor or to a women's health clinic as soon as possible. In 1997, a home test for AIDS became available to encourage more people to get tested early. You apply a secretion sample to a card that you mail to a laboratory. Then, after a period of time, you call the lab for the results by giving the number of the card you submitted. There is no way the results can be traced to a particular person.

Latex condoms are the only way to prevent sexually transmitted infection. The diaphragm does not stop them, nor does the pill or spermacides. Male condoms, when properly used, prevent transmission of gonorrhea, chlamydia, herpes virus, HIV, and the human papilloma virus. Unfortunately for women, many men refuse to wear a condom and are likely to punish a woman for insisting on one. Like my patient, Angela, many women want to believe their men are faithful.

Another recent development has been the increasing use of oral sex among teenagers as a way to avoid STIs or pregnancy. (A study of sex practices in 1994 found that most women under 35 had both given and received oral sex. In the same study, only a few women over 50 had ever had oral sex.) Many young women mistakenly believe that if they have oral sex they are protecting themselves from pregnancy and AIDS. While you won't get pregnant, you can still get a sexually transmitted infection. Open sores or recent dental work make the mouth susceptible to infection. Savvy teens, however, are learning to use condoms for oral sex, too. (Some actually come in flavors.)

While a male condom will protect your partner from acquiring an STI from you, a female condom will protect you from acquiring most or all of his STIs. Female condoms are now available, but they are expensive and we do not yet know how effective they are in preventing HIV. Woman-controlled contraceptive products that prevent transmission of HIV are being developed. The FDA is also lobbying for enforcement of product labeling guidelines that would accurately and effectively convey the product's relationship to the prevention of HIV/AIDS.

In the meantime, practice safe sex, get to know your body so you can tell when something is wrong, and have regular checkups.

·· 10 ··

Eating Disorders of Adolescence

Eating too much or too little accounts for serious nutritional disorders among adolescents. Both anorexia nervosa and obesity, opposite extremes, are life-threatening. One can cause sudden death, while the other kills gradually by increasing the risk of mortal conditions like heart disease and diabetes.

WHEN THIN KILLS: ANOREXIA NERVOSA AND BULIMIA

Anorexia nervosa and bulimia have reached an epidemic proportion in the Western world; more than a million girls in this country suffer from these disorders. Their prevalence among women is nine to ten times greater than in men. The Commonwealth Fund survey (1997) found that adolescent girls in particular were at risk for eating disorders. One in six girls in grades five through twelve said she had binged and purged. Eighteen percent of high school girls reported that they had binged and purged, while only 7 percent of high school boys said that they had. In the past these eating disorders were thought to affect upper-middle-class white girls only, but they have now been diagnosed in all classes and races.

A recent study at Stanford University revealed that in the past thirty years eating disorders have become more widespread in this country and other developed countries. It is now estimated that 10 percent of college students are affected—and 90 percent of those affected are women. The pressure to be thin is assumed to be the reason behind the disorders. Teenage girls who are slightly overweight seem to be at the highest risk, and these disorders sometimes begin after failed efforts to diet.

Some girls become binge eaters, eating large amounts of food and gaining weight. Others become bulimic—they wolf down large amounts of food and then "purge" themselves with laxatives or vomiting. In others, a more rare disorder, anorexia nervosa, develops. These girls shun food altogether in a compulsion to lose weight. And while they become dangerously emaciated, they still believe they are overweight. In 10 to 18 percent of these cases, the disorder proves fatal. Only about 10 percent are cured with antidepressants and psychotherapy.

The anorexic girl looks like a concentration camp survivor, and she is in just as much physical danger. She starves herself, frequently to the point of death, because she is convinced she is overweight and fears gaining even an ounce. There might or might not be binges of overeating followed by self-induced vomiting. Menstruation stops because of the drop in estrogen production that accompanies dramatic weight loss. The loss of estrogen might lead to bone deterioration.

Bulimia is a milder variant of anorexia that was brought to worldwide attention when the late Princess Diana revealed her own bulimia. Recurrent episodes of binge eating are compensated for by self-induced vomiting; purging with laxatives, diuretics, or enemas; and prolonged episodes of fasting or excessive exercise. Before Princess Diana was able to get medical treatment for her condition, she was criticized by the royal family for her bizarre eating habits. With bulimia, weight loss is not as profound as with anorexia. The bulimic may actually retain normal or above-normal weight. It is not unusual to see a combination of obesity and bulimia in a young girl.

According to current studies, 18 percent of college-age women binge and purge with some regularity. About 10 to 18 percent of girls affected by anorexia nervosa die in this country. This might be due to cardiac arrest, abnormal heart rhythm due to profound electrolyte and water depletion, or because the stomach or esophagus has been torn by so much retching and vomiting. Laxative abuse can lead to *pancreatitis*.

An entire industry of health professionals is trying to deal with these diseases, and despite more sophisticated attitudes and more knowledge, it is still difficult. The American College of Sports Medicine has labeled anorexia and bulimia, and other compulsive eating problems, as "disordered eating."

These disorders are much more common in women because our society—and especially competitive areas like gymnastics and ballet—has placed an inordinately high value on how women look. The average disordered eating occurs in about 1 in 100 in the white middle-class population. (In classical ballet, it is estimated to be 1 in 5.) One young woman was asked to lose about five pounds, but no more, by the head of a ballet company, who believed the loss would improve her performance and "line." The girl took the advice but did not stop at five pounds. She became anorexic and died.

One of my patients, Suzanna, summed up bingeing in a letter she wrote me years after her adolescent experience. She remembered her feelings well.

"I recall my feelings of self-dislike and emotional insecurity beginning at 13. I had always dreamed of becoming a dancer, first a ballet dancer, then a modern dancer. I had always been thin and energetic. My parents were very supportive and provided me with all the necessary opportunities to train so that I could achieve my dream. Around this time my body began to change and take on new proportions. Everything I ate or even looked at seemed to stick to my hips and buttocks. I no longer fit the body image of a classical ballet dancer with tiny features and legs longer than my torso. At this time I changed my focus to modern dance. The freer more expressive movements seemed to suit my turbulent temperament at this time."

Suzanna later went away from home for a summer. "When I was away that summer, I had thinned down considerably, but once I returned, I again began to gain weight. I tried to control my weight initially by trying to control my appetite, but later resorted to bingeing and laxatives. My parents tried their best not to be critical about my eating habits, but could not refrain. My eating was the only thing I felt I had control over in my life, and although it made me very unhappy to be fat, eating gave me satisfaction and fulfillment."

Another telling comment she made was, "I was also unhappy about my face, skin, and features and felt that they contributed to my unattractiveness to men. I truly did not know how to make myself happy."

BINGEING AND OBESITY: MORE THAN JUST WILLPOWER

More than 58 million adult Americans (32 million women and 26 million men) are at least 20 percent or more over their desirable weight. We are the fattest nation on the planet. The number of obese adults continues to rise. It went from 25 percent in 1980 to 33.4 percent in 1991. Americans are about eight pounds heavier on average than they were fifteen years ago.

If you gain twenty-two pounds or more after the age of 18, you are at increased risk of dying young from heart disease, cancer, and all causes. According to a 1996 study reported in the *American Journal of Medicine*, more than 280,000 deaths a year are attributable to "overnutrition."

As many as a third of people who are obese are binge eaters, and two thirds of them are women. Studies have shown that binge eating begins in the teen years or the early twenties. Ironically, it usually begins after a woman has successfully lost weight with a diet. The diets followed are usually extreme, with certain foods and the number of calories severely limited, leaving the dieter feeling hungry and emotionally deprived. Such diets rarely can be sustained.

A woman will fall off the diet by bingeing on one of the restricted foods, which leads to a feeling of guilt. Now she feels she cannot control her impulses, and the resulting anxiety causes her to seek comfort in food. She becomes caught in a vicious cycle of eating and fasting. To the binge eater, food is what alcohol and drugs are to other addicts.

Obesity is at least twenty times more common than the self-starving disorders like anorexia and bulimia. While the public is horrified by the pictures of self-starving adolescents, it casts a permissive and bemused eye on the ice-cream-and-burgers-gorging teenager. It is precisely in adolescence and the early twenties that our basic exercise and eating habits are formed. Our weight around puberty and adolescence sets the subsequent pattern. Chubby kids have a tendency to grow into fat adults.

A researcher at the Rockefeller University discovered that obesity depends on both the number of fat cells and on the size of each fat cell. In his investigation, he discovered that with weight loss and gain, the fat cells either shrank or swelled with additional fat, but their number remained more or less the same as that acquired in adolescence. Once the number of fat cells has become established, there is no way of decreasing that number. Even liposuction decreases the number of cells only temporarily. As every crash dieter knows, it all comes back. Unfortunately, while the number of fat cells will not decrease after adolescence, they can most certainly grow and expand. Overweight young women sometimes become morbidly obese adults. Few live to an advanced age. It is possible, though difficult, for even a chubby teenager to develop healthy eating habits and keep weight down, too.

While young women need to understand the dangers of being overweight or underweight, they also need to consider their body type and the genetic disposition to certain body types. Ideal weight is different for everyone; we talk about how to find your ideal weight later in this chapter.

A Gallup survey in the late 1990s revealed that most people realize that obesity is not good for their health, but few had any specific idea about causes for obesity or specific knowledge about what could be done about it. Obesity is defined by the National Center for Health Statistics as being 20 percent above your ideal weight. If you are 10 percent over your ideal weight, you are overweight but not obese. Obesity is a gradual, cumulative condition caused by a number of factors including metabolic rate, genetic predisposition, and diet, as well as cultural, social, and economic conditions. It is a chronic condition like diabetes or drug addiction.

We know from research, for example, that women in lower socioeconomic groups suffer more obesity because they are less aware of proper nutrition, have less access to good health care and education, and have less access to quality foods. One study revealed that overweight adolescent girls had completed fewer years of school, were less likely to be married, and had higher rates of household poverty than women who were not overweight. Marketing of "junk" foods, those with high fats, high calories, and low price, is aimed largely at the poor. One of the most powerful risk factors for obesity is growing up in a poor environment, according to one recent study.

Obesity varies widely according to race, too. Some Native Americans, such as the Pima Indians, are at a higher risk of becoming obese. One third of white women are estimated obese, compared to nearly half of all African American and Mexican American women. Some investigators have identified the combination of being female, poor, and black, Hispanic, or Native American as the "triple threat" for weight-related problems in this country.

It is ironic that in poor and third-world countries, where people subsist mainly on grains and vegetables, there is much less obesity and the diseases caused by it. But as nations become westernized and eat more of the wrong kinds of calories, the obesity follows. Japan, for example, was always regarded as nutritionally sound because the level of fat in its diet was a low 10 to 15 percent. Rice, vegetables, and fish were staples. In the last twenty-five years of the twentieth century, however, fat consumption has increased to the levels usual in Western countries. This has resulted in a problem of childhood obesity. Similar trends are apparent in other Asian nations.

Discrimination against obesity is a form of prejudice that is accepted by most of society. An Italian study of schoolgirls aged 13 to 16 revealed that 78 percent of normal weight girls considered obesity a social stigma—and 62 percent of the overweight girls agreed with them. They were considered less active, less attractive, less healthy, weak willed, having poor self-control, and with inferior physical abilities. In school, the obese child received lower academic ratings than the handicapped or deformed child. Employers often feel they are justified in refusing to hire obese people because their size or weight will somehow interfere in the performance of their job, even though this is the same kind of discrimination as sex or race. One woman, the director of a small art museum, felt very guilty about turning down a very heavy woman for a curating job for which the woman was obviously qualified. She shook her head sadly and said, "You know, I just don't think our clients will take her seriously. She doesn't project the kind of image we need. Besides, she takes up so much space; in the cramped quarters, she may knock off some of our treasures to the floor."

Most people believe that anyone who is overweight lacks the willpower to take off the weight. But few realize that the pathologic mechanisms that lead to an imbalance between caloric intake and energy expenditure are not yet understood. Metabolism, genetics, and endocrine abnormalities all play a role in the total picture. The genetic cause is thought to be a human equivalent of the mouse obesity gene, which might form part of a signaling path to the brain center. New research with mice is leading to discovery of genetic reasons for rare cases of extreme obesity.

The Appestat: Your Appetite Control Center

In the past, the rate of metabolism was thought to be controlled exclusively by the thyroid gland. Now we understand that the metabolism rate is constantly being adjusted by the appetite/weight-controlling center in the hypothalamus, called the "appestat," or AC, which stands for Appetite Control Center and is situated near the gonadostat (see chapter 1). Normally, there is a balance between the fat cell mass in the body, the AC, appetite, eating, and body weight.

In obese persons, however, the hypothalamic appestat seems to have its own ideas as to what one's ideal weight should be. If your AC perceives your weight as being below your weight set point, the appestat sends out signals to slow down the rate of metabolism and increase your appetite. Your energy output drops, and you become sluggish. Energy is conserved even while performing standard tasks such as walking or sitting. So instead of inducing a state of satiety, your appestat leaves you feeling unsatisfied. You eat more and your body stores more calories until your weight is brought up to the level preferred by your appestat, which has obviously not read the latest fashion magazine or watched "Melrose Place." When weight goes above the set point, your metabolism speeds up, the appestat curbs your appetite, and—Presto!—you lose weight to approximate the appestat's ideal. It is very difficult to gain or to lose weight past the set point. You are literally working against an immovable resistant barrier. This is the most recent theory. Not everybody subscribes to it.

What sets the appestat's set point and why are set points different among various people? Genetics has a lot to do with your body's set point. Identical twins raised in different environments frequently achieve similar adult weights. Perhaps the high set point of the hypothalamus of our cave-dwelling ancestor had an evolutionary advantage. Between buffalo and deer kills, there were long stretches of hunger and famine for cavemen and cavewomen. The hypothalamus slowed down their energy after the feast because that energy had to last until the next hunt. The caveman and cavewoman fell asleep after the feast and slept until hunger woke them up and pushed them to hunt and gather once again. The contemporary man and woman frequently feel sleepy after a large meal. But we do not go out and hunt anymore, or wait weeks for our next meal. We just get up from the couch and go to the fridge.

Fat is addictive, like salt and alcohol. Even though fatty foods ease hunger, the fat cells and the brain do not always get the message. Fat is stored by the body. It is not burned immediately the way a high-carbohydrate meal could be. It takes three to seven days of eating lots of fats to increase fat oxidation. There is no limit to the number of pounds of fat we can store. We simply put it on the hips or abdomen or thighs and let it sit there.

Fatty foods are dense with energy. Lots of calories get packed into a small quantity of food. For example, there are 100 calories in one pat of butter, whereas it would take four tomatoes or a pound of carrots to equal 100 calories. One gram of fat provides nine calories compared to four calories from the same amount of sugar or protein. Increasingly, there is more fat in our foods, especially fast foods.

Cholesterol and Body Fat in Girls

Few young people are aware that their arteries begin to clog up in childhood. An autopsy study of teenagers who had died in accidents revealed that fatty deposits and lesions were already present in their arteries. The high cholesterol levels of the blood showed up as early as age 15. This study, reported in a 1997 issue of a leading cardiovascular journal, was the first such study to include young women. In the past, studies were done only on soldiers killed in wars. The study added evidence to the theory that even though women begin getting heart attacks later than men, they still must alter their diets early in life.

A high cholesterol level in a teenage girl might not be related to the amount of body fat she has, according to a study reported in 1997 in the American Heart Association journal *Circulation*. Findings of the study indicate that the proportion of body weight that is fat is unrelated to cholesterol levels in girls, but for boys the two are closely linked. The study looked at 678 children from age 8 to 18 for four years. About a quarter of the children had high cholesterol. This is the first time the differences in girls and boys were studied, and investigators want to learn how the sex hormones, diet, and other factors such as exercise affect cholesterol levels. It is hoped that this will lead to new ways of treating obesity and high cholesterol in children.

Women can safely have a higher cholesterol rate because we have more high-density lipoproteins (HDL), the good cholesterol, and low-density lipoproteins (LDL), the bad cholesterol, included in the total. Estrogen provides us with a higher level of the good cholesterol than men have. Their testosterone gives them more of the LDL. (Refer to chapter 24 for more about cholesterol.)

A teenage girl with high cholesterol, under conventional wisdom, would be told to lose weight. According to the new findings, this could be a mistake, because losing weight will not necessarily affect the cholesterol level. Children with high cholesterol levels generally become adults with high levels, but the levels of children fluctuated significantly. More than one screening is needed for a true picture.

Finding Your Ideal Weight: Body Mass Index (BMI)

Two measurements help us detect serious overweight. The first measurement is the body mass index (BMI). To find your own BMI, first square your height (in inches). Then divide your weight (in pounds) by the squared height and multiply the result by 705. The resulting number is somewhere between 20 and 30, with a BMI between 21 and 22 being optimal.

$$\text{BMI} = \frac{\text{Weight in pounds}}{\text{Height in inches, squared}} \times 705$$

For example: If you weigh 150 pounds and you are five-foot-five, or 65 inches, your BMI would be 25. If you lose 25 pounds, your BMI would be an optimal 20.

Investigators have found that there was no elevated risk of heart disease in women with a BMI below 21. Women with BMIs between 22 and 24 had their risk increased by 30 percent. The risk was 80 percent greater in women with BMIs between 25 and 29. Among women with a BMI over 29 the risk was double that of women with optimal BMI. While in men only massive obesity is a major risk factor for heart disease, in women even mild overweight increases the risk of heart disease.

Hip/Waist Ratio: Apple or Pear?

Another measurement, the waist/hip ratio (WHR), might be even more useful. Death from coronary heart disease is more strongly related to the ratio of the waist circumference to the hip circumference than to the BMI. This is based on the finding that the fat most associated with health risks is in the upper body (waist). The fat in the buttocks and hips, the site where most women usually store fat, does not carry as much risk for coronary heart disease as does the apple shape, where the hips and legs are thin but weight is above the waist.

Both types of obesity are risk factors for coronary heart disease and diabetes, but the apple shape, with its central obesity, is more serious, and also is associated with high cholesterol, hypertension, and breast and endometrial cancer.

To check your WHR, measure the circumference of your waist halfway between the bottom rib and the hipbone, and divide it by the largest circumference at the level of your hips. This is your WHR. In an obese woman, a WHR below 80 indicates peripheral obesity, or a pear; a WHR above 89, central obesity.

TREATING EATING DISORDERS

Eating disorders are chronic conditions and are extremely difficult to treat. They are also considered a form of mental illness. Unfortunately, programs to inform young women about the perils of eating disorders have not been very effective as yet. The longer bingeing has been going on, the more difficult it is to treat. There are programs of counseling and treatment at various eating disorders clinics throughout the country. Treatment that incorporates nutritional counseling, medication, and psychotherapy is the most effective.

Anorexia nervosa and bulimia must be treated by a team that includes a psychiatrist and a principal physician, preferably an internist/endocrinologist. An "unrepentant" anorexic might need to be hospitalized for refeeding. Treatment of the anorexic includes energetic refeeding, antidepressants, appetite-stimulating medications, and psychotherapy for the underlying issues of control and anger. The bulimic can usually be treated on an outpatient basis by a psychiatrist.

Refer to chapter 1 for information about selecting a principal physician who will then coordinate the treatment team.

ONE POUND AT A TIME: LOSING WEIGHT WISELY

The health care community is now taking weight control seriously. However, only a small percentage of the overweight people ever seek help from their physicians when they want to lose weight. Being overweight is a very emotional issue, and while we all know that losing weight can help us look and feel healthier, it is not that easy to do. Your doctor might not feel comfortable talking about weight either. Indeed, there are plenty of overweight doctors!

Obesity is a chronic health condition that should be discussed and treated just like any other chronic condition. Ask your doctor about reasonable goals and diet plans as well as sensible ways to increase activity. There are also medications that might be appropriate for you. Curing obesity involves a multicomponent plan over a long period of time. It can involve diet, activity, behavior modification, medication, and in extreme cases, surgery.

The emphasis in treatment of obesity has shifted from the goal of weight loss to a goal of continuous, lifelong habit of exercise, rejection of sedentary lifestyle, and achievement of physical fitness. *Whichever way you lose weight, you still can be one of the 20 percent who don't regain it!*

A recent survey by the University of Pittsburgh School of Medicine and the University of Colorado Health Sciences Center revealed that ultimate success in maintaining weight loss among people who had been obese since childhood involved some kind of strategy for limiting food intake.

Some counted calories, while others considered fat grams. Most of them ate more often—small meals five times a day—and they mostly ate at home. They also increased their exercise level. The common factor with these dieters was that they understood the long-term commitment they needed to make and they were willing to make it. What prompted them to diet in the first place? The majority traced it to a very specific event. They had been hurt by a negative comment, had seen an unflattering photo of themselves, or had faced serious medical problems.

Treatment options include do-it-yourself programs based on information from diet books; group approaches, such as Overeaters Anonymous; nonclinical programs, such as Weight Watchers; and clinical programs that provide medical care and more aggressive therapies, such as very-low-calorie diets, medication, and surgery.

If you are significantly overweight, you might require support from your physician and your family and friends as well. In many weight-control programs, such as Weight Watchers, the participants support each other by reporting weekly in a group any setbacks and victories they had. Obesity is not a problem you can solve alone.

Anita was chubby as a child, and during adolescence she gained an inordinate amount of weight. An athletic 18-year-old girl, she weighed in at 200 pounds when she came to see me because of back pain. The burden of her excessive pounds had eroded many of her spine joints, and her X-rays revealed chemical osteoarthritis of a degree usually not seen in a person thrice her age. Anita's back prevented her from engaging in many of the sports she loved. She had to lay off tennis and running. She even experienced discomfort walking.

I told her that her spine joints were many times older than her chronologic age because she was carrying twice as much weight on these joints than she was supposed to. Upon hearing the news, Anita was determined to lose weight. With the help of a nutritionist, she went on a moderately low calorie diet. Under close supervision and with a combination of weight-bearing and non-weight-bearing exercises, she succeeded in getting rid of the excessive ballast. When she reached 150 pounds her back pain cleared, and she resumed running and tennis. She continued to slowly lose weight until she was at her desired weight of 135. She maintained this weight for many years.

Unfortunately, not every adolescent girl is as successful as Anita. In my experience, to a young girl, the prospect of eventually developing complications of diabetes and heart disease does not seem real enough to overcome the desire to eat.* Sometimes it takes an immediate prob-

---

*There is frequently a strong need of denial: "But I am eating so little, almost like a bird! You don't believe me," and the girl bursts into tears. Of course, the bird needs all that energy to fly, and it eats many times its own weight daily. But the irony of this excuse escapes her. And it is not just the food but the energy expended in exercise and daily activities that count. The bird needs all that energy to fly, and its metabolic rate is much higher than ours.

lem such as pain to motivate someone to begin the tedious process of a weight-losing diet. It also takes a strong girl to respond with affirmation and determination to the "tough love" approach from her doctor. Many girls get discouraged and depressed and "relieve" their depression by uncontrolled eating.

Diet Pills and Their Side Effects

Diet pills—amphetamines—were banned from use in 1968 because they were being abused as recreational drugs, or "uppers." Amphetamines depressed the appetite but also speeded up the heart. They kept you so hyperactive you had no desire to sit still long enough to eat!

Amphetamines and their analogs, available over the counter (Dexatrim, Accutrim), stimulate the central nervous system, suppress the appetite, and increase the metabolic rate. They are addictive, however, and might also increase heart rate and elevate blood pressure. In some people amphetamines can cause a "high" followed by a very unpleasant "down" state (depression). In general, their effect on appetite is only fleeting, and I have used them sparingly in my practice.

"Starch blockers" and "fat blockers" are supposed to prevent calories from being absorbed by the intestine. In reality, however, they produce a number of unpleasant side effects and are seldom used long enough to be effective. The abuses involved in these drugs put the kibosh on medication as a form of weight control.

The newer diet pills raise the level of serotonin, a substance involved in transmitting nerve impulses in the brain, producing a sensation of satiety as well as affecting the mood of the person. Many of the antidepressive medications work by inhibiting the clearance of serotonin from the nerves in the brain. Fenfluramine and Redux (dexfenfluramine) not only inhibit the clearance but also release additional serotonin. Both drugs, and especially Redux, were found to be associated with a lung disease called primary pulmonary hypertension (PPH) that has a 45 percent mortality rate and were recently taken off the market. Redux might also cause brain damage; both Redux and fenfluramine are off the market now.

A more gentle drug, phentermine, inhibits the clearance but does not produce additional serotonin. Some persons who took a combination of fenfluramine-phentermine (so-called fen-phen) over a long time developed heart valve disease, and the fen-phen combination has also been taken off the market. It is thought that it is the fluramine in the combination that is responsible for this side effect. Phentermine is still available.

In 1998 sibutramine (Meridia) was approved by the FDA panel. This drug appears to act on the appestat center conveying feelings of fullness. It also allows serotonin a longer stay in the body but does not release additional serotonin. Meridia also inhibits the clearance of norepinephrine (an adrenalinelike substance) that raises blood pressure and increases pulse rate. In clinical studies, Meridia did not help diabetics lose weight, and there were many dropouts from the drug protocol.

Another 1998 approved diet drug—orlistat (Xenical)—works through inhibiting an enzyme, lipase, in the intestines. Lipase facilitates absorption of fats from the intestine to the bloodstream. Xenical allows about 30 percent of the consumed fat to be excreted in the stool. A recent double-blind, placebo-controlled, two-year trial of Orlistat plus diet in 1187 obese adults was reported in 1999 as having significantly promoted weight loss, lessened weight regain, and improved some obesity-related disease risk factors.

There is a concern about long-term vitamin depletion as Xenical inhibits absorption of vitamin D, E, beta-carotene, and K. Other side effects include gaseous, oily spotting and occasional fecal urgency (sudden need to move the bowels with or without success). There seems also to be a slight tendency to kidney stones (no symptoms) in the research subjects on this drug.

While these drugs are more effective than diet alone, all the weight losses attributed to them were dependent on the combined use of a reducing diet. They are ineffective in many people and hazardous to some.

Because there have been no long-term studies of the drugs' effectiveness, it is important that you discuss this candidly with your doctor and do some research on your own as well. You can get medical information from your public library, medical library, and the World Wide Web.

On the horizon are new possibilities for drugs based on the normal mechanism that usually controls eating and weight in healthy people. This mechanism, discovered by Rockefeller University scientists, involves *leptin,* a natural substance produced by the fat cells. When leptin levels increase they inhibit the appetite center in the brain (see the section on appestat discussed earlier in this chapter), producing the sensation of satiety. Genetically obese mice who lack their own leptin stop eating and lose weight when injected with leptin.

However, another strain of obese mice produces plenty of leptin but lacks leptin receptors in the brain; these animals do not respond to leptin treatment. It is not known if obesity in humankind is due to lack of leptin or lack of leptin receptors. A number of pharmaceutical companies are frantically searching for substances that would stimulate the leptin effect in humans. But the clinical application of this discovery is still some years away.

Fad Diets: Never Out of Fashion

Diet books are never out of print. The diets change from year to year, however, according to the latest fad. We will get thin if we eat only grapefruit, or if we eat only meat, or if we have only liquid. When a diet deprives you of your basic daily nutritional requirements, it interferes with your body's ability to function.

Very-low-calorie diets usually involve prepared powder meals, such as Slim-Fast and Optifast, consisting of a mixture of amino acids and limited amounts of essential fatty acids. These diets require total dedication by the patient and frequent monitoring by the physician and should not be undertaken without proper professional supervision and mineral and vitamin supplementation. Unless body salts are carefully monitored potassium deficiency might prove fatal. Unless uric acid is checked at intervals, a rise in the blood level of uric acid can evoke an acute attack of gout, a form of arthritis, due to deposition of uric acid crystals in some joints, typically at the base of the big toe.

Oprah Winfrey, the popular talk show host, lost a great deal of weight in the 1980s with a liquid diet, and when her TV viewers saw the results, they rushed out to try it themselves. The problem for Oprah and everybody else was they gained back the weight. Oprah now expounds on a sensible balanced diet and lots of exercise to keep weight down.

One of my patients, Melody, was so obsessed with food that she actually dreamed about sumptuous meals laid out on the dining room table or spread on the lawn in the back of her house. She constantly browsed through food magazines and wrote down recipes, which she cataloged onto her computer. Melody was a young mother with two children who had given up her job as a flight attendant to raise her children. Before she was 30 years old, she weighed 200 pounds and had diabetes and high blood pressure. Melody had to lose weight quickly because of these conditions, so I put her on a controlled liquid diet, Optifast.

The medical program for this kind of diet has three stages: weight loss, consolidation, and maintenance. The first stage brings on very fast weight loss and must never be done without your doctor's guidance. You feel full of energy and need less sleep, but when you go back on food you can go into a depression. This is why it must be gradual. The consolidation phase is the introduction of a small amount of food each day, just breakfast or lunch, and checking your weight daily. If you eat supper instead during this stage, you might gain weight. Eating late means you go to sleep soon after eating and the food is not metabolized.

Melody's weight came down to 160 pounds on the diet, and her blood pressure went down and her diabetes disappeared (see chapter 19 for more about diabetes and diet). She committed herself to the other stages of the program and did not regain the weight. She continued to eat her meals early, and she increased her exercise.

One of my most successful obesity patients was a psychiatrist, aged 50, who was overweight. She went on a liquid diet (Optifast) supplemented with vitamins, and massive doses of mineral potassium during the first, "active," phase of her therapy. Having lost 50 pounds within several months, she was placed on a consolidation regimen, the liquid diet plus one "regular" modest meal a day, either breakfast or lunch, not dinner. She lost weight more slowly and eventually added one more meal at a time to her daily routine as part of her maintenance regimen. She remained at her desired 145 pounds, without the help of the liquid diet and without diet pills.

Liquid diets are dangerous and must not be undertaken except under close supervision of a specially trained physician. Some patients lose scalp hair despite careful professional supervision. Fainting spells are not infrequent especially in older and massively obese persons. Deaths have been ascribed to a low potassium in the heart muscle and to a cardiac abnormality called long QT interval. These dieters need to be monitored with periodic electrocardiograms.

About 80 percent of people who successfully lose weight regain it within a few years. Many obese people have a long history of weight cycling—losing weight and then gaining it back. At one time it was thought that weight cycling was riskier than remaining at the high weight. But this theory has been recently disproved. In other words, trying to lose weight, even given the yo-yo effect, is better than staying obese.

Your Best Bet: Lifestyle Adjustment

Low-calorie diets (not to be confused with the very-low-calorie liquid diets described above) work only in conjunction with behavioral therapy, exercise, restructured eating habits, and emotional support such as joining a Weight Watchers program. Otherwise, you always feel hungry.

My first rule for weight loss is get a doggy bag! Whether you are at home or at a restaurant, before you begin to eat, remove half of everything on your plate and put it away for tomorrow's lunch.

Changing everyday habits can help a great deal with mild overweight. For example, eat a full breakfast, shift your main meal to lunch, and have a light supper. There was an old maxim that we should eat breakfast like a queen, lunch like a princess, and supper like a beggar. This is still good advice! Breakfast cranks up your metabolism. Without breakfast, you linger on at the slow, nighttime metabolic rate. A woman who subsists on black coffee during the day and eats a full dinner out every night might wake up repeatedly during the night and go to the refrigerator and to the cupboard for cookies or ice cream. This is called the "nighteating" syndrome. Never go to bed on a full stomach. The food might keep you awake and, not being metabolized to support activity, might all become stored as fat.

The basic principle of behavioral therapy is self-monitoring. Record your behavior; maintain diaries of foods eaten, portion sizes, caloric content, time and place of eating, what you were thinking and feeling, and what has compelled you to overeat. Also record your physical activity. The diary can be kept just for you, or you can review it with a doctor or therapist who is helping you lose weight.

Some women do this themselves. They write down the number of calories and stop at the maximum. Or, they do it the other way around, record the maximum number to be consumed for that day and then plan their meals to fit that number. This is much the same as Weight Watchers, but Weight Watchers is even more effective because it includes a balanced diet around the number of calories needed, as well as emotional support.

The techniques of stimulus control help you limit exposure to food and increase the opportunity to exercise. For instance, when feeling an urge to eat, run a mile instead. The strength of your legs is directly related to your cardiovascular fitness. Exercise your arms, also important to cardiovascular health, by pushing yourself away from the table and lifting weights. Separate eating from other activities such as watching television or reading. Eat more slowly, chewing the food thoroughly. Regular exercise is constantly emphasized. A 1999 study of obese women demonstrated that a program of diet when combined with either aerobic exercise or increased lifestyle activity resulted in a consistent weight loss and improvement in their cardiovascular risk profiles. Lifestyle changes include walking briskly, walking the dog, digging in the garden, raking leaves, riding an exercycle, playing catch, swimming laps, polishing furniture, and mopping the floor.

Put a picture of a fat woman on your refrigerator. When you are depressed or unhappy, look at that picture before you open the refrigerator, and try to find another way to cope other than by eating. Binge eating is more common in women when they are depressed, no matter their age. A study of more than 1,000 obese women and men at the Duke University weight-control center revealed that women binge when they are unhappy, while men are more likely to overeat when they are at happy social occasions.

Eating is more fun than it used to be. Dining out is much more than about the food itself than in the past. With the general reduction of socializing in bars and with alcohol in the "enlightened" 1990s, entertainment began to revolve around food and eating. Chefs command high salaries. There is an entire television cable channel devoted to the joys of cooking and dining. Cookbooks frequently become best-sellers.

The renewed interest in eating is partly due to renewed medical interest in nutrition. The general public is more versed on cholesterol, the benefits of fruits and vegetables, and low-fat diets. The interest in food, once common only in places like France, where it approaches a religion (and people are thinner, by the way), has spread to our shores. We are now getting away from the plain meat-and-potatoes style, where steak was a sign of affluence (rather than a sign of a heart attack), to a more diversified palette. We have discovered exotic vegetables and fruit, and pork has become a "lean" meat. We might be eating better, but we are still eating too much.

WHERE TO GET HELP

The following organizations can provide you with educational materials or refer you to a clinic in your community.

- The Anorexia and Bulimia Association, 212-501-8357
- Eating Disorders Awareness and Prevention, 206-382-3587
- National Center for Overcoming Overeating, 212-875-0442
- The Eating Disorders Clinic, McLean Hospital, 617-855-3410
- Eating Disorders Center at Cornell Medical College, 212-583-1000

•• 11 ••

Substance Abuse: Cigarettes, Drugs, and Alcohol

Irene had a short life. She began smoking when she was 11 years old and was dead by 42. My heart broke as I witnessed her struggle to survive lung cancer. She was so brave and valiant. And her death was so unnecessary! I was a resident in a competitive teaching hospital, and I identified strongly with Irene's professional struggles in a man's world. A daughter of a construction worker and a grammar school teacher, Irene went to college and graduate school on scholarships so she could become an architect. She entertained me with outrageous stories about her trip up the corporate ladder.

Irene's struggle also marked a turning point in my personal life. In the days before cigarette smoking was considered a public health hazard, doctors received many complimentary products, among them cartons upon cartons of cigarettes. (The irony of this still astounds me!) My husband, a chemical engineer, smoked then. I begged him to stop, but the cartons kept coming and he kept smoking. I shared with him my anxiety and sorrow over Irene's cancer and my sadness upon seeing her leave behind her husband and two young children. My husband continued to smoke cigarettes.

On the evening of Irene's death, I was in the hospital cafeteria with my husband and several of my fellow residents. When I was paged by the Pathology Department that the postmortem on my patient was about to begin, my husband joined me and the other residents in the autopsy room. When the extent of Irene's tumor, a gray mass that had collapsed the lung, which itself was black from the carbon particles inhaled as smoke, was exposed, my husband took one look and left the room. Back in our apartment, he gathered all remaining cartons of cigarettes and dropped them into the incinerator chute. He never smoked again.

150

Forty years later, I am still seeing the ravages of the single most preventable cause of death in the world.

- One of every six deaths is related to smoking.

- Thirty percent of all cancer deaths are related to smoking.

- Fifty percent of cardiovascular deaths of women younger than 65 are due to cigarette smoking.

- The use of tobacco is linked to cancers of the lung, mouth and throat, esophagus, pancreas, bladder, breast, and cervix.

- The American Cancer Society has found that women who are heavy smokers suffer almost three times more from bronchitis and emphysema, a condition characterized by a progressive breakdown of lung tissue with resulting difficulty in breathing, air hunger, disability, and death.

- Women who smoke during pregnancy have babies that, on average, weigh seven ounces less than babies of nonsmoking mothers.

- SIDS (sudden infant death syndrome) occurs more often in babies of smoking mothers.

- Babies of smokers show nicotine levels equal to adult levels, and these babies go through withdrawal in the first days of life.

- Women who smoke are twice as likely to lose their vision, even after they quit.

TOBACCO: THE GATEWAY INTO SUBSTANCE ABUSE

Tobacco is an equal opportunity killer. In 1987, lung cancer surpassed breast cancer as the leading cancer killer of American women. For American Indian women, it is the leading killer of any disease, according to a 1988 study in the Dakotas. Over the last decade, more men than women have stopped smoking. Twenty-six percent of women age 18 to 44 smoke on average eighteen cigarettes a day. The number of teenage girl smokers has doubled in the same ten years.

Tobacco company marketing almost guarantees that young people will begin smoking. In a landmark court case in 1997, an executive of one cigarette manufacturer finally admitted that, yes, the industry does target young people—and, yes, tobacco is addictive. While the Marlboro Man and Joe Camel hooked the boys, the Virginia Slims cigarette campaign told young women, "We've come a long way, baby."

Nicotine is more addictive than most narcotics. By stimulating release of endorphins from the brain, nicotine induces a feeling of well-being and reward, reduces hunger and anxiety. Frequently nicotine addiction leads to other addictions, to alcohol, heroin, and cocaine. It is the so-called gateway into substance abuse.

Anyone can become addicted to nicotine, but it is especially risky for people with "addictive" personalities. The personality profile of addiction-prone individuals includes the following features: rebelliousness, low tolerance to stress, difficulty in delaying gratification, impulsiveness, low self-esteem, a sense of alienation, and a lack of commitment to social goals, also a predisposition to anxiety and depression. These are also characteristics of the adolescent.

Kids smoke because they think it is cool, when in reality they are being manipulated by the tobacco industry's formidable marketing power. Peer pressure is a big factor. Girls say they will quit later when they have a family. Naturally, some of them do, but few realize the extent of the damage to their health and how difficult quitting an addiction really is. In 1995, more tenth grade girls than boys said they smoked in the last month, according to a University of Michigan survey. The number of eighth grade girls who smoked jumped from 13 percent in 1991 to 21 percent in 1996. Among high school seniors, 32 percent said they smoked in the last month. This is up from 27 percent in 1991. A greater proportion of the girl smokers came from the ranks of successful or well-adjusted students than did boys, according to the study.

Overall, there was a 400 percent increase in smoking among the young at the end of the twentieth century. According to studies by the Harvard School of Public Health and the World Health Organization, tobacco will have killed more people by the year 2050 than any other single disease. It is already the largest health burden in history.

The Poisons in Cigarette Smoke

When research scientists wish to induce cancer in animals on purpose, in order to test drug treatment, they use the same chemicals that the smoker inhales from a burning cigarette. Of the more than 4,000 chemicals that have been identified in tobacco smoke, many are known carcinogens. In 1992, the Environmental Protection Agency (EPA) placed tobacco on the list of class A carcinogens, in the same category as asbestos and benzene. Here's a partial list of what's in the "bouquet" of tobacco smoke:

- carbon monoxide

- ammonia

- polycyclic aromatic hydrocarbons (very toxic)

- hydrogen cyanide

- vinyl chloride

- nicotine

Passive smoke, the so-called sidestream smoke, affects everyone exposed to the smoke of others. Wives of smoking husbands have at least double the rate of lung cancer and heart attacks than wives of nonsmokers.

Wanda, a patient who began smoking at 13, always tried to rationalize her addiction by telling me that her mother, who died of lung cancer, had never smoked. I had to remind her that her father smoked three packs a day and that women exposed to passive smoke also have an increased risk of getting lung cancer.

"But my father died of a heart attack, not lung cancer," she insisted. Wanda was a slim, attractive schoolteacher with a husky voice, a smoker's voice. What started as a teenage rebellion at 13 remained with her through her life, and it shortened her life by decades.

Best Is Never to Start

As with any addictive substance it is better never to start than to try to stop after you have been hooked. I have found several techniques useful in discouraging my adolescent patients from starting this pernicious habit. Some of the techniques are relevant to the doctor's office, others are applicable to anybody. You can use many of the strategies below when dissuading your youngsters from smoking:

1) I mark the folders of my smoking patients with a large label saying SMOKES. When asked I explain to the girl that this sign alerts me to anticipate more episodes of bronchitis in that patient and her family. I celebrate with my patient the day I can remove the label forever.

2) When the girl says: "Everybody smokes" I cite statistics that actually only about 20% do. Kids who smoke usually overestimate smoking rates among their peers.

3) "But my friends do"—requires another response. I paint before the girl the image of lemmings who when following the crowd hurl themselves in a lethal jump into the sea. "Do you want to be a sheep or a leader?" I point out that peer pressure can be used for beneficial ends rather than for harmful ones. I try to awaken the girl's pride in resisting the harmful pressure. I also bring up possible motivational reasons not to smoke. She may abstain from smoking if she looks forward to dancing with nonsmoking partner who might dislike her tobacco breath. If she aspires to athletics I point out that smoking will cut down on the ease of her breathing and ability to run fast. That smoking will fill her face with wrinkles (a few photos of women smokers will do fine) and discolor her fingernails.

4) Is it really cool? I pull out a cigarette ad and point out that there is really no connection between the cigarette and the glamour of the depicted model. Once the girl sees through the advertiser's guile she is more likely to resist it.

5) If the girl looks to the cigarette as a way to lose weight I attempt to enroll her in an exercise program (chapter 5) and good eating schedule (chapter 4).

Ask Your Doctor to Help You Quit

Because more adolescent girls than boys start smoking, the American Medical Women's Association has created the Task Force on Smoking Prevention and has been training brigades of its medical student members to talk with high school and grammar school children on the dangers of smoking. If we tell an adolescent that Evelyn, who started smoking at 11, only lived to 42, they would say, "Oh, well, 42 is ancient! That won't happen to me. Why worry about that now? I'll quit in a few years." Not everyone succeeds in quitting an addiction. I have seen people hooked up to oxygen because their emphysema was so acute they could not breathe. Yet, they will insist on smoking a cigarette when the oxygen mask is removed. Some smokers, failing all other quitting methods, sign themselves up—for $3,000—for an in-hospital program at the Mayo Clinic to help them kick the habit.

Girls gain more weight when they quit than boys, a major factor in preventing women from quitting smoking. This issue needs to be taken seriously, especially among teens, who are so concerned about appearance that they risk death by bingeing and purging themselves of food. The body's metabolism is speeded up by smoking tobacco, and when this stops, an average weight gain of 10 pounds can occur in some women. More exercise can help offset this, and chapters 4 and 5 have more information about diet and exercise and maintaining an ideal weight.

It is not easy to quit smoking, but at least one third of those who try hard do succeed. The most important factor is the resolve to quit, to understand the reasons for quitting, and to prepare for situations that might precipitate a relapse. There are many medical and behavioral treatments for quitting. Quitters have been helped by hypnosis, acupuncture, gradual withdrawal, and with nicotine patches and chewing gum. Some have done it cold turkey, the way my husband did after seeing Irene's cancer, but I think it is more difficult for women to quit this way.

Nicotine gum is now available without prescription. Gum gives you the nicotine without the harmful smoke, and it does not get into your lungs. Most recent smokers need to chew about thirty pieces of this gum a day. The potential side effects are a sore jaw, mouth irritation, heartburn, nausea, sore throat, and, very rarely, heart palpitations.

Nicotine gum has not been tested for safety and effectiveness in children and adolescents, however.

Nicotine patches became available over-the-counter in 1996. The instructions appear on the package insert; still, ask your physician for any special instructions that fit you best. The early patches went out of favor for a while because many people abused them by continuing to smoke while wearing the patch. This caused heart problems because the amount of nicotine going into their system was too great. There are several types of patches and gums available. Talk with your doctor. There are no long-term studies on the effects of patches on young women.

Behavioral Methods. Many hospitals and some chapters of the American Cancer Society sponsor clinics and support groups to help people stop smoking. There are also many private organizations such as Smokenders. Call the American Cancer Society in your community to find out what is available.

Hypnosis. This must be administered by a skilled practitioner. Some psychiatrists specialize in hypnosis. Several of the local branches of the American Medical Women's Association have a referral system that can provide you with the names of qualified professionals. If the local AMWA branch does not have this service call the local County Medical Society. For hypnosis to be effective, you must learn the technique of self-hypnosis, which is part of the treatment taught by the hypnosis professional. Anti-anxiety drugs like buspirone might be of help.

Acupuncture. Acupuncture has helped some women stop smoking. This method, too, must be administered by qualified professionals.

Coping with Nicotine Withdrawal

Most heavy smokers experience withdrawal symptoms upon stopping cold turkey. The withdrawal symptoms might consist of anxiety, difficulty in concentration, irritability, insomnia, constipation, and excessive hunger. Quitting is easier for men, from what I have observed.

While your body is recovering from smoking the withdrawal symptoms usually diminish within three to four weeks, but it might take as long as a year to lose the desire and craving. If you smoked for many years, you might always miss it, but gradually it will become less important, less prominent in your consciousness.

Withdrawal causes an increased amount of nasal and chest secretions for about a month. You might cough more often than while smoking. And this phenomenon might give some smokers an excuse to return to smoking again. Wanda complained that whenever she quit she coughed up gray sputum.

Tobacco smoke has a drying and anesthetizing effect on the mucous membranes of the respiratory passages. Cells that line the lower respiratory passages (the throat, larynx, trachea, and the bronchi and bronchioles) have fine hairs called *cilia* that act like tiny brooms. In a normal lung they constantly wave and sweep foreign particles such as dust and bacteria out to the mouth and throat, from where the intruders are efficiently eliminated by coughing or swallowing. In addition, tiny glands in these passages produce a normal secretion that lubricates the passage and facilitates the coughing up of such particles.

Tobacco smoke paralyzes the tiny brooms and destroys the cells and glands. With the natural defenses neutralized, dust and bacteria fall unimpeded deep into the lung and set up an inflammation and scarring in the lung itself, thus hindering the exchange of carbon dioxide for oxygen, which is the basic function of the lung. That scarring renders portions of the lung nonfunctional, a process we know as emphysema.

Once you stop smoking there is reawakening of the normal natural defenses. The glands begin to secrete and the cilia begin to sweep. You start producing sputum and more coughing. This might lead to an erroneous conclusion that the quitter is getting worse. This is a temporary event. After a few weeks, the excess sputum and cough subside and you start feeling much better.

It is amazing how much better many smokers feel after stopping. Within days, the carbon monoxide level in the blood decreases and the oxygen level increases. After two years of not smoking the risk of a heart attack drops sharply and approaches that of a normal nonsmoking person in about ten years. The risk of cancer returns to normal after about ten to fifteen years. And, of course, spouses and infants are healthier as well.

Over the years, I never stopped asking Wanda when she was going to quit smoking. She always gave me the same smile, as if pacifying a pesky child.

"Soon, very soon," she promised. Then, one day, in the throes of a coughing fit from particularly severe bronchitis, Wanda admitted to trying all known methods of quitting. They just did not work, and she did not want to gain all that weight, she complained.

"I am not sure what my problem is," Wanda said one day. "I can swallow food but it does not go down. It gets stuck down here." She pointed to the middle of her chest. After a few tests, we discovered what I had suspected. Wanda had cancer of the esophagus, the tube that connects the throat to the stomach, a common cancer of smokers. It was too late to cure Wanda's cancer, and all we could do was alleviate the pain. She had lost a great deal of weight and had to be hospitalized. During a visit one day, I commented on the absence of the bedside ashtray.

"Yes. I have given up smoking. It is difficult but not that difficult." She smiled weakly. "You were right. You win!" I swallowed hard. I had not won. I had lost the battle along with her. I was struck by the sad irony of the situation: she might as well have smoked in her deathbed if it gave her pleasure. It would no longer make a difference.

BINGE DRINKING

Alcoholism is a disease that begins with a habit, which becomes an addiction. It can take years for a social drinker to become an alcoholic or, under the right conditions, it can happen much sooner. Alcohol, often combined with drugs and cigarettes, quite simply, beats up the body. Women are at greater risk than men because of smaller blood volume and liver, and because there are lower levels of alcohol dehydrogenate in the stomach. This means it takes less alcohol to get a woman drunk than it does a man. Drinking is also responsible for birth defects such as fetal alcohol syndrome (see chapter 14 about pregnancy).

Binge drinking is as common to teenagers as binge eating. From a chartbook of selected facts on women's health, the Commonwealth Fund Commission on Women's Health defined binge drinking for eighth graders and high schoolers as five or more drinks in a row at least once in the previous two weeks. For college women, it is defined as four or more drinks in a row at least once in the past two weeks. The American Alcoholism Association studied 140 campuses for the consequences of binge drinking in 1994, and the Centers for Disease Control and Prevention has also gathered national statistics.

While 24 percent of eighth graders consumed alcohol, 14 percent participated in binge drinking. Of high school seniors, 47 percent reported drinking alcohol, and 23 percent reported binge drinking. While the number of college women who drank was slightly less than high schoolers at 45 percent, the number reporting binge drinking increased to 39 percent.

Most adolescents, if they do not use alcohol or drugs themselves, know someone who does. The more affluent young people from suburban areas seemed to abuse alcohol and drugs more than others, according to some studies.

Alcohol abuse leads to long-term risks like depression and liver and cardiovascular damage. Short-term risk are auto accidents and becoming a victim of sexual violence, both more likely when a woman has been drinking. Drinking is also responsible for a large share of deaths by automobile accident among young people. For example, among American Indian women between 15 and 34, the incidence of fatal auto accidents is three times higher than for other groups of women.

I had a patient who had been a binge drinker since her college days. Now, in middle age, the bingeing had persisted, although it happened less often. Astrid was an interesting woman, an artist who was married to an art dealer. On the occasions when she drank, she could not stop. If she and her husband entertained at home, she usually avoided the wine or cocktails she served her guests. In other environments, however, she was for some reason more vulnerable. The bingeing and the marriage were sadly intertwined. When Astrid was drinking, she verbally abused her husband, and he in turn chose these times to show his contempt for her. He often encouraged her by making her another drink.

Astrid was taking antabuse, a medication that causes a reaction, makes you nauseated if you drink while you are taking it. Unfortunately, Astrid did not always take the drug when she should, and her husband also refused to be part of the treatment, which included counseling. Well, as it turned out, Astrid was also hypertensive, and one day her husband found her unconscious on the floor of their apartment when he came home. He assumed she had passed out drunk and decided to leave her there until she dried out.

When one of Astrid's daughters came to visit and found her mother on the floor, she took her to the hospital. Astrid had not been drinking at all that time. She had had a stroke, and because she was not treated right away, the stroke left lasting damage and Astrid was never able to speak or walk again. (See chapter 28.)

"RECREATIONAL" DRUGS

Sex, drugs, and rock and roll was the anthem of the 1960s, when young people (today's baby boomers) rebelled against the establishment and openly used drugs, including marijuana, heroin, and LSD. In the 1980s cocaine use became popular among the upwardly mobile young, and crack cocaine became the street drug of choice, cheaply made and easily available. In the late 1990s, heroin made a comeback. Illegal drugs, like legal tobacco, are a multibillion-dollar industry. And the United States is the biggest consumer of illegal drugs on the planet.

Recreational drugs, like alcohol, can wreak havoc on the central nervous system. Excessive amounts can cause seizures, degeneration of the brain, dementia, and peripheral neuropathy. Infections are another risk: intravenous drug use can cause bacterial infection of the spinal cord and brain, and is a special risk for HIV.

Cocaine causes constriction of blood vessels in the brain, heart, and other organs. If you use cocaine regularly, you are at risk for a stroke, brain infection, or brain hemorrhage, as well as psychiatric disorders. In the nineteenth century, cocaine was widely touted as a wonder drug, and it was a primary ingredient in Coca-Cola. The newly developed amphetamines replaced cocaine, but once the danger of "uppers" was known, cocaine came back. It can injure your heart muscle, resulting in a heart attack, cut off oxygen supply to a fetus if you are pregnant, and cause a stroke.

Millions of young (and old) people still smoke marijuana because they believe it is not addictive. However, it is generally considered the introduction to hard drugs. Recent studies prove that people who regularly smoke marijuana in large amounts might experience changes in their brain chemistry similar to changes experienced by users of cocaine, heroin, amphetamines, nicotine, and alcohol. This study, reported in a 1997 issue of the journal *Science,* adds support for the idea that all addictive drugs interfere with the same brain circuits in varying degrees.

Heroin is an opiate that relaxes us and creates a sense of euphoria. It can also relax the respiratory system to the point of death. Cocaine, on the other hand, is a stimulant. It also produces a euphoria, but it increases agitation, anxiety, and paranoia. It can cause abnormal heart rhythm and stroke.

Addictive drugs increase our feeling of well-being, a job normally carried out by the brain chemical dopamine. Dopamine levels doubled in some experiments with animals given marijuana. This increase was similar to other studies using heroin. The brain's ability to produce dopamine can diminish over time, so we need greater amounts of recreational drugs to replace this ability. This, together with another brain chemical responsible for controlling stress, causes the withdrawal symptoms. When an animal is under stress or stops taking addictive drugs or alcohol suddenly, corticotropin-releasing factor (CRF) levels rise. This is what makes people edgy, anxious, and unable to cope when they are going through withdrawal from drugs.

Treatment for Drug Abuse

As the century ends, we are in conflict about the medical use of marijuana as a painkiller for people with terminal disease such as cancer. At the same time, it is estimated that 100,000 people in this country turn to drug rehabilitation centers every year to get off their marijuana habit. This contradiction, or double standard, it seems to me, would make dealing with the problem of drug addiction that much more difficult.

In addition to the catastrophic social problems, addiction to alcohol and drugs is a serious medical problem. It is critical to get appropriate medical help. You need supervised medical detoxification and rehabilitation.

In general, detox is a short-term stay to "dry out" and is immediately followed by a longer-term rehabilitation with lifelong follow-up and maintenance. Addiction is treated like the chronic disease that it is. Ask your doctor for help in locating proper treatment.

There are clinics in almost every city and town in the country, from the famous Betty Ford Center in Southern California to the more reachable ones that operate in affiliation with hospitals and other organizations and provide affordable treatment.

Alcoholics Anonymous (AA) is still the tried-and-true source of help for alcoholics, and drug programs such as Narcotics Anonymous (NA) follow the same principle of joining other people with the same problem, acknowledging that you have a problem, and supporting each other in an effort to get off drugs or alcohol.

Information is available from your local hospital, library, and phone book—and from these organizations.

- National Clearinghouse for Alcohol and Drug Information, P.O. Box 2345, Rockville, MD 20847-2345; 301-468-2600

- Alcoholics Anonymous

- Al-Anon

- Narcotics Anonymous

··12··

Sexual Violence

Violence against women is epidemic in the modern world. It begins with female fetuses aborted in countries where only boy children are prized and girl children are sold into slavery and prostitution or are raped by their own fathers. Once girls reach childbearing age in some cultures, they literally become baby-making factories and have no other value except to keep themselves hidden from view and obey their husbands. Violence against women takes up a whole spectrum—from gender bias and sexual harassment to rape and murder.

Domestic violence—mostly against women—is so endemic in American society that the American Medical Association has finally declared it a public health hazard along with alcoholism and drug and cigarette abuse. According to the 1997 Commonwealth Fund survey, one in four girls had wanted to leave home because of violence. More women receive injuries at the hands of their intimate partners than any other single cause. This violence against women only recently became a federal offense with the Violence Against Women Act of 1994 (see chapter 21).

Violence is the extreme of deviant behavior, and it is growing at a dangerous rate among adolescents. Homicide is rampant among adolescents of both genders and all races. We are familiar with the fact that homicide is the leading cause of death among young black American males, but it is also true for young black American women aged 15 to 34. The risk is four times higher than for white girls the same age. In 1990, homicides accounted for 55 percent of all deaths among black males and 27 percent of deaths of balck females age 15 to 34.

SEXUAL ABUSE AND INCEST

Regardless of age and demographics, girls and women are more likely to be sexually assaulted by a relative or acquaintance than by a stranger.

161

Eighty percent of rapes are committed by someone the girl or woman has known and trusted: a relative (father, stepfather, uncle, brother), a date (a recent acquaintance or a longtime "friend"), or a fiancé or husband. And when the men get away with it, it makes women feel they must be to blame. A past history of incest in childhood or adolescence leads to depression and is correlated with suicide attempts. Irritable bowel syndrome (see chapter 26) is common among women who have been sexually abused. Overall incidence of incest is difficult to ascertain.

Rape within the family household and incest are seldom reported, although that is beginning to change as more support systems are developed to help women deal with this. Date rape is reported rarely, but surveys suggest that one in five women might be sexually assaulted in a dating relationship. Chapter 21 is devoted to the health issues of violence inflicted by intimate partners.

In a study of 100 incestuously abused girls, 21 percent were abused once, but 51 percent were abused one to seven times a week. In 21 percent, the incestuous relationship lasted one day, but in 59 percent it lasted between one and ten years. The perpetrators were biological fathers in 30 percent, fathers or father-surrogates in 53 percent, stepfathers in 20 percent, the mother's boyfriend in 2 percent. If a girl survives her childhood without being abused, she still must face the possibility of abuse when she begins dating boys or men who believe they can shove girls around or demand sex whether the girl wants it or not. This is rape. Nearly one in ten high school girls reported (to the 1997 Commonwealth Fund survey) abuse by dates or boyfriends; 8 percent acknowledged date-forced sex. A third of the abused girls said they had never told anyone about that rape.

Even in a marriage forced sex is rape. Naturally, it is rarely reported. Marital rape usually occurs within a pattern of violence and intimidation of the continued domestic violence.

A recent study demonstrated that having been sexually abused as a child is a risk factor for subsequent early sex and adolescent pregnancy. Another study correlated a history of sexual abuse with unexplained pelvic pain later in life.

RAPE HAPPENS EVERY FIVE MINUTES

The rape of women and children has been a scourge of human society since time immemorial. Rapes committed by soldiers during wars are clear examples of the impersonal rage and exultation in power that lie behind the act. During World War II thousands of Korean women were forced into brothels used by the Japanese military. More recently, women in war-torn Bosnia-Herzegovina were systematically raped by soldiers.

According to the National Crime Victim Center, a woman is raped every five minutes in this country. That means that each day more than 300 women and children are raped. About 683,000 women were raped in the United States in 1990. Most rapes go unreported and lead to posttraumatic stress disorders, as well as emotional and physical health problems that can last a lifetime.

In my years of medical practice I have seen what rape does to women—many women. I remember one patient, Mona, an attractive, divorced mother of three who was gang-raped by her social acquaintances at a Park Avenue party after they got her drunk. Her immediate response was to blame herself for being so naive, to worry about what her children would think if they found out. Mona came for medical treatment, but she never reported the rape or pressed charges. It took years before she went to another party, and even more years before she was able to go out on a date with a man.

Another patient, Patricia, had been raped by a man who broke into her apartment through the fire escape window. Just out of college, Patricia had come to New York to work for a book publisher. She moved into a tiny studio apartment in a brownstone on Manhattan's Upper West Side. Patricia was excited to begin her life as an independent, self-supporting woman. She wrote ecstatic letters home to rural Indiana. Everything about her job was exciting; meeting all those hyperactive people with ideas, the elegant offices, a glamorous life in the fast lane.

Her apartment was small but clean, and the only window, at the fire escape, looked out on a small park, teeming during the day with children playing. But at night it was quiet and she could concentrate on her work, which she always took home. There was a metal gate for the window to provide protection, but Patricia, not yet street-smart, never used it. She did not want to block her view of the park. Before dawn one night she was awakened by a hand clamped on her mouth, a knife blade at her throat, and a strong arm pinning her down. The stranger raped her over and over again. In the darkness, Patricia could barely see the outline of his face. She struggled first and thought of biting his hand, but remembered that she had read this would inflame the violence and he might kill her. She kept quiet and the attacker finally left through the same window he had entered.

For a while, Patricia lay in bed, petrified, afraid to scream. After a while, she broke out in a cold sweat and began to cry and shake violently. Her body hurt, her throat was burning, her vagina was in flames. She was frightened, helpless, and alone. What should she do? She must get help. The thought of contacting her boss, a woman in her thirties, seemed inappropriate. She felt that somehow she, the victim, would be blamed for the incident and perhaps be fired. She phoned her only friend in the city, an older woman from her college who had been living in the city for the last few years. Awakened from a deep sleep, Lenore was stunned but quickly suggested that Patricia call 911, the police, and go to an emergency room nearby. Lenore said she would be right over to help.

Patricia worried about her family back home and did not want to go public. She wanted to see a private doctor, a woman doctor, so Lenore brought Patricia to me the next morning. The shock and fear were obvious under the remote monotone of her voice when she answered my questions. She said no, she would not be able to identify him; the light was poor, it would be futile, and it would only prolong her agony. I explained to her that thanks to prominent local women legislators and prosecutors, the police have undergone sensitivity training and all precincts have specially trained rape officers. There is a protocol to follow. The emergency rooms are equipped to handle and collect evidence such as sperm for future legal actions. Patricia resisted. She had already showered and taken a douche to rid herself of any traces of the event. I wanted her to report the crime, get it on the record, but all I could do was let her know how I felt and what was available to her.

Patricia had bruises all over her neck, breasts, and torso, and lacerations in her vagina. I took the appropriate smears for detection of STIs and to check her blood for possible pregnancy. (I saved some serum for other tests should they become necessary.) I was still hoping Patricia would change her mind about reporting the crime. I urged her to see a rape crisis counselor or psychiatrist for supportive therapy, and I gave her several names and phone numbers. Her calm exterior would eventually crack, and I needed to try to help prevent a very likely posttraumatic stress disorder.

Six months later, when she returned for a checkup, Patricia told me she had seen a psychiatrist for several visits. She still could not walk near her previous apartment without shuddering, and had found another in a building with twenty-four-hour protection. Her body had healed, but her psyche had not. She had nightmares, no appetite, and had lost weight. She absolutely avoided dating men. Under a controlled exterior, Patricia was hiding her anxiety and depression.

WHAT TO DO IF YOU ARE RAPED

Was Patricia right in refusing to report the rape to the authorities? Many women heal faster if the incident is not publicized. Others feel that it is their duty to help apprehend and remove from circulation the menace to other women. Others, still, are so angry that they desire vengeance. Every woman is different. And although it is better to report the incident and get medical and psychological help, no woman should be forced to do this if she is not willing.

The rape survivor's feelings and wishes should be explored. It is important at first to urge her to go through a procedure of collecting evidence and documenting all information necessary for apprehension and conviction of the rapist. If evidence has been destroyed, the chances of apprehending the rapist and pursuing legal action are diminished.

Get Help

As soon as you can, call 911. Most police now understand that you are a victim of a violent crime and will help you.

Collect Evidence

Do not shower or douche. If you remove your clothes, put them in a plastic bag and seal them. Gather evidence from the scene of the rape— anything used as a weapon, something that might have the rapist's fingerprints, torn or bloody clothing.

Tell Someone

If you don't want to call the police, call a rape crisis counselor. Ask the telephone operator to connect you with the nearest center available. If the rape remains your secret, you are less likely to recover emotionally. There are rape crisis centers in most cities. Police, emergency officials, and hospitals can connect you with such agencies. So can women's organizations and women's centers, which are often listed in the phone book. There are women's crisis hot lines in every community. Ask your telephone operator or call your state coalition against domestic violence. All have resources for rape victims, too.

Telling the Story. It might be very difficult to talk about a rape, but health care workers need to ask you very particular questions so they can help. Questions include:

- When did the attack occur?

- What did you do since the attack?

- Did you shower or bathe, urinate, or have a bowel movement?

- Did you change clothes?

- Did you brush your teeth or use mouthwash?

(Any of these activities might alter the evidence to be collected.)

- Were you hurt?

- Did you lose consciousness?

- What happened?

- Was there vaginal, oral, or anal penetration?

- Did the rapist ejaculate?

- When was your last menstrual period?

- Were you using any form of contraception?

- Are you at risk of becoming pregnant?

- Are you aware of having any sexually transmitted infection?

- Are you taking any medication?

Health care workers are trained to help crime victims cope immediately after a violent attack, to help bring them back to an emotional norm, and possibly to stave off posttraumatic shock syndrome. Women who are beaten or raped suffer the same trauma as victims of war and concentration camps.

The immediate psychological effects of rape are emotional shock, disbelief that it actually occurred, and a deep sense of loss of control. Whatever her outward appearance, a woman who has been raped is profoundly disturbed, frightened, and angry. Unless she has immediate supportive counseling, the effects of the violence will create sleep, eating, and mood disorders; chronic anxiety; depression; sexual dysfunction; phobias; and even suicide attempts.

In addition to trauma and violence, the complications of a sexual assault are physical injuries, sexually transmitted infections, or pregnancy. A rape victim can be tested for AIDS, but ironically, even if the rapist is caught, the victim is not entitled to know his HIV status and he can legally refuse to take the AIDS test!

Medical Examination Following Rape

A physician would have to ask permission to use an evidence kit during an examination of a rape victim. The evidence kit is a box containing cotton-tipped applicators for collection of sperm, several envelopes and containers, labels, a comb to check pubic hair for sperm, and an orange stick for fingernail specimens. The kit must not be left unattended because that would invalidate it in a court of law.

Parts of clothing might have to be kept as evidence, and the rape survivor must undress over a white sheet, which is used to collect any loose debris that might be used as evidence.

Doctors will look for injuries to the head, neck, throat, and buttocks, as well as the genital area. Seminal stains on the body can be seen under an ultraviolet lamp, and are collected with a cotton-tipped applicator moistened with saline.

The mouth is inspected for trauma, and an applicator is used to swab the oral cavity and transfer specimens to a slide. If oral intercourse occurred, a culture of the throat would be tested for gonorrhea.

Blood is drawn to determine the presence of syphilis and preexisting pregnancy. Once preexisting pregnancy has been ruled out, a morning-after pill can be offered to protect against pregnancy. Blood is tested for HIV with permission and after counseling. Medications to stave off any possible STI infection might be given.

Defensive Tactics Against Rape

We cannot prevent rape. We can only learn how to try to defend ourselves and possibly prevent serious injury or death.

Any date could turn into a date rape, so before going home with a man be sure to tell someone where you are going and with whom. Let the man know that you have done so. If any date begins to cross the line or pressure you for intercourse, let him know immediately that you don't approve. Look for an escape route and leave as quickly and as safely as you can.

Be aware and live defensively. Avoid walking alone late at night. Always make sure your home is secured. Never allow anyone to follow you into the building. Whenever possible, travel in a group, preferably in a mixed group. There is some safety in numbers, although a premeditated attack by a gang could neutralize this defense strategy.

Here are more protective strategies:

- Carry a whistle with you—or scream "Fire," which is more likely to mobilize people than screaming "Police."

- Run if there is a safe haven near you.

- Stall the attacker by speaking calmly and rationally to him.

- Urinate or vomit if possible.

Fighting is the last resort, especially if he has a weapon. However, women who react quickly (within the first twenty seconds, when the body releases adrenaline into the blood) have a better chance of avoiding rape.

Once you feel that you have no chance of avoiding the rape, do nothing. Some women chose to ask the rapist to use a condom to avoid pregnancy or the spread of disease. This request has sometimes later been turned against the woman as a proof that she consented to sex.

Keep alert. Try to pay attention to anything that can help you identify the man later. When you can, write down the facts about the rape and the rapist.

PHASE II

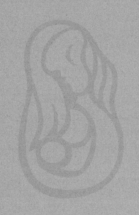

THE ADULT WOMAN

AGES 20–45

· · · ·

INTRODUCTION:
THE BALANCING ACT

The adult phase in a woman's life begins when adolescence ends and lasts until menopause begins, roughly between the ages of 20 and 45. However, this cycle is fluid at both ends. Some adolescents mature early, even suddenly, to assume adult responsibilities and reproduce. At the other end of young adulthood, women might begin to show signs of menopause as early as the thirties or as late as the fifties.

This period is generally the healthiest period of a woman's life. It is as if nature endowed the potentially reproductive period of our lives with the best possible health to protect the survival of our species. Consider your good health in this phase of your life as a gift of nature to you and your future generations. Safeguard it carefully.

The development of more effective methods of contraception as well as safe and legal abortion have enabled women to expand their world. They are better able to plan their reproductive lives according to their aspirations for education and career, while still keeping an eye on their biological clocks. However, the same forces that have liberated us and allowed us more choices have also burdened us with more work.

Young, working, married women with children are the most highly stressed of any age group. There is good and bad stress involved in this balancing act. If you like your job and are well paid, and you can afford to pay for some things to make your life easier, such as household help and eating out, you can feel very fulfilled. If you are not affluent, or if you have a job you do not enjoy, you might find the burden exhausting. Much depends upon the support you get at home, too. If the other members of your household do not shoulder their fair share and instead expect you to do it all, then your resentment just adds to the stress. Single mothers are often happier because they do not have expectations of getting help from a partner, and the children themselves often share the work to be done.

A 1997 survey sponsored by Wyeth-Ayerst found that although women in their twenties were successfully navigating their lives to fulfill personal and professional goals, 57 percent felt they were under a great deal of pressure most of the time. They felt stressed out, burnt out, maxed out. More than 79 percent said that their work balanced their lives and gave them a sense of accomplishment. Almost half said they tried to keep up with health and medical issues by reading such news in books and newspapers. Women surveyed were divided into categories such as "nurturer," "decider," "waffler," and "achiever." Those in the "balancer" category, accounting for 13 percent of the women, were in their late twenties and believed that a woman could achieve anything she set her mind to. Balancers were also highly dedicated to physical fitness and emotional health. Most of these women were also satisfied with their sex lives, the highest percentage of all the categories.

In my patients, I have found the most complex balancing act displayed by married working women with high expectations. Part of the stress is the political pressures of their jobs if they are high achievers, or their dedication to giving more than 100 percent of themselves, as many women in the helping professions do.

Women feel guilty when they are away from their children all day, and many take on even more responsibility to assuage this guilt. They schedule more family events, elaborate birthday parties for their children, and vacations that require enormous planning. Men, even those who share the responsibilities and duties of home and family, rarely feel this kind of guilt. Women are unable to close off their minds to what they've left at home, even while they are most involved at work. The balancing act must have smooth, routine edges so that the additional stress brought on by emergencies such as a sick child, failure of the baby-sitter to show up, a death in the family, the sudden onslaught of urgencies at work, or the loss of a job can be handled rationally.

In many homes, both partners contribute to housekeeping and child rearing, but this can often backfire. A young physician I knew, Irene, made elaborate plans with her fiancé before getting married.

"I want to be a physician and take care of patients," she told her fiancé.

"Good for you! I want to be an architect and build soaring buildings. And I will be proud to have a doctor for a wife. I love you, you love me, we can work it out. We will need to depend on each other to survive. Let's make up a list of chores that need to be done in a small city apartment and see how we can divide them up."

They were married the day of Irene's graduation from medical school. Robert had one more year to go. Irene got through her internship and residencies. In the first year of her fellowship in cardiology, she had her first baby, a son. In her second year of practice (in a small group near the hospital) she had her second baby, a daughter. Robert, now employed by a prestigious architectural firm in the city, a good husband and father, kept his bargain and shared the chores with Irene.

However, there were still many problems related to the "executive" duties of running the household—the planning, hiring, and supervision of the nanny and domestic helper; planning the children's nursery school; strategizing the delivery of their children to and from school. These were the jobs Robert did not want to get involved with. It was Irene who took up the slack when there was an emergency or if a child was ill. She was the first line of defense. Robert pitched in, but she had to ask for his help.

Overworked women share many physical and psychological symptoms of stress leading to overload. These symptoms are often vague and withheld from their families or doctors because of embarrassment. Women often do not want to attribute anything in their lifestyle to problems, preferring the doctor find a physical cause.

I saw Irene professionally over the years for minor respiratory and urinary tract infections and was impressed by her stamina and optimism. Her husband's steady support, emotional and practical, was a crucial element in her happiness. Her medical practice was doing well, and she was up for promotion at her hospital.

After the birth of her second child, Irene developed a pain in her neck when she turned her head, and her throat hurt, although when she came to see me there was no sign of a throat infection. She also complained of palpitations and insomnia. What Irene had was subacute thyroiditis, a viral infection that causes an inflammation of the thyroid gland in the neck.

Irene appeared under constant stress, running from one responsibility to another—office, hospital, home, children. She compared herself to a juggler who depended on very good luck not to miss a flying plate. She wistfully remarked that she would have liked for Robert to assume more of the major "executive" functions. The nanny was sick one day and Irene had to stay home. The domestic worker had quit and Robert steadfastly refused to look for another one. Irene was being sent to another city to learn a new technique in interventional cardiology. It was a great honor and responsibility for Irene to be delegated for such an important job, but how was she to arrange the home situation so that she could be absent for a whole week? She felt like a general with very few troops. Robert said: "Let the cleaning of the apartment go for a moment! Who cares if there is a little dust here or there."

However, Irene could not let it go. Was she obsessed or guilt-ridden? Before her departure for the course, she cleaned and scrubbed the small apartment till her knuckles were raw. She was dead tired and went to bed semiconscious. Then the baby fussed during the night and Irene got up to soothe her because, after all, she was not on call for the hospital, and it was her turn for the night duty. No wonder she was somewhat worn out at the edges. With the thyroiditis barely responding to the medication, Irene still was trying to shoulder all her responsibilities squarely.

Doctors are notorious about neglecting their own health. Women doctors are the worst. By trying to be "superwomen" they storm through their various duties and multiple roles until they collapse in exhaustion.

"Take Robert's advice and leave the dust be," I told Irene. I had given her an anti-inflammatory medication and suggested that she might enjoy a week of "vacation" from the household. Although the course she was taking was hard work and intensive learning, at least it would be a change and she wouldn't be expected to be in charge, as she was at home.

The focus of this section of the book is on how the multiple roles of adult life affect a woman's physical and emotional health. Planning pregnancy before you get pregnant is important to assure optimum health for you and your baby. You will also find information about nutrition and fitness during pregnancy, childbirth, and postnatal concerns such as breast-feeding and returning to work.

There is information about reproductive diseases such as endometriosis and gynecological cancers, breast health, and the autoimmune diseases such as lupus and rheumatoid arthritis, which are more common in young women and are sometimes misdiagnosed or diagnosed too late for effective treatment. Women are more prone to several other chronic and debilitating diseases during this time, such as diabetes, the fourth leading cause of death among minority women. Another concern during this period is domestic violence, which affects one in four women in this country and is even more of a threat if you are pregnant.

During this phase of life, a woman's health is usually at its peak, but so might be her workload, and it is important to understand how this affects the immune system. Chronic fatigue syndrome, the so-called yuppie flu, hits hard during this time. Young women are more prone to major depression in their twenties and thirties than they are later in life.

Dr. Ruth Benedict, a professor of Margaret Mead, once remarked that the reason there were so few geniuses among us was that women had no wives. It is remarkable that, with all our impediments and limitations, there were a number of creative minds and even geniuses among women. Marie Curie Sklodowska, Dr. Mary Putnam Jacobi a century or more ago, Indira Gandhi, Dr. Rosa Lee Nemir, Margaret Thatcher, and Dolly Parton in our century have "done it all": they achieved high standing in their chosen professions and a happy family life. It is very difficult, but it is possible.

Irene took the course her group was sending her for. While on the plane she had the time to think of a solution to her domestic problem. She simply had to get some help. Her mother was gainfully employed full-time in California. Grandparents were no longer living. There were no aunts, and no mother-in-law. Irene and Robert moved to a larger apartment with a spare room for a live-in house-keeper. They advertised in several newspapers and Robert carefully checked the candidates' references. They were fortunate with their ultimate choice. Mabel helped them with the children and the house. They were also fortunate in that they were able to afford a larger apartment and the hired help.

·· 13 ··

Planning for Parenthood

A larger and larger number of women in the last few decades of the twentieth century are putting off parenthood until they accomplish their work and financial goals, since many believe that an unplanned pregnancy would have a negative effect on their lives. They want their children when they are ready for them, whereas a generation ago babies were wanted as soon as possible after marriage.

Today's savvy women know about planning the date they want to get pregnant, but few women, with or without their partners, visit their primary physicians or an internist before they get pregnant. They should. It is important to map out a course of prenatal care, not only with your obstetrician but also with your principal physician, so you can be your healthiest before you get pregnant.

With wise medical counseling, a couple, or a woman planning to have a child on her own, can identify any possible health risks to the child and herself. This is also the time to find out about any possible genetic risks, review your family's health history, and learn how any condition you have, such as diabetes or asthma, can affect you during pregnancy. Additionally, you can evaluate genetic risks such as an Rh negative blood factor and have a thorough physical exam to find out if you need to correct any possible vitamin deficiency that can cause birth defects in your child.

If you have hypertension, diabetes, anemia, allergies, thyroid or rheumatic heart disease, you need to understand the chance that your child will inherit these disorders. For example, if you are diabetic, you will need to follow a strict diet while pregnant because the levels of sugar and insulin in your own blood affect the baby's, too. If you have a tendency to get clots in your legs—thrombophlebitis—tell your doctor; with this heritable condition there is an increased danger of miscarriage.

If you are obese with a body mass index (BMI) greater than 29 (see chapter 10) your baby is at risk for serious congenital malformations; the time to lose weight is before becoming pregnant, not after.

If you have used drugs or smoked, it is a good idea to detoxify yourself before you become pregnant. Smoking increases the risk of tubal pregnancy. By the time a fetus is seventeen days old its organs have begun to develop, and by then it is too late to rectify the effects of drugs, alcohol, or other substance abuse. Make a trip to the dentist, because gum disease has also been implicated in causing low birth weight babies, and untreated periodontal disease might be responsible for a large share of premature births for which other causes cannot be found.

Some other health issues to consider are whether or not you have had previous babies that were underweight; if you have had frequent conceptions, such as more than two within the past two years; a history of spontaneous abortions; or a stillborn child. If you are less than 90 percent of the ideal weight for your height, or you are anemic, these conditions should be corrected before you become pregnant.

EVALUATING HEALTH RISKS TO PREGNANCY

Genetic Risk Factors

Genetic counseling is especially important if you are over 35 and there is any family history of Down's syndrome, Tay-Sachs disease, or thalassemia. The latter is more common in people of the Mediterranean regions of Asia and Africa. One in twelve Ashkenazi Jews carries the gene for thalassemia, Tay-Sachs, and Gaucher's disease. Cystic fibrosis occurs in one in twenty Caucasian Americans. Not all of these can be identified with commercially available tests, but only with DNA testing if the family history is positive.

Congenital Birth Defects. About 3 to 4 percent of babies have a major congenital abnormality. Of these, 5 percent are chromosomal, such as in Down's syndrome; 10 percent are due to *teratogens* (drugs and other substances that injure the dividing DNA and cause malformations), and 20 percent are genetic. The most common chromosomal irregularities are Down's syndrome, which affects one in every 800 live births; Turner's syndrome, one in 2,000 female births; and Klinefelter's syndrome, one in 500 male births. Over 80 percent of abnormalities are of unknown cause. Parents should never blame themselves for any congenital birth defect.

Sickle-cell Disease. Sickle-cell anemia is common to one in ten African Americans and people of Middle Eastern descent. Pregnancy is a serious burden for women with this genetic disorder, which is caused by a mutation of the hemoglobin gene. There are crises during pregnancy with severe abdominal, chest, back, leg, and arm pains and the risk of fatal blood clots in the lungs.

The Rh Factor. Regardless of your blood type, you might be missing an antigen known as the Rh factor. About 15 percent of Caucasians lack this antigen, and less than 5 percent of Asians and Native Americans are Rh-negative. If you are Rh-negative and your baby's father is Rh-positive, your baby's red cells might be rejected by your own immune system and the baby will be in trouble. When an Rh-positive baby gestates in an Rh-negative mother, the baby's Rh-antigens on the surfaces of the red cells cross the placenta and evoke an immune response in the mother. Her antibodies, in turn, upon crossing the placenta, destroy the fetal red cells. The fetus becomes anemic and might be stillborn. There are ways to prevent this with Rh immunoglobulin at twenty-eight weeks into the pregnancy, and another dose shortly after childbirth.

Spina Bifida. If one of your sisters had a neural tube defect, an anomaly that prevents the spinal bones from properly forming, you have an even stronger reason to take folic acid during your pregnancy and perhaps even before pregnancy. There is more information about this in the next chapter.

If You Have Had a Sexually Transmitted Disease

Blood and urine tests, as well as a complete pelvic and rectal examination, are vital before you get pregnant. You might be unaware of having a sexually transmitted infection or believe you are no longer infected. An STI needs to be treated *before* you get pregnant. Most infants who develop neonatal herpes are born to mothers who had no signs or symptoms around the time of delivery and no history of prior infection. If the mother has active lesions of herpes at the time of labor, a cesarean section is usually performed to avoid exposure. A newborn infected with maternal herpes at birth might suffer from infections of the brain and possibly die unless treated promptly. Gardnerella vaginitis (see chapter 9) increases the risk of prematurity and low birth weight.

Dormant gonorrhea in the mother can be transmitted to the baby and cause blindness (gonorrheic conjunctivitis and keratitis). This is the reason all newborns routinely get an antibiotic salve applied to their eyes upon emerging from the mother's birth canal. Prompt treatment before pregnancy will prevent this illness altogether.

HIV-infected pregnant women might be unaware of symptoms but can still transmit the disease to their babies. Legal and ethical controversies exist about compulsory HIV testing of all pregnant women. The conflict between safeguarding the civil rights of the woman and the rights of the unborn baby has not been resolved. Now, that timely medical treatment of the mother during pregnancy can prevent transmission to the fetus, it is even more important to know if the woman is HIV infected.

The Effects of Substance Abuse

If you smoke, your baby smokes, too. Smoking deprives the baby of oxygen and increases the risk of placental rupture and miscarriage. Nicotine and chemicals used in cigarettes are found in the fetal amniotic fluid. Smoking is the cause of nearly half of all low birth weight babies born in this country.

If you have used drugs or alcohol, it takes time for the body to be detoxified. Your baby receives everything that you ingest, so if you drink alcohol or use drugs, your baby will do the same. You need to stop alcohol and drug use completely, and then allow a certain period of time to elapse before getting pregnant so that all the toxic substances can be flushed from your body. Many women experience aversion to alcohol during pregnancy and might suffer from reactions to drinking they had never experienced before.

A pregnant woman's drinking can lead to the *fetal alcohol syndrome,* characterized by a low birth weight baby, premature delivery, and congenital irregularities (anomalies). Fetal alcohol syndrome causes neurological abnormalities, facial deformities, and failure to thrive. Babies take this burden with them all the way to adulthood, and generally have an IQ of less than 70.

In addition to fetal alcohol syndrome, drinking during pregnancy can cause problems to your heart, liver, and brain, and this will, naturally, affect your baby as well. There is also the risk of falling when intoxicated and harming the baby.

Hard drugs like heroin and cocaine, in addition to causing birth defects, cause your baby to be born with the addiction, so in the first few critical weeks of life the baby will suffer withdrawal symptoms from the drug. The baby will be extremely irritable and difficult to manage. It is horrible to watch an infant experience excruciating withdrawal symptoms from drugs. Heroin causes many complications, including spontaneous abortion and stillbirth, placental rupture, and premature birth.

Rubella: The Boomerang Disease

Rubella, once commonly known as German measles, all but disappeared between 1969 and 1988 because all babies were vaccinated. The trend did a sudden turnaround in 1989, and rubella cases doubled. This was caused by the failure to vaccinate all susceptible young women. With the increase in rubella cases, there was naturally an increase in congenital rubella syndrome. Even if you were vaccinated, however, it is possible to be reinfected with rubella.

There is no specific treatment for rubella, so it is critically important to be vaccinated before you become pregnant and to wait at least three months after vaccination to become pregnant. You will not be able to be vaccinated during the first trimester of pregnancy, and you cannot receive any live vaccines at all during the entire pregnancy. So it is a good idea to find out what you need before you get pregnant.

Rubella can infect children and adults, and it is usually a mild infection—fever, rash, and enlargement of the lymph nodes at the back of the neck, or just below the skull, are common symptoms. If you get rubella when you are pregnant, however, you transmit the virus to your baby, and this results in severe congenital malformations. The infection incubates for twelve or thirteen days before presenting itself as a fever, usually for a day. Then a slightly elevated rash begins on the face and lasts three to five days. Cervical lymph nodes (in the neck above the collarbone) might also be swollen.

If the baby with congenital rubella does not die, it is born with multiple defects of the brain, eyes, heart, liver, and immune and endocrine systems. The baby is also at risk for deafness, cataracts, mental retardation, and a long list of other conditions. The illness is more severe if it is contracted in the first trimester, resulting in death in 40 to 80 percent of cases. There is less damage in the second trimester. Any woman who suspects she might have rubella should seriously consider terminating the pregnancy.

Cytomegalovirus (CMV) Infection

Cytomegalovirus (CMV) is a member of the herpes virus family and is the most common congenital infection worldwide. From one third to one half of pregnant women who get this infection transmit it to their babies. There are 40,000 cases a year in this country, and the condition occurs in 1 percent of all newborns.

About a third of these babies die, and most of those who survive have hearing loss or mental retardation. Of those who show no symptoms at birth, as many as 15 percent will develop neurological problems, hearing loss, and reduced intelligence. Most severe cases show jaundice and other complications throughout the system that will show up in testing.

CMV can be transmitted through infected secretions sexually or by blood transfusion. There are usually no symptoms. About 10 percent of patients develop something similar to mononucleosis. In rare cases, it causes fever, occasional hepatitis, pneumonia, meningitis, and a type of anemia.

About 60 percent of women of childbearing age have antibodies that protect them from this infection. However, in a small number of women, this protection might change during pregnancy. Nobody knows why. It is thought that perhaps many hormones produced by the placenta, especially those related to ACTH (adrenocortical stimulating hormone), suppress the immune system.

There is no vaccine to prevent CMV, and pregnant women are not routinely screened because it adds extra time to an office visit. Women who might be at risk, such as pregnant day care workers and those with small children at home, should wash their hands frequently and avoid handling children's secretions by, for example, wiping their noses with tissues. Women with more than one sexual partner should use condoms or avoid intercourse.

Abortion is not usually recommended because the risk of severe disease in the baby is low. However, if a woman gets the infection during her pregnancy, an ultrasound test might be able to detect congenital abnormalities.

The Effect of Medications

Review with your principal physician any medications you take, even those sold over-the-counter. Even such things as occasional asthma medications, which contain iodine, could cause an abnormal enlargement of the baby's thyroid gland (a fetal goiter). Cough medications contain up to 25 percent alcohol and can be as harmful as drinking too much. The use of ACE inhibitors, for example, can cause renal problems in the fetus. Fetal abnormalities can result from epilepsy medication and blood thinners like Coumadin. The latter can cause mental and physical retardation in the baby as well as fetal stroke.

Some medications cross the placenta and enter the baby's blood supply, while others do not. Every drug that crosses the placenta affects both you and your baby. The Food and Drug Administration lists drugs with proven fetal risks in categories from A to X, with A as the safest. Ask your doctor for this list, then you can evaluate together any risks to you by matching your medications against this list. Sometimes, it might be necessary to use a drug in the B or C category if the benefits far outweigh the risks.

The physical changes in pregnancy can also alter the way medications are absorbed, excreted, and bind with proteins in your body. Ask your doctor about any medications you routinely take, such as aspirin or cough medications.

NEVER TOO EARLY: PRECONCEPTION AND PRENATAL EXAMINATIONS

If you plan to have an obstetrician deliver your child, consider visiting the obstetrician before you become pregnant. Tell him or her who your principal doctor is and what, if any, medications and conditions you have that might affect pregnancy. A good obstetrician will check with your principal doctor (internist, family practitioner) to be sure you have had the required blood tests, a Pap smear, and so forth.

In any case, a pelvic exam and checkup with either of these doctors is required before you get pregnant. Also, your blood should be typed as well as tested for many things, including anemia, white blood count, rubella, hepatitis B virus, sexually transmitted infections, and HIV (with your permission). Urine should be checked for white blood count, for sugar to rule out diabetes, or for a kidney problem. Cervical secretions should be tested for sexually transmitted infection. A Pap test is taken to screen for cervical cancer.

Subsequent visits to your doctor during pregnancy will include a urine sample and a weight check. After twelve weeks, the doctor will begin to listen for the baby's heartbeat. An internal exam is made to assess the size and position of the uterus and the baby. There is more about prenatal testing in the next chapter.

Choosing an Obstetrician and a Birthing Place

Nurseries are usually the happiest parts of any hospital, with their brightly decorated corridors and cheerful staff and visitors. It is easy to overlook some of the important aspects that you cannot see.

Ask about their capability to handle whatever complication might arise in the birthing process: that is, if the baby is born with a distress of some kind, or if you develop complications such as hemorrhage or an embolism of the lung. Visit them before you decide. Most maternity centers are happy to give prospective parents a tour of the facilities and answer any questions.

Explore the cost of prenatal care, hospital care, birthing rooms, and the use of the neonatal unit. Check your medical insurance to see how long you will be able to stay in the hospital and be covered. In the late 1990s there was a public uproar when certain managed care health plans (HMOs) would not pay for more than twenty-four hours in the hospital. This has been changed to forty-eight hours in most states, but that still might not be enough if you or your baby requires extended care because of a complication.

Traditional obstetrical care is administered by an obstetrician (70 percent) or a family doctor and a hospital, but midwives are being utilized more in maternity centers in hospitals as well as in birthing centers. A midwife is a registered nurse with at least two years of extra training in obstetrics. Midwives work in birthing centers or hospitals, and many hospitals require that an obstetrician be available if complications develop. There are many, many current books available about pregnancy and childbirth to help you sort through the options.

Many women and their partners attend classes in the weeks and months before childbirth to make the process less painful, and also to get ready for a shared experience. The classes are meant to teach you and your partner the stages of pregnancy, childbirth, and nursing, and to help you master special breathing techniques that will help you relax during the birth. If you are not married, you can choose a friend—of either sex—to be your coach for the lessons. That person will be with you during the actual birth and will coach you in the breathing and relaxation techniques while your baby is being born.

Many people believe they will not need any painkiller if they do this. Some women do achieve this, but many do not, and there is no reason not to give yourself the benefit of both natural childbirth and the help of a modern drug to lessen the pain if it becomes necessary.

OVERCOMING INFERTILITY

In the past, potential parents unable to have children had only one choice: adoption. With the advances in reproductive medicine, we now have clinics around the country dedicated to helping parents achieve natural childbirth, at almost any age, through the use of fertility drugs and in vitro fertilization. But the costs are extremely high.

Some conditions that cause infertility, such as endometriosis, can be reversed with proper treatment (see chapter 16), but many cannot. Sometimes, after comprehensive testing, there is no apparent reason for the failure to get pregnant. It is estimated that about one in every six couples has a problem conceiving a child. It might become more difficult for a woman to conceive in her late thirties or forties because the number of eggs released is reduced as we age.

According to a recent California study of the rapidly growing number of women having children after age 40, almost all of the women had healthy babies; however, the first-timers had the highest rates of complications.

Reproductive medicine is a rapidly changing science, and the following is simply a "shopping list" of the kinds of procedures that are available. Many of these may have changed by the time you read this.

Fertility Drugs

If there is a problem with ovulation, fertility drugs are prescribed. These drugs work on the hypothalamus to stimulate the release of follicle stimulating hormone (FSH) and luteinizing hormone (LH) from the pituitary so that an egg can be released from the ovary. Often, a drug can cause several eggs to ripen at once, so-called "superovulation." This is why we hear of women having triplets or more after being on fertility drugs. However, if the pregnancy "takes," ultrasound and blood testing can monitor for the presence of multiple births so that the pregnancy can be terminated if desired, or the superfluous and often less advanced embryo can be eliminated. The procedure, which to many appears inhumane, actually duplicates a process that not infrequently occurs naturally when a defective twin is aborted and only the healthy baby is born.

While fertility drug schedules are becoming more sophisticated and effective, superovulation—the overstimulation of the ovaries—may be associated, according to some researchers, with an increased risk of borderline ovarian cancer. Superovulation with resulting multiple births has recently been questioned from the ethical/societal view point in our cost-effectiveness–targeted system; the babies are usually small and premature, and require heroic and costly measures to keep them alive.

Artificial Insemination (AI)

This is a procedure by which sperm from your partner, or from a donor to a sperm bank, is inserted into the cervical os at the time of ovulation. Success depends on the quality (numbers of healthy and motile sperm cells) of the semen, presence of a healthy egg in the Fallopian tube, and proper timing of the procedure. The sperm must be motile to swim up through the cervix, uterus, and "countercurrent" into the Fallopian tube to impregnate the egg. Artificial insemination has been successfully used for more than twenty years.

In Vitro Fertilization (IVF)

An egg can be removed from a woman's pelvis after it has ruptured from the ovary and then be fertilized in the laboratory with the male sperm. The egg is then placed back in the woman's uterus. This is a common procedure in fertility clinics all over the country, used when there is an obstruction in or an absence of the Fallopian tubes.

Surrogate Mothers

Using another woman's womb to carry an embryo to maturity and delivery remains a controversial issue. An in vitro fertilized egg of a woman and her partner is implanted into another woman. This is also called a donated embryo transfer. Another version is when the egg is taken from the surrogate mother, fertilized with the man's sperm, and then implanted back into the surrogate mother. Many legal complications have arisen because in some cases the surrogate mother did not want to give up the baby after bearing it.

Gamete Intrafallopian Transfer (GIFT)

This procedure eliminates the need for a third party. Two to four egg cells can be extracted from a woman by laparoscopy. These cells are mixed in the laboratory with thousands of sperm from the male partner. Then, using a laparoscope, a catheter is introduced into the woman's Fallopian tubes. The sperm and eggs are injected into the tube, where the egg can be impregnated in its natural environment. This takes about an hour and can be done in outpatient fertility centers. This method is used successfully in cases of endometriosis, low sperm counts, and unexplained infertility.

Zygote Intrafallopian Transfer (ZIFT)
This procedure is a variation of GIFT, except that the transfer is made after the egg has been fertilized. *Zygote* means "fertilized egg," while *gamete* applies to eggs and sperm. Multiple births are common with both these procedures.

Ask your principal physician or gynecologist for a referral to a center that specializes in "technologically facilitated reproduction," and do some research on your own as well. Technologically assisted reproduction is a costly and time-consuming process that carries a high emotional price tag as well, so you need to know as much as you can about such a place before you begin the process.

Find out what their audited rates of success are for women under and over 40. Some centers will take women over 50, and with the 1997 birth to a woman of 63, there is a great deal of conflicting opinion about age limits. Most practitioners agree it does not hurt a woman to give birth after menopause, but some believe it is harmful to the child to have such an aged parent. Others claim a mature woman is a better mother than a 15-year-old with no resources or education.

The center should have an embryologist and endocrinologist on staff. The embryologist studies the development of the human embryo and can determine when the embryo is ready for implantation. The endocrinologist assesses the hormonal environment that is best suited for the implantation and carrying out the pregnancy.

Costs range into thousands of dollars for each attempt, and many couples require more than one attempt. Most medical insurance companies do not cover this.

··14··

Having a Healthy Pregnancy

Pregnancy is a normal, healthy event, and for most women it is a happy time. Women's bodies are built to accommodate babies. Ribs move up, the pelvis expands, and other organs move aside, although not always without rebelling at the tight squeeze. Breasts, the digestive system, skin, blood vessels, muscles, and bones, as well as the emotions, all react to the pregnancy. As the fetus grows from the microscopic embryo to a six- or eight-pound baby, distending your uterus and abdomen, a number of things will happen that, although entirely normal, can worry you.

Most women experience few complications with pregnancy, but as they grow larger, they do feel discomfort. Much of this depends on your body type and size, as well as your lifestyle. For example, you can expect to urinate more frequently because of the growing pressure on your bladder. There is nothing you can do about this, and you certainly should not stop drinking fluids. You might notice your hair is thicker, and you might have occasional leg cramps, or a tingling sensation in your fingers or toes.

HOW THE BABY GROWS

The egg is fertilized while in the Fallopian tube, so it is already an embryo when it gets to the uterus, where the hormones estrogen and progesterone have prepared a protective implantation "cradle" for it. The fertilized egg becomes implanted in the uterus and grows quickly within the fluid-filled amniotic sac, with a placenta that attaches the baby to the wall of the uterus. The placenta consists of three separate networks of blood vessels: the maternal component, the fetal component, and a network of tiny blood vessels (capillaries) in which the maternal

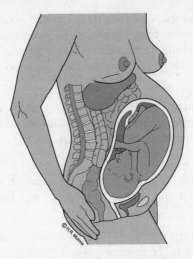

Figure 13. Pregnancy near term,
with baby's head engaged in pelvis.

blood and fetal blood mix. This is where the fetus derives all its nourishment. After eight weeks, the embryo becomes a fetus. Here's how it develops:

• **First month:** A simple brain and spinal cord develop, and the circulatory and digestive systems begin to form.

• **Second month:** An umbilical cord connects the embryo to the placenta. The cord provides oxygen, food, and water to the developing fetus. The heart begins to beat and the brain becomes more complex. Spots appear where the eyes will be. Arms, legs, and major internal organs can be identified.

• **Third month:** Eyes, eyelids, fingers, and toes, as well as vocal cords, begin to form. The fetus is now the size of a tennis ball.

• **Fourth month:** Now the fetus can suck its thumb, and it has eyelashes and eyebrows. The heart can be heard with a special device called Doppler ultrasound. The baby's heart beats twice as fast as the mother's, and the baby is about five inches long.

• **Fifth month:** During this month, the mother will feel a quickening, or flutter, as the fetus turns around. Fine hairs known as *lanugo* and a greasy substance called *vernix* cover and protect the tiny body, which weighs about one quarter of a pound.

• **Sixth month:** Weighing about two pounds, the fetus can now kick and punch, cough and sneeze, and hiccup. It also responds to loud or sudden noises.

• **Seventh month:** Personality, intelligence, and temperament begin to emerge as the brain develops. Although the skin is wrinkled, fat begins to form under the skin. The lungs are formed but do not yet function. The baby is about a foot long and weighs just over three pounds.

• **Eighth month:** Now the baby moves down to the pelvis, head-first. The bones begin to harden but the skull plates have not yet joined, in order to maintain some flexibility. The baby is sixteen inches long and weighs about five and a half pounds.

• **Ninth month:** The baby has nails, and if a boy, the testicles descend. The lanugo and vermix disappear, and the baby gains about an ounce a day.

• **Term:** At full term, forty weeks, a baby is about twenty inches long and weighs from six to nine pounds.

PRENATAL TESTING

If there is any reason to suspect complications or problems with a pregnancy, a variety of tests is available. With or without problems, most women will have an ultrasound early in the pregnancy to find out if the baby is okay, and very often to find out if it is a boy or a girl. The ultrasound deflects sound waves and forms an image on the video screen while a hand-held transducer is moved across your abdomen. The reflection of the sound waves forms a picture on the screen of the fetus, suspended within the sac filled with amniotic fluid and attached to the placenta by the umbilical cord. The test is often done at different times to ascertain the changing size, maturity, and position of the fetus.

The **alpha-fetoprotein** test is a blood test useful in determining proper development of the fetus. A high level of the alpha-fetoproteins is a sign of a spinal cord or brain abnormality, such as spina bifida, in which the bony skeleton protecting the neural tissue fails to close over it correctly. A low level of alpha-fetoproteins could indicate Down's syndrome, a chromosomal abnormality.

The **Triple Screen** refers to three tests performed on the mother's blood. The first is the alpha-fetoprotein test described above. The second test is serum human chorionic gonadotropin (hCG) that is elevated in Down's syndrome. The other marker in the triple screen is unconjugated estriol (uE3) a steroid that is manufactured by the placenta; Down syndrome is associated with a low serum uE3.

Amniocentesis is recommended if a previous baby had a birth defect, your blood test was abnormal, or you are over 35, because you have a higher risk of delivering a baby with Down's syndrome. This test, performed between the fourteenth and eighteenth weeks, involves a needle inserted through the lower abdomen into the amniotic sac surrounding the fetus. A small amount of fluid is withdrawn, and the fetal cells are examined under the microscope for chromosomal abnormality. The baby's gender is clearly evident, as well, because the cells show either a pair of X chromosomes for a girl or XY for a boy. Amniocentesis poses a 1 in 200 risk of miscarrage.

Chorionic Villus Sampling (CVS) is a biopsy of the fetal portion of the placenta for chromosomal examination. Since the test can be performed at ten to twelve weeks of pregnancy, the result is available earlier than with amniocentesis and before considerable bonding occurs. Some women prefer it, even though the risk of miscarriage is slightly higher than with amniocentesis.

Fetal monitoring is offered in the last ten weeks of pregnancy to check on the baby's well-being if complications are suspected. A device is strapped to your abdomen that continually records the baby's heartbeat and movements, as well as the baby's response to uterine contractions. Sometimes internal monitoring is needed. The amniotic sac is ruptured and the recording electrode is placed on the baby's scalp. The test is used to detect fetal distress during labor.

EATING FOR TWO: PRENATAL NUTRITION

Poor nutrition of a mother before and during pregnancy alters the long-term functioning of a child. Unfortunately, improved nutrition after birth cannot erase the effects of poor nutrition before birth. Whatever you eat or drink—or breathe—goes to your baby via the bloodstream and placenta, so it is especially important to understand the needs for balanced nutrition and vitamins and minerals. If you are a vegetarian, you need to be certain you are eating balanced meals and getting enough protein and other nutrients from vegetable sources to get you and your baby through a healthy pregnancy.

More than twenty-four international studies in a variety of population categories showed that undernutrition caused underweight babies and a large placenta. A small baby has a higher risk of heart attack later in life, as well as six times the risk of becoming a diabetic. When a small baby has a big head, it means the brain was getting blood first but the body was starving.

During the first trimester of pregnancy many women suffer from morning nausea and vomiting. If you are suffering from morning sickness, you might not want to eat, but if you do not, the baby will deplete your own supply of nourishment. Eating a few crackers or dry toast before getting out of bed may help. Drinking fluids between meals rather than with meals prevents getting too full and then vomiting. It helps to eat six small meals a day, rather than three large ones. Don't go for long periods without food. Choose bland foods rather than spicy, fried, or greasy ones.

The average pregnant woman needs about 2,400 calories a day (about 300 more than when not pregnant). And these should be nutrient-rich calories, not the empty ones found in sweets and fast foods. Fiber is needed to prevent constipation, which is quite common in pregnancy and might lead to the development of hemorrhoids. Cereals and grains provide trace minerals, vitamin E, fiber, and B vitamins. Plenty of fluids—at least eight glasses a day—is recommended. (Avoid coffee and colas with caffeine, which can harm the baby the same way they can hurt you, by speeding up your heart and keeping you awake. Refer also to chapter 4 about nutrition.) Your daily food intake should look something like this during pregnancy:

- 3 to 4 cups of milk or milk products, such as yogurt and cheese

- 6 to 7 ounces of either meat, fish, poultry, eggs, dried beans, or lentils

- 1 to 2 cups of green, leafy vegetables

- 2 to 3 cups of orange juice or other sources of vitamin C

- 1 cup or more of other fruits and vegetables

- 6 slices or ounces of breads, cereals, or grains

Vitamin and Mineral Supplements

The most effective way to get all the vitamins and minerals you and your baby need is from foods themselves. However, pregnant women often take a multiple vitamin and mineral supplement to be sure they get enough folic acid, iron, and calcium. Too much supplementation, however, can be toxic. Vitamin A, which is not water soluble, can be toxic in large amounts, and studies have shown it to cause birth defects if taken in megadoses. Always check with your doctor before taking supplements.

Iron. You need thirty milligrams of elemental iron a day. Sources are liver and red meats, seafood, green leafy vegetables, and whole grains. If your doctor prescribes supplements, take iron supplements with meals and with vitamin C for better absorption. Side effects could include epigastric pain, constipation, and gas.

Calcium. Most women also require a calcium supplement during pregnancy and lactation, although this is now debated by some medical authorities, so check with your doctor. If you do not get enough calcium for both you and the baby, the baby's needs are met first at the expense of the stored calcium in your bones. Any depletion of your body's calcium levels can put you at risk for osteoporosis later. If you are lactose intolerant, a supplement is needed, unless you can get enough calcium from yogurt.

See chapter 4 for more information about these nutrients.

Folic Acid. Despite public awareness campaigns to enlighten women about the need for folic acid and its role in preventing birth defects, more than half the women of childbearing age are not well informed on this subject, according to a 1997 survey. The majority of the American population cannot name a specific food that contains folic acid. (Sources of folic acid are green leafy vegetables such as spinach, and citrus fruits. Whole-grain breads are also good sources, as are liver, kidneys, and nuts.)

A study in the *Journal of the American Medical Association* showed that the only women who had enough folic acid to prevent birth defects were those taking supplements. Studies show that taking supplements for the first six weeks of pregnancy can reduce the risk of neural tube birth defects by more than half.

An earlier study, in 1995, by the March of Dimes Foundation, revealed that nearly half the women surveyed had never heard of folic acid and that only 15 percent were aware of the recommendations of the Public Health Service. Because of this lack of awareness, the Food and Drug Administration is now requiring manufacturers to include folic acid in enriched breads and other products made from grains.

Folic acid—or folate, as it is also known—was first identified in 1941. It helps the body build red blood cells, and while it is primarily noted for its importance in preventing neural tube defects, recent studies suggest it might also reduce risk of heart disease (see page 363 in chapter 24) and certain types of cancer. It is needed for DNA synthesis and to avoid spina bifida, defects to the brain and spinal cord. Such defects cause stillbirth and infant death, and they remain a severe handicap to those babies that survive.

If you had a previous pregnancy with neural tube defect, you need to begin taking folic acid at least a month *before conception*. The Centers for Disease Control issued a guideline in 1991 that women who had prior births with these defects take four milligrams a day for at least a month before conception, and continue through the first three months of pregnancy. The following year, the U.S. Public Health Service recommended that all women of childbearing age take 400 micrograms. They estimated that if women did this, the rate of these birth defects would be cut in half. Most women from 19 to 50, it was estimated by the U.S. Department of Agriculture, consume only half the ideal amount.

Because of the beneficial effect of folic acid on prevention of heart disease, why not, having started taking it during pregnancy, continue this supplement for the rest of your life?

How Much Weight Should You Gain?

It is normal to gain between 15 and 20 pounds during pregnancy. The developing baby accounts for about 38 percent of the weight gain. The rest is for blood (20 percent), enlargement of the breasts, womb, and buttocks (20 percent), and the placenta (9 percent).

If you are underweight, you should gain more, because if you do not get enough nourishment, both you and your baby can suffer from malnutrition. Overweight, on the other hand, is conducive to the development of diabetes and hypertension. It is wise to maintain a healthy, low-fat diet and avoid a sedentary lifestyle.

I once had a patient named Emily who had severe problems with her first pregnancy because of her unwillingness to exercise as a teenager and young adult. Emily came from a wealthy and rather old-fashioned family in South Carolina, and her mother was so distressed at Emily's height—she grew to be six feet tall—that she actually took her to an endocrinologist to see if something could be done medically to shorten her daughter. Emily's mother wanted to stunt her daughter's physical growth, but what she actually did was stunt her daughter's self-esteem by making her feel like an outcast, an ugly duckling among elegant swans. She went from being a smart and witty child to a sullen and withdrawn teenager who rebelled against the requisite tennis lessons and horseback riding of her mother's circle. She never walked or ran. Dancing was the worst—after all, wasn't she taller than all the boys? In those days, tall women did not think of themselves as "vertically gifted." Emily slouched. And she got heavy.

Emily did eventually come into her own as an adult, although a very shy one. She fell in love, married, and got pregnant. Because she was so physically inactive, Emily gained too much weight during pregnancy. I knew if she did not get moving, she would grow to be enormous.

When Emily and her husband came in for preconception counseling, I knew I would have to get through to Emily about her sedentary lifestyle. I examined her thoroughly to be sure there was no thyroid or other innate condition that would cause weight gain.

In the third month of her pregnancy, Emily appeared in my office with a swollen and tender right leg, which proved to be the site of extensive phlebitis involving deep veins of both calves and her right thigh. This is not an uncommon complication of pregnancy in overweight sedentary women. The placenta produces large amounts of estrogen, which at high levels can cause blood clotting. The pregnant uterus presses down on the pelvis, causing obstruction of the pelvic veins.

I had to admit Emily to the hospital to start applying hot moist compresses, elevating her legs and placing her on anticoagulants. Her obstetrician and I decided on heparin, a blood thinner, because other medications might cause birth defects. We administered the drug subcutaneously, via injection under the skin. With intensive treatment, Emily's phlebitis subsided, and from strict bed rest she graduated to hot moist soaks and elastic stockings. Ultrasound confirmed that the baby was okay. At home, Emily would have to give herself injections of heparin and begin a careful program of exercise and walking. She was checked periodically by me and the obstetrician, as well as by a vascular consultant, who recommended she take the medication until she went into labor.

FITNESS AND EXERCISE DURING PREGNANCY

Emily delivered a healthy son, but the complications of her pregnancy convinced her that she would not be able to handle another pregnancy unless she got herself into shape. She actually learned how to play tennis, and does this regularly; she also works out in a health club.

Exercise is important to you and your baby. When you exercise, your baby gets more oxygen and more blood. Exercise should be done prudently and appropriately—you do not want to exercise yourself into early labor. Always let your doctor know what kind of exercise you are doing, so he or she can keep that in mind while monitoring your pregnancy.

Regular exercise at least three times a week is better than occasional exercise. The best exercises are swimming and walking, to strengthen back muscles. Water exercise is excellent during pregnancy, especially if your bones or joints ache from the pressure of the extra weight. Dr. Jane Katz, an Olympic swimmer and a professor of physical and health education at John Jay College of Criminal Justice in New York City has devised a series of safe and effective exercises for pregnant women that were published in her 1995 book, *Water Fitness During Your Pregnancy.*

Women who are used to being active often feel guilty when they have to slow down during pregnancy. We still don't have much data to support concerns about exercise during pregnancy because it has only recently been studied.

Dr. James Clapp, of the Metro Health Center in Cleveland, studied a group of well-conditioned recreational athletes who continued regular exercise during pregnancy. Dr. Clapp found that 15 to 20 percent of women considering pregnancy are engaged in strenuous, prolonged physical activity such as aerobics, circuit training, stair climbing, and running. In the initial 380 pregnancies, the women who ran or performed aerobics had fewer spontaneous abortions. Continued exercise did not initiate premature labor, but delivery occurred five days sooner. Women who exercised regularly needed fewer medical interventions such as forceps or cesarean section on delivery. They also had babies with less fat mass, cord entanglement, or heart patters. And the babies had higher Apgar scores (Apgar testing is a system of rating a baby's physical condition and alertness at birth).

Here are a few things to keep in mind about exercise during pregnancy.

• Kegel exercises can strengthen the pelvic muscles and provide better support for the uterus. These simple exercises can be done anytime and anywhere (see chapter 31). They involve flexing the muscles that control the flow of urine. Try to stop and start the flow of urine to make yourself aware of these muscles. Then you can contract them and hold the contraction for a few seconds twenty to thirty times a day.

• Do not exercise while lying on your back. This reduces the blood flow to the fetus and makes it more difficult for the baby to breathe. Move slowly and avoid jarring motions.

• Don't get overheated. The ability to dissipate heat is improved by both training and pregnancy. Pregnant women sweat sooner and have better ventilation. But if you overheat to the extreme, such as by relentless running in very hot weather, you can cause a spontaneous abortion. Drink plenty of water and don't get overtired.

• Avoid serious athletic competition early in the pregnancy.

• Avoid scuba diving and any action that risks blunt or penetrating abdominal trauma such as horseback riding, hang gliding, or being hit with a hockey stick.

PREGNANT AT WORK

When my two babies were born the world was a different place. Far fewer women were full-time professionals, and medicine, especially, was a man's world. I was blessed with a supportive husband, and we did truly work as partners to manage our careers and our family and household.

When my first son was born, in 1953, I was a resident at the New York Hospital. I worked all through my pregnancy, and while my colleagues paid little attention, my patients were very close and caring. I felt lots of love from them when they wanted to know how I was feeling, and if the baby kicked a lot, and had we chosen any names yet.

Two years later our second son was born (on Labor Day!), and during that pregnancy I was chief medical resident for the outpatient department. Again, I felt admiration and concern from my patients. One of them was a man with bone cancer who did not have long to live. He was determined to see his daughter married and begged me and my husband to come to the wedding. Normally, I would not get involved in a patient's private life, especially when pregnant, but it seemed so important to him that I made an exception and agreed. I also think that because his doctor was pregnant, it made that doctor more human. That was a long time ago, but one day this past year I was walking along a street in Florida, and a woman came up to me and said, "You were at my wedding!" It was my patient's daughter.

Today, most women work right up until the time they deliver unless the pregnancy is complicated by some condition that requires special treatment. If you work around toxic substances or fumes or radiation, you need to consider taking a leave of absence while pregnant. Everything you inhale, as well as what you eat and drink, affects your baby. A recent OSHA (U.S. Occupational Safety and Health Administration) survey found that nearly 8 million workers in America are potentially exposed to one or more occupational asthmogens. This means they are breathing in substances that trigger asthma and respiratory problems. The largest number of such asthmogens affect people working in the garment industry, followed by the transportation equipment and food and related products industries. Factories might expose you to chemicals that could cause neural tube defects. Everybody's threshold for side effects is different. A whiff might not hurt most people, but if you are pregnant it might hurt you or your baby.

If your job involves lifting, such as a doctor or nurse might encounter in moving a patient, don't do it without help. If you work in an intensive care or dialysis unit of a hospital, or take care of the mentally retarded, you could risk TB, hepatitis, or CMV (see page 180). A fetal CMV infection might cause mental retardation, deafness, and cerebral calcification.

TRAVEL PRECAUTIONS

There is no reason you cannot travel during a normal pregnancy, but think ahead for any possible risks to you or your baby.

Most domestic and foreign airlines will not allow pregnant women on board in the last month of pregnancy because the high altitudes and inadequately pressurized cabins might cause you and the baby to suffer a reduction of arterial oxygen. If you fly at high altitudes, you should have supplemental oxygen.

On a long flight, sitting for many hours could cause your legs to swell. Be sure to get up and walk around periodically. Ask for an aisle seat so you can do this easily. Also, wear your seat belt low so it is not constricting the baby.

Airport security checkpoints—magnetometers—are not harmful to the baby.

If you know you are having twins (or more), or if there is a history of hypertension or bleeding, consider postponing distant travel in case you need medical care. Keep in mind that vehicular injuries are the major cause of death in travelers, so wear your seat belt. It is also a good idea to carry your medical records, especially a prenatal record, with you.

Contaminated food and water can cause diarrhea and electrolyte depletion. When traveling, especially to foreign countries, drink only bottled water you know to be safe. If you do get sick, be sure to let any doctor know that you are pregnant, because some antibiotics or other medications might be harmful to the baby or you.

Immunizations

Consider carefully any travel to countries where malaria is present. Severe complications of malaria, including acute renal failure, are more common during pregnancy. The disease can retard the baby's growth or cause its death. Wear long-sleeved clothing and keep mosquito netting around your bed at night. Use topical insect repellents, and spray the house, too. Ask your doctor to recommend particular products.

In some countries your choice of treatment for malaria might be limited, and some drugs used can be harmful to you and the baby. Travel to countries in East Africa and Thailand, where malaria is common, should be carefully considered.

If you are traveling to remote areas you might need a tetanus booster (every ten years) and possibly a diphtheria booster. Some vaccines to avoid or use only with your doctor's permission include:

• **Malaria:** It's best to avoid this vaccine in the first trimester and avoid live vaccines entirely.

• **Typhoid:** This vaccine is composed of killed bacteria and can cause fever.

• **Cholera:** This vaccine causes fewer reactions than typhoid vaccine but offers less protection. Unless you are working in an area of cholera epidemic, avoid this one.

• **Yellow fever:** This is a live vaccine to be avoided, even though teratogenicity (ability to produce congenital abnormalities) has not been proved. If you travel to a country where this vaccine is required, ask your doctor to write a letter exempting you from it.

- **Hepatitis A:** This disease is commonly acquired by travelers during two- or three-week stays in developing countries. The infection is associated with premature births and with making the pregnant woman sick. There is now a vaccine for hepatitis A, but I don't know if it is safe to be vaccinated during pregnancy.

- **Hepatitis B:** This immunization is not routinely given to travelers unless they are exposed to blood or body fluids of an infected person.

Where to Get Information

Because regulations might change, always find out before you travel. The U.S. Centers for Disease Control (CDC) has a "yellow book" with health information for travelers. You can get this from the U.S. Government Printing Office in Washington, D.C. The CDC also maintains a travel health phone line at 404-332-4559. The World Health Organization also has a book, *International Travel and Health,* available from the WHO publications center in Albany, New York. Medical practitioners themselves formed an organization in 1989 called the International Society of Travel Medicine, which offers health advice to the travel industry. Find out if your travel agent has the latest update on health risks.

COPING WITH THE DISCOMFORTS OF PREGNANCY

Morning Sickness

Morning sickness is one of the early symptoms of pregnancy in many women. This is nausea and vomiting that occurs when the stomach is empty, thus the name. This usually goes away by mid pregnancy, but not always. Eating small meals of easily digested foods several times a day might help. Dry crackers can be nibbled during the day to add sustenance.

Gastrointestinal Problems

While morning sickness usually disappears by the third month, other digestive conditions can occur later as the fetus grows and takes up more abdominal space. Eat small but frequent meals, so you don't make yourself feel full and uncomfortable. Avoid spicy and fried foods. The feeling of fullness and acid burning in the throat and chest happens when the sphincter muscle at the lower end of the esophagus relaxes and fails to prevent food from backing up. This condition—called the *gastroesophageal reflux,* or, simply, *reflux*—is common during pregnancy and usually disappears after childbirth. This condition is also common in older women and bears no relationship to having had it during pregnancy (see chapter 26).

Constipation and Hemorrhoids

These problems plague many pregnant women—11 to 38 percent—because of the pressure of the fetus on the bowel loops and a general, hormonally conditioned slowing of the digestive passage. Hemorrhoids are enlarged and weakened veins near the anus. The baby's head presses on these veins, and the veins swell, causing tenderness, itching, and occasional bleeding, especially if you strain during a bowel movement. Avoid this by drinking plenty of fluids, eating enough fiber, and getting regular exercise. Hemorrhoids can be treated with local medications available in drugstores, but mention this problem to your obstetrician, who might suggest other medical treatment. Hemorrhoids usually disappear several weeks or months after the delivery.

Mouth and Teeth

A variety of discomforts from losing teeth to gum disease can occur during pregnancy, mostly due to the hormonal changes. An estimated 60 to 75 percent of women experience *gingivitis,* an inflammation of the gums, because of hormonal changes that disturb the immune system's natural response to bacteria in the mouth. This needs to be taken care of at the time, because it will not just go away after the baby is born. Sometimes purplish blue growths appear between the teeth and bleed easily when you eat or brush your teeth. Many women notice that their teeth feel loose. This could be partly caused by mineral changes in your body that affect the tissue binding your teeth to the jawbone. This usually disappears after pregnancy. In very rare cases, women who experience extensive morning sickness can lose tooth enamel due to the reflux of gastric acid.

Fatigue

Fatigue and need for sleep are frequently exaggerated in early pregnancy. On the other hand, some women cannot fall asleep and stay asleep. Vivid dreams are not uncommon in pregnancy, although we cannot explain this. Avoid sleeping pills, especially during early pregnancy, when fetal organs are forming. Remember, your baby receives everything you ingest, so you will put the baby to sleep with drugs, too. If you cannot sleep, relax in a warm bath, do some exercise, and try drinking a glass of warm milk at bedtime. Because of the changes in your body's contour, it might be more comfortable to sleep on one side with one leg supported on a pillow. Lying flat on your back can make it hard to breathe and might contribute to backache.

Breast Soreness

In pregnancy, your breasts swell and become engorged and tender. The nipples and the surrounding areas become darker and, late in pregnancy, might leak colostrum, a yellow liquid that is a highly nutritious precursor to milk. Colostrum is rich in antibodies that protect the baby from infection. Wash this away with warm water and gentle soap. You will need a larger-sized bra, but make it a comfortable bra with good support and wide shoulder straps that will not cut into your shoulders. It is important to examine your breasts during pregnancy to look for nodules, cysts, or tumors, and to make sure your breasts are symmetrical. If a nipple is inverted, stimulate the areola to force the nipple into its proper position (see chapter 17).

Fluid Retention

The hormones secreted by the placenta frequently lead to fluid retention and swelling (edema) of feet, hands, and face. Elevate your legs to avoid the swelling of your feet. Elevate your head on a pillow or two to prevent facial edema. Cut down on salt, which stimulates more fluid retention.

Varicose Veins

Veins in the legs and vagina are dilated and sometimes become tender. Avoid standing for long periods of time. Walking is better than standing. Wear special knee-high support stockings. Longer elastic stockings will constrict the veins around your knees when you bend the leg or sit down. Keep moving your toes and heels to promote circulation. Floating in water, and exercising in water, can also minimize the edema.

Skin Changes

Stretch marks might appear on the sides of the abdomen, but these usually fade after pregnancy. These are light pink or purple initially, and they eventually fade to white. Most often, stretch marks are found on breasts, thighs, abdomen, and hips. There is no cure for these marks, although they can be lightened with laser treatments or Retin-A. You might develop patches of brown pigmentation on your hands and face called *chloasma* because of the surplus of estrogen and progesterone you are producing. These marks fade away after childbirth. *Linea nigra* is the dark pigmented line running down the middle of the abdomen from chest to pubic bone. It disappears after childbirth.

Backaches

Backaches are common in pregnancy. Because your center of gravity shifts while carrying your baby, the extra weight in front of you can pull your spine forward into an unnatural position. Backache is also caused by the relaxation of ligaments and joints that occurs in preparation for delivery.

Increased Libido

Because you are producing more estrogen, you might also feel sexier. For some women this is canceled out by morning sickness or other discomforts, or by a partner's changing attitude about her pregnant body. Most of the time, there is no reason to abstain from intercourse during pregnancy. If you have had a spontaneous miscarriage in the past, then avoid vaginal penetration in the early months. In later pregnancy, around the eighth month, once the baby's head descends, penetration could rupture the membranes. However, except for the early and late stages of pregnancy, there is no reason not to enjoy sex. Once the baby gets big, you might want to change your position during intercourse, for the sake of comfort.

Emotions

Psychologically, pregnancy—and especially the first pregnancy—is a time of great change. When the pregnancy is desired, profound happiness is part of the picture. However, there is also anxiety and apprehension about the physical challenges ahead, the labor, the new responsibilities, and sometimes financial uncertainty. Your fluctuating emotions can affect your bonding with the baby, which begins some time in mid-pregnancy, especially if the sex of the baby is known.

Some people, often both partners, also sing or play music to the baby, or talk in soothing voices to the baby while gently massaging the abdomen.

COMPLICATIONS OF PREGNANCY

Sometimes a pregnancy can be complicated by a preexisting condition or a sickness acquired during the pregnancy. There are sometimes complications like miscarriage, preterm labor, or premature rupture of the placenta, which we cannot explain. Call your doctor if you notice any of the following:

- Vaginal bleeding, which might be a sign that the placenta has separated or the precursor of a possible miscarriage.

- Increase or change in the character of vaginal secretions, which could indicate infection or a premature rupture of the membranes.

- Cramps, severe abdominal pain, or backache.

- Swelling of the body, headache, or blurred vision, all of which are sometimes indicative of hypertension, or preeclampsia.

- Fever or chills.

• Cessation of the baby's movements for 10 hours or longer after the seventh month.

Urinary Tract Infections

Pregnancy can sometimes change the alignment of the bladder and the ureters—two long tubes that connect the bladder to each of the kidneys—and the urethra—the short tube that connects the bladder to the outside through the urinary meatus (see chapter 3 for explanations and illustrations of anatomy). These alignment changes make you more vulnerable to both lower urinary tract infections (urethra and bladder) and upper urinary tract infections (ureters and kidneys). In pregnancy, the urethra might be pushed closer to the anus, and fecal bacteria can more easily invade the bladder. *Urethritis*, an infection of the urethra, and *cystitis*, a bladder infection, are common in pregnancy.

An infection that spreads from the bladder to the kidneys is serious and can cause severe pain in the area of the ribs in your back and the spinal column. High spiking fever is associated with shaking chills. Pus and blood might appear in the urine. An uncomplicated *pyelonephritis*, a kidney infection that can affect one or both kidneys as well as the pelvic tissue, can sometimes be treated in the office or clinic. However, in a pregnant woman it requires hospitalization and intravenous treatment. Fever alone might cause miscarriage. Some antibiotics must be avoided because of their effect on the baby, and the woman needs to be closely watched. To prevent this serious infection, the pregnant woman must redouble her efforts to keep the urethral meatus, the vulva, and the anus clean by wiping from front to back (see the section on personal hygiene in chapter 3).

Toxoplasmosis

If a woman gets an infection called toxoplasmosis when she is pregnant, her baby could be born with birth defects. *Toxoplasma gondii* is a one-cell microorganism that lives in cats but can infect other animals, including cattle and humans. This disease is acquired through contact with a cat or cat feces or through eating contaminated raw or rare meat. The infection spreads through the body in the bloodstream and can cross the placenta and infect the baby.

Toxoplasmosis might be entirely without symptoms—you might have been infected at one time or another without your realizing it. Nonspecific "viral" or flulike symptoms or an acute mononucleosis-type condition such as fever, sore throat, and swollen and tender lymph nodes might occur. In people with suppressed immune systems, such as those with AIDS, toxoplasmosis can cause encephalitis, which is an inflammation of the brain.

I remember attending a lecture given by the famous heart surgeon Christian Barnard in the 1970s at Cornell Medical College. It was scheduled for six P.M., and after a full day of classes, the students needed some food to keep their energy up for this lecture. They all went to a local "greasy spoon" for hamburgers, and more than a dozen of the students came down with toxoplasmosis within the week. The infection was caused by rare hamburger meat contaminated with *Toxoplasma gondii*.

Congenital toxoplasmosis occurs in less than 1 percent of all live births in this country. On average, one third of babies are affected if their mothers acquire toxoplasmosis while they are pregnant. The baby is more likely to get the disease in the second or third trimester of pregnancy. However, the fetal infection acquired earlier in pregnancy is more severe and can result in spontaneous abortion. If the baby survives, he or she could develop eye infection, sometimes resulting in blindness; seizures; mental retardation; pneumonia; hydrocephalus (water on the brain); or bone marrow suppression.

This is why pregnant women should be tested for toxoplasmosis. The tests for the infection are not 100 percent accurate, and new tests are being developed to detect the organism in the amniotic fluid. If the infection occurred early in pregnancy, abortion should be considered because of the severity of the potential birth defects.

Meanwhile, keep away from cats and their litter trays during pregnancy, and don't indulge in raw meats such as steak tartare. If you do get toxoplasmosis while pregnant, your doctor will undertake intensive antimicrobial treatment.

Lyme Disease

If you are pregnant during the summer months, be especially cautious about walking around in areas that might be infested with deer ticks. Lyme disease occurs if the tick remains attached to your body for at least twenty-four hours. Because deer ticks are so tiny, they are not as easily detectable as the larger dog ticks. They might look like black pinheads around unprotected areas of your body (groin, armpits, behind the ears). Every sojourn in the country, especially from May to July, must conclude with a thorough shower and inspection of the body for new "blackheads."

Lyme disease is manifested in three stages, very much like syphilis. First, within three to thirty-two days of being bitten, a ringlike rash might appear. Within two days or two weeks, the infection spreads from the skin to the heart, central nervous system, muscles, and bones. The last stage, months or years after infection, includes chronic arthritis and neurological conditions such as Bell's palsy, which causes a temporary paralysis of one side of the face. Skin conditions might also develop.

If this happens during pregnancy, the infection can cross the placenta and infect the fetus. There are no long-term studies, but some isolated cases have been recorded. A Wisconsin woman developed the ringlike rash while she was pregnant, and later developed arthritis that was resolved with treatment. However, her baby was born with widespread cardiovascular problems and died within thirty-nine hours of birth. Autopsy revealed the disease in the kidneys, spleen, and bone marrow. There have been stillbirths, and babies born with two or more fingers or toes fused together.

Your best bet is to avoid heavily wooded areas altogether during pregnancy. If you cannot avoid them, then wear long sleeves and long pants and check your skin for ticks every night. If you find a tick, save it so it can be identified.

If you are bitten by a tick, antibiotics can be given for ten to fourteen days to try to offset the infection.

Asthma

As many as 4 percent of pregnancies are complicated by asthma. Additionally, if you have asthma and become pregnant, it can either get worse or better during pregnancy. We don't know exactly why this is, but it's possibly due to hormonal fluctuations or pressure of the growing fetus on the lungs.

When you have a concurrent chronic illness such as asthma while you are pregnant, it is vital to have your principal physician—or the specialist who treats your asthma—communicating with your obstetrician. Many women stop taking their asthma medications when they are pregnant because they believe the medications will harm the baby. In fact, the opposite might be the case. If asthma is not kept under control, the baby might not be getting enough oxygen.

At a conference in 1997 of the American Lung Association, American Thoracic Society, it was discovered that during pregnancy, while more than 9 percent of women had asthma, less than 4 percent used their asthma medication during pregnancy.

Most asthma medications are safe during pregnancy. Your doctors might advise periodic monitoring with sonography and monitoring your baby's heart during the later stages of pregnancy.

Hypertension

Hypertension can appear for the first time in pregnancy, or the onset might precede pregnancy (refer to chapter 28). In either case hypertension must be carefully controlled by a specialist. Occasionally hypertension in a pregnant woman is part of a syndrome called preeclampsia, explained on page 206.

Checking blood pressure is part of most routine physical examinations, and this is one more reason to have a complete physical checkup before you get pregnant. If your blood pressure is elevated, it should be brought down before you get pregnant, either with medications or lifestyle changes outlined on page 435.

Breast Cancer

Many women have had healthy pregnancies after having breast cancer. It is more of a problem if you discover the cancer while you are pregnant. There are no definitive studies, but it is estimated that fewer than 5 percent of women who get breast cancer are pregnant. This requires careful evaluation and consideration by breast cancer specialists and your obstetrician and principal physician. What you can do also naturally depends upon the stage of pregnancy.

Treatment of breast cancer (see chapter 17) depends upon the type and stage of breast cancer, and there are several options available. Surgery such as a *lumpectomy,* which removes only the tumor, could probably be done during a pregnancy using local anesthesia. However, *mastectomy,* removal of the breast under general anesthesia, would be too risky for the baby in the first trimester.

Radiation treatment would also be extremely risky to the baby in the first trimester while the fetus is forming. Consideration of an abortion should probably be discussed with your doctors.

Chemotherapy is a systemic treatment that sends cell-killing drugs to the entire body. It would kill not only the cancer cells and cause side effects, but your baby would suffer as well. Some women have waited until their babies were born to begin chemotherapy.

Any woman at increased risk for breast cancer, such as those with a family history, should ask her doctor about getting a mammogram before getting pregnant. Once pregnant, especially in the first trimester, having a mammogram would put the fetus at risk from radiation.

Diabetes

Diabetes in pregnancy must be very carefully controlled to safeguard the health and the lives of both the mother and the baby. An endocrinologist should be sought to manage this condition and work together with the obstetrician and the principal physician.

Domestic Violence

When I was a first-year medical student in Poland, I used to study with a friend in her small apartment. One day the building super's wife ran up to us crying and screaming. Her husband had beaten her up again and she was now going into early labor. Neither my colleague nor I had ever delivered a baby or seen one delivered. We called for a midwife, which was the only way to get the woman some help right away. The baby was delivered right there, and it was completely malformed. It did not cry, it had problems with its heart, it had six fingers on one hand and six toes on one of its tiny feet.

The midwife did all she could, but the baby died that afternoon. It never had a chance. The woman had been beaten regularly by her husband, who was often drunk. He always punched her in the stomach. That evening the super got drunk again. He thought he had an excuse: His baby had died!

There is no doubt in my mind that it was violence that caused the baby's ugly malformations and eventual death. And that episode left a powerful memory with me.

About half of all abused women are abused when they are pregnant, and a quarter of the pregnant women seen in clinics and hospitals have been assaulted by their violent partners. The physical effects of violence during pregnancy are especially profound. You are twice as likely to miscarry and four times more likely to have a low birth weight baby. A study by the March of Dimes revealed that *more babies are born with birth defects as a result of violence against their mothers than from all the other diseases and illnesses combined for which we now immunize pregnant women.* If you are physically abused, you are at risk for a ruptured uterus, a detached placenta, hemorrhage, miscarriage, and early labor. Your baby could be malformed, permanently disabled, or killed before it is born.

If your spouse or partner becomes violent when you are pregnant, get help immediately, because the violence will very likely escalate as the pregnancy progresses. The problem rests with the abuser, who is caught up in a common syndrome of men who need to exert dominance and control. You need help from people who are familiar with this so that you can remain safe.

Ask your doctor or hospital emergency room to connect you with a crisis center or domestic violence advocate who can help you remain safe from the violence. All states and many metropolitan areas have networks of help for women in abusive relationships (see chapter 21 for more on the health risk of domestic violence).

Miscarriage

A miscarriage, or spontaneous abortion, usually cannot be prevented. It is frequently due to an abnormality of the placenta or fetus, but does not necessarily mean you cannot have children in the future. Early warnings are bleeding, cramps, lower abdomen and back pain, and a vaginal discharge. Headache, blurry vision, fevers, and chills can also be symptoms. The amniotic sac will rupture. About 15 percent of miscarriages happen in the first trimester. After week sixteen, the chance of miscarriage is less likely, but the risk increases with the mother's age.

Preterm Labor

Preterm labor is labor before thirty-seven weeks, or more than three weeks before the baby is due. About 75 percent of perinatal deaths are caused by preterm labor, but there have been many advances in neonatal care units, and sometimes the mother can be given medications to relax the uterus so the contractions will stop. There is a higher risk of preterm labor if you are having twins (or more!).

Preeclampsia

Preeclampsia can be caused by a rise in your blood pressure during the third trimester, vascular constriction, and edema. It occurs in about 7 percent of pregnancies. Women with prepregnancy hypertension are at risk of developing preeclampsia. Women with preeclampsia are admitted to the hospital for bedrest and blood pressure control. Preeclampsia can lead to abnormalities in the fetus and seizures in the mother. When seizures occur, it is no longer preeclampsia but eclampsia. The best treatment for both eclampsia and preeclampsia is delivery of the baby.

TERMINATING A PREGNANCY

American women no longer have to leave the country to get a legal—and supposedly safe—abortion. Now you can go to your doctor or hospital in any state and get a legal abortion. The earlier an abortion is done the safer it is, and most are done within the first twenty weeks of conception.

Drugs

A large dose of estrogen, or extra amounts of birth control pills (two pills followed by two more in twelve hours), can be used to prevent pregnancy within forty-eight to seventy-two hours after intercourse. This is sometimes known as the morning-after pill (see chapter 8 for more information about oral contraceptives).

Medical Abortion

Methods include the use of mifeprestone (RU-486), an oral progesterone antagonist, in combination with an intravaginal prostaglandin misoprostol. Or the use of intramuscular methotrexate, a preferential blocker of rapidly multiplying cells—such as those of an embryo—in combination with intravaginal misoprostol.

Partial Birth Abortion

The labor is medically induced and the head of the immature fetus is destroyed upon emerging from the birth canal. In 1997, Congress attempted to outlaw this procedure but was unable to override the president's veto.

Dilatation and Evacuation (D&E)

This is the most common procedure for the majority of abortions during the first fourteen weeks. This is much like a D&C (see below), except that instead of the curette, the spoonlike instrument, a suction curette, called a vacurette, pulls the lining from the uterus. This is known as suction abortion or vacuum curettage, and it takes about one minute.

Dilatation and Curettage (D&C)

Once the cervix is dilated, a metal curette with a sharp-edged spoon is introduced into the uterus to scrape the surface (see chapter 16 for more on this procedure).

Intraamniotic Infusion

If the pregnancy is too advanced for a D&E or a D&C, then a variety of medications are introduced into the amniotic sac after some amniotic fluid is withdrawn. These medications destroy the fetus and bring on contractions within twelve to twenty-four hours; the dead fetus is then delivered. There is still controversy about this procedure, because it is done when the fetus has already developed many features of the person he or she would have become.

Talk with your doctor before you get an abortion, and find out about support groups or special counseling for before and after. Although most women believe abortion is their right—and we do, too—it is still not an easy thing to do, and is not a recommended method of birth control. Many women feel depressed for long periods afterward, and it helps to talk with others who have experienced it or have treated women who have been through it.

·· 15 ··

The Miracle of Giving Birth

Today, childbirth requires only a day or two in the hospital, rather than several days, as in the past. However, some HMOs tried to shorten the stay to twenty-four hours—and created a public uproar until the federal government got into the act and declared that they must pay for at least forty-eight hours following childbirth.

While childbirth is a normal process, it is a truly strenuous and stressful one that can leave you in a weakened condition. In addition, if you go home too soon, and you or your baby develops even a minor complication that is not resolved in the hospital, it could cause more serious complications. There is a certain amount of time needed to monitor the mother and child to be sure no complications have occurred, and forty-eight hours might sometimes not be enough.

STAGES OF LABOR AND DELIVERY

In the last weeks of pregnancy your body is getting ready for delivery, and the uterus goes through a sort of dress rehearsal, or false labor. The upper part of the uterus contracts, pushing the baby down at the cervix, which dilates. It is false labor if the contractions are irregular and do not get closer together, or if they stop when you change position.

About twenty-four hours before the real labor begins, a mucus plug is expelled from the cervix; it can show up as blood leaving the vagina. Once contractions begin, time them. If they last thirty to seventy seconds, come at regular intervals, and do not go away, time the intervals and call your doctor or midwife. Don't eat anything once labor begins. When your "water," the amniotic fluid sac protecting the baby, breaks, it is a sure sign that delivery is imminent.

First Stage

Contractions last forty-five to sixty seconds and come a minute or two apart. The cervix is dilated. This is measured with the number of fingers that can be inserted into the os, the opening of the cervix. You might feel slightly nauseated now, but it is not yet time to push down on the baby.

Second Stage

The cervix is fully dilated to four to five fingers and the baby is being pushed out. This stage could last for two hours or longer. Tough physical labor includes contractions of a minute or a minute and a half coming every two to five minutes. It helps to coordinate pushing with the contractions and to rest and practice deep breathing in between. (This is what the breathing and relaxation classes were all about.) You and your partner or coach breathe together. When the baby's head is pushed down and bulges in the pelvic floor, it might go back and forth between contractions, or it might retreat. When the head's crown becomes visible, don't push or you might break the cervical tissue and the skin.

An *episiotomy*—an incision in the perineal area between the vagina and the rectum—might be done to prevent tearing and excessive stretching of the skin (see below). You will feel a stinging or burning sensation as the baby's head is born. The umbilical cord is checked to make sure it is not wrapped around the baby's neck. The head is turned to the side and mucus might be suctioned off the mouth of the baby. The shoulders are now lined up with the vertical axis of the vagina, and with the next contraction, the baby slips out. The episiotomy is sutured with stitches after birth.

Third Stage

The placenta, often called the afterbirth, is expelled up to thirty minutes later by contractions of the uterus that are less painful than the previous ones. The obstetrician must check to be sure the placenta is fully separated from the wall of the uterus. Otherwise postpartum hemorrhage might occur.

Today, most fathers stay with their baby's mother throughout labor and delivery rather than pace up and down in the hospital corridor as they did decades ago. If a woman is a single mother, without a male partner, often a friend or her own mother can be present.

NATURAL AND ASSISTED DELIVERY

Natural childbirth does not mean painless childbirth. Childbirth hurts, but the degree of pain varies with each woman. You can always ask for pain medication, so do not feel you are a failure if you are screaming for pain relief. Most women get whatever it takes to help them through the ordeal. An *epidural block* is an anesthetic injected into the fluid around the spinal cord. A *pudendal block* is injected into the vagina and rectum as the baby is born. This is the safest anesthesia. General anesthesia, which puts you to sleep, is used only with a C-section, which involves abdominal surgery.

Induced Labor

Oxytocin (pitocin) is a drug that causes contractions. Labor might be induced if a mother has not gone into labor after the forty-second week. It is sometimes also used if contractions are weak. It is not unusual, especially for the first-pregnancy delivery, for the contractions to be weak and ineffectual, and the labor might be protracted, perhaps for days. Pitocin might be used in this circumstance to increase the strength of the contractions and shorten the duration of labor.

Episiotomy

An episiotomy is an incision, traditionally performed by the obstetrician in the last stage of labor, in the perineum, the area between the vagina and the anus. This is done to relieve the pressure of delivery and to prevent general stretching and weakening of the pelvic support muscles. The sudden force of the baby's head descending might tear the pelvic floor muscle and cause intestinal and bladder problems. It can also weaken the ligaments that hold up the uterus in the pelvis and cause a *prolapse* of the uterus—that is, the uterus falls down into the vagina, and sometimes even to the outside of the vagina. The effects of unrelieved pressure of labor can manifest themselves years after childbirth, and especially after menopause, when the healing and invigorating effect of estrogen is missing. Urinary and fecal incontinence can be a serious complication.

Some obstetricians and midwives believe that routine episiotomy is not necessary. They believe that a gentle massage of the perineum can relax the pelvic floor muscles to make them more flexible. This controversy is not yet resolved, because no randomized controlled study of that preventive has ever been made. According to a recent cohort study (a type of research that is less meaningful than a randomized interventional trial) fecal incontinence that is due to weakness of the pelvic support structures was higher in women several decades after having undergone episiotomy than in women who experience childbirth without episiotomy. Ask your doctor what his or her feeling is on this issue, and do what you are most comfortable with.

Forceps Delivery

If the baby's head is larger than the size of the pelvic opening, forceps are used to assist in the delivery. Shaped like two large spoons that support the baby's head, forceps are used to ease the passage of the baby through the birth canal. They may be necessary if the contractions and the abdominal pressure exerted by the mother pushing are not strong enough to expel the baby, or if the baby is too big. In some cases a cesarean section, described below, might need to be performed instead.

Cesarean Section

When the baby cannot be born through the vaginal birth canal, it must be removed surgically through the abdomen. This is also done when a vaginal delivery might be risky. For example, if the head is too large or if the baby is not positioned properly or is in some kind of distress. In the past it was believed that once you delivered a baby this way, all your subsequent babies would have to be delivered by C-section. It was thought that the scar after the first C-section would prove too weak to support subsequent labor. However, later evidence has proved this to be untrue in most cases.

Among women who had a second C-section, maternal complications were twice as likely. As with any other invasive procedure, there is danger from possibly introducing infection, or the anesthesia risk.

Along with hysterectomy, C-sections were one of the most overused and unnecessary surgical procedures performed in this country. As women have begun to take charge of their health care, the use of these procedures has declined. Today they are considered elective, used mainly for low birth weight babies to minimize perinatal mortality, and if the baby's head is too large for the pelvic outlet.

POSTNATAL CARE

All women are different after delivering a baby. Some are prostrate for days, while others are up almost immediately taking charge of their babies, their households, and their jobs. One of the magical things about how our bodies are designed is that we can recover from such intense pain and forget it almost instantly. If this were not true, perhaps no woman would go through childbirth more than once.

Be careful, however. Trying to do too much too soon after childbirth can knock you down. One of my patients, who felt so good after delivery that she refused to stay in bed, even in the hospital, later went home to her two other children and husband, and organized a big celebratory dinner party for their large extended family. Even though she had lots of help, she was on her feet constantly. She also felt so good without the bulkiness of the pregnancy that she did not let herself heal from the ordeal of delivery. She began to hemorrhage, and as a result was forced to stay in bed for a week.

Normally, some minor bleeding and spotting is expected for at least two to three weeks postpartum. But if the woman hemorrhages she might have to have a D&C in case some of the placenta is still attached to the uterine lining.

If you decide not to breast-feed, the doctor usually prescribes large oral doses of estrogen, which suppress lactation. The estrogen can cause further enlargement, caking, and pain of the breast over the following week or two. Then milk production stops and the breast returns to its usual condition.

If you had an episiotomy, sit in a warm bath three or four times a day for the first week or two to decrease the pain of episiotomy and hemorrhoids. Hemorrhoids are common during pregnancy (because of the pressure of the baby on the pelvis) and especially during delivery (because of all the bearing down). It's even a good idea to take warm sitz baths after a bowel movement to prevent infection of the episiotomy.

Use menstrual pads rather than tampons after delivery so you do not introduce infection. Abstain from intercourse while you are bleeding. Sexual intercourse should wait for six weeks after delivery, and preferably until after the follow-up visit with your doctor. Use birth control when having intercourse, because you can get pregnant before your regular menstrual period has started up. Breast-feeding is not a dependable birth control method. Ask your obstetrician for birth control that will not interfere with breast-feeding if you plan to nurse the baby.

Postpartum Sex

Most physicians advise women to abstain from intercourse for four to six weeks after childbirth. The most common penalties for disobeying this injunction are tears in incisions (episiotomy or C-section) and uterine infection caused by bacteria on the sperm. The October 1998 issue of *The Postgraduate Medical Journal* carries a report of fatal complication of early intercourse (within eight days of giving birth) in two young women; the deaths were caused by air emboli; apparently, the air was forced into the uterus during the intercourse and entered the blood vessels that had been torn during delivery. Such an air bubble can be fatal if it reaches the brain or lungs.

Postpartum Blues

The sudden drop of estrogen levels after childbirth leaves most women with the blues for three to four days after delivery, but the condition is unrelenting in the estimated 15 percent of new mothers who go into a deep depression. Many physical discomforts combine to affect mood, too. You might be feeling exhausted, bruised, stretched, and stitched from the hard work of labor. You might have cramps as the uterus shrinks back to its normal size. Your bladder and bowel might be sore, especially after an episiotomy, and vaginal bleeding can last for weeks.

On top of that, you might be called upon to function as usual at home after an early discharge from the hospital.

Most of this goes away within two or three months as you adapt to your new life and your wonderful new baby. However, if symptoms persist, such as those described in chapter 20, get professional help. In rare cases, postpartum psychosis presents a medical emergency with severe agitation, insomnia, paranoid ideas, and even hallucinations. This is a warning sign of danger to mother and child.

The tendency to treat all depression with antidepressant drugs needs to be countered here, because the condition is precipitated by the sudden drop in the level of estrogen. Treatment with estrogen supplements might be a better way to restore emotional equilibrium. Indeed, estrogen has been used at Cornell Endocrine Clinic for many years. Recently, a controlled study from England reconfirmed the effectiveness of estrogens in postpartum depression until a woman's own menstrual cycle gets reestablished. However, you might need to stop breast-feeding if you do take these medications. If you suffer from postpartum depression you need to be cared for jointly by a psychiatrist and an endocrinologist, and both your doctors need to communicate with each other.

BREAST-FEEDING

There are well-known advantages for you and your baby when you breast-feed. Mother's milk is easier for the baby to digest (infants often do not have the enzymes to digest cow's milk). The baby gets more iron from your milk, and stronger immune system protection. This comes from the colostrum, a yellowish fluid that precedes the milk from the breast. Colostrum contains less fat than human milk but many more antibodies to infections that the mother had been exposed to in her life. Soon after delivery, first colostrum and then milk begin to be secreted. Milk production is stimulated by repeated squeezing of the nipple and suckling by the infant.

Because babies are never allergic to their mothers' milk, they develop fewer allergies later in life. If you nurse four months or longer, your baby is less likely to develop Crohn's disease, diabetes, childhood leukemia, and lymphomas. Breast-fed babies are also less likely to become fat adults.

The benefits to you include (in addition to the special bonding) reduced risk of breast and ovarian cancer, obesity, and osteoporosis. The uterus returns to normal more quickly if you are nursing, because the suckling causes contraction and shrinking of the uterus to its normal size.

Ducts and milk-secreting cells increase in number when pregnancy begins. By sixteen weeks into the pregnancy, you are ready to produce milk. Nipples and areolas become more pigmented, ready to feed a premature infant. The alveoli fill up with colostrum. Once the baby is born, his sucking stimulates the collecting cells. The reflex goes through the nerves to the brain and pituitary gland and prolactin stimulates cells to produce milk. Oxytocin stimulates the ducts to pass the milk along.

The usual hygienic measures of keeping the nipple clean and dry should be adhered to during pregnancy and even more rigorously while nursing because the breast is susceptible to infection. Acute inflammation and even breast abscess can develop. Then breast-feeding must stop while the mother is placed on antibiotics.

Sit in a comfortable position and put a half inch of the areola in the baby's mouth. The baby might nurse ten minutes or so at each breast. If the baby nurses six times a day and sleeps well in between, he or she is probably getting enough milk. Another clue is if the baby urinates six times a day and gains weight.

If you are breast-feeding you need an extra 500 calories a day, including two to three ounces of protein-rich food such as turkey, tuna, cheese, cooked peas, and beans, and plenty of milk.

When you go to work, or if you will be away, you can always express some milk for your baby to have later. Before using the breast pump, wash your hands and wipe your nipple with plain water. The first teaspoonful or two of milk should be discarded because it might contain bacteria. Many mothers also alternate with formula if they find providing enough milk a superhuman effort.

Your baby will probably let you know when he or she is emotionally ready to be weaned. This is usually at about six months of age, although in the past a year of breast-feeding was considered appropriate. Most women stop after two or three months because of the time constraints of work, family obligations, and busy lifestyles. Milk production will cease in five to ten days once you stop, but you can feel discomfort for a few days. This can usually be handled by periodically applying cold compresses to your breasts, taking Tylenol, and wearing a tight bra. Avoid any stimulation of your nipples, and don't express any more milk.

If you drink or smoke it will interfere with nursing. Alcohol inhibits oxytocin and tobacco blocks the prolactin. Barbiturates and some medications also interfere.

The LaLeche League can provide you with comprehensive information about breast-feeding. Ask your obstetrician for the phone number of the chapter nearest you.

··16··

Conditions of the Reproductive System

Most women at some time or another experience abnormal pelvic pain, vaginal discharge, bleeding, or other problems in the reproductive tract. Most of these conditions are benign, but because they can cause discomfort and are troubling symptoms, it is critical to be alert to changes and to always get regular pelvic checkups. Anytime you have an unusual discharge or other symptoms that you believe are not normal, get a medical examination and have the discharge specimen tested to be sure of the cause. It is important that the initial diagnosis be correctly made by a trained health professional and that a sample of the secretion be tested by a medical pathologist.

Routine pelvic exams should be a regular part of health care. The annual physical, including the pelvic, for most women includes a Pap test for the early detection of cervical cancer. If you are sexually active, or have a new partner, ask your doctor to check you for sexually transmitted infections.

The importance of an annual Pap test cannot be overemphasized. It is the early warning that cellular changes are taking place. While not all changes mean cancer, they do mean that surveillance is necessary, and treatment could very well prevent cervical cancer. If your Pap test comes back abnormal or suspicious, you should have another test done and sent to a different laboratory. There is a high level of error because of the sheer volume in numbers in these tests. A lab technician might examine more than 100 specimens—cells mounted on slides under the microscope—a day. Each slide has hundreds of thousands of cells and must be examined for patterns and abnormalities. ThinPrep, AutoPap and Papnet are three new more expensive technologies that increase the accuracy of cervical cancer screening.

THE COMMON CANDIDA: YEAST INFECTIONS

Candida infection of the vagina and vulva, also called *vulvovaginal candidiasis* or *vaginal moniliasis*, is the second most common cause of abnormal vaginal discharge. Most of us know it as the yeast infection. Typically, it causes itching, burning, stinging, irritation, rawness, or simply pain known as *vulvodynia*.

Candidiasis discharge might be only scant, but is easy to identify. It resembles crumbly cottage cheese and is brilliantly white against the red background of the inflamed vulva and vagina. The diagnosis of candidiasis is usually made by microscopic examination of the secretions. A more precise diagnosis is made by culture.

The overwhelming majority of superficial yeast infections occur in the vagina, but sometimes appear as red patches in the "kissing" body surfaces such as groins, undersides of the breasts, and inner surfaces of heavy thighs. Candidiasis can also involve the mouth and throat ("thrush" is sometimes seen in newborns whose mothers carry the infection), the esophagus, and the skin.

Yeast infections are sometimes misdiagnosed as *cystitis*, an infection of the urinary bladder, which has similar symptoms. These two conditions often coexist, but failure to diagnose properly could result in treatment that will be ineffective. Cystitis is treated with antibiotics, which will only exacerbate a yeast infection. An antifungal agent is needed for yeast infections.

Some doctors and alternative medicine practitioners believe that chronic candida infestation with its toxins, or an immune response to the infestation, might be related to or be responsible for many vague and not yet well understood syndromes, such as the chronic fatigue syndrome, multiple sensitivities syndrome, and interstitial cystitis. This hypothesis has not been proven; however, in a person with a badly damaged immune system, such as a woman with an HIV infection, candida can become deep-seated, and even life-threatening, carried by the bloodstream to other organ systems in the body, most commonly the kidneys, eyes, skin, liver, spleen, and lymph nodes.

Candida is present almost everywhere. Its growth, however, is usually kept in check by "good" bacteria. But this protection can break down when conditions change. For example, if we are taking antibiotics for bronchitis or some other infection, the medication kills off the protective bacteria and changes the balance of power. Generally, it is a good idea to eat yogurt, which contains the good bacteria, when using such antibiotics. The growth of candida is favored by any of the following:

- A moist, warm, sugar-rich environment of secretions and sweat.

- A high blood sugar level because of diabetes or a high-sugar diet.

- An absence of the competing "good" bacteria, which are destroyed by antibiotics. This is why we sometimes get yeast infections after taking antibiotics for bronchitis or other infections.

- Overweight and obesity.

- Pregnancy.

- Use of oral contraceptives.

What to Do About Yeast Infections

Once you have had an accurate diagnosis by a physician, you can usually tell when the infection has recurred if you remember all your usual symptoms correctly and if the physician okays the subsequent use of the medication.

Currently available medication consists of vaginal gels, creams, or suppositories, all of which are an enormous improvement over painting the vagina and vulva with a solution of *gentian violet*, which is what was done in the old days. Although effective, this treatment was very messy and colored the underwear purple. It is rarely used today and only when all other treatment fails.

Over-the-counter medications, such as miconazole (Monistat), clotrimazole (Lotrimin) and fluconazole (Diflucan) preparations, are heavily marketed in magazine and television ads. Powders and creams are used when candidiasis infects or inflames the skin folds, such as under the breasts. Oral medications are sometimes added to vaginal treatment when the infection proves resistant.

When using intravaginal medication, douche beforehand to remove secretions and discharge that can set up a barrier between the medication and the vaginal tissues. The medication should be introduced deeply into the vagina with the applicator supplied. The best time to use such intravaginal medication is at bedtime, to allow longer contact between the medication and the yeast-infected tissues. In the morning, douche again to remove the secretions resulting from the interaction between the medication and the yeast infection. Dry yourself with a clean towel. Bacteria and yeast live quite comfortably on a damp towel and can be easily spread if you use a previously used towel.

If candidiasis persists despite treatment, ask your physician to rule out conditions such as diabetes that might predispose you to the yeast infection. Your doctor might be able to prescribe more potent antiyeast medications.

Preventing Yeast Infections

If you are susceptible to recurrent yeast infections, ask your doctor about stronger medication, and try the following:

- Observe meticulous personal hygiene.

- Wash the vaginal area using a douche or bidet.

- Never sit around in a wet swimsuit.

- Do not wear tight or nonabsorbent underwear or panty hose.

- Cotton panties are preferable to nylon because cotton allows air to circulate.

- Change your underwear after horseback riding, bicycle riding, and intercourse.

- Use cornstarch to soothe dry (never wet) skin after bathing. Do not use talcum powder, which has been associated with a risk of ovarian cancer.

- Periodically have yourself tested for diabetes.

- Avoid concentrated sweets such as sugar, candy, chocolate, cake, and ice cream.

- Avoid broad-spectrum antibiotics.

CYSTITIS

Although cystitis is a disease of the urinary rather than the reproductive tract, it is a common occurrence in sexually active women. It used to be called the "honeymoon disease," because frequent and intense intercourse often prompted the infection. While frequent and intense sex no longer waits for the honeymoon, it does make you vulnerable to infection because bacteria from the vaginal area and rectum can be pushed into the urethra and get into the urinary bladder.

Urinary tract infections are fourteen times more common in women because we have a much shorter urethra, the opening of which to the outside is continuously contaminated by germs, and bacteria enter the urethra during sexual intercourse.

Cystitis is most common in young women—especially pregnant women—and then again after menopause because the diminishing estrogen levels reduce the levels of natural protection in the vagina (refer to chapter 31 for more information about how to diagnose and treat cystitis).

PELVIC INFLAMMATORY DISEASE (PID)

When bacteria travel through the vagina into the uterus, Fallopian tubes, and upper genital tract, they can cause an inflammation in the tubes, ovaries, and surrounding peritoneum, the lining of the pelvic structures. It was once thought the only way PID was acquired was through sexual intercourse, but we know now that it can also be introduced by the string attached to an intrauterine device (IUD). Frequently, you do not know you have PID until it is in an advanced stage, with abdominal pain, lower back pain, fever, and a puslike vaginal discharge.

An infected Fallopian tube might evolve into an abscess, and when it also involves the ovary, it is called a tubo-ovarian abscess. The infection causes scarring of the tubes that ultimately blocks the passage of sperm and egg. PID is one of the major preventable causes of infertility. The other cause, not as easily preventable, is endometriosis.

PID is treated with oral or intravenous antibiotics and possibly surgical drainage of an abscess. Skillful plastic surgery performed through a lapararoscope, or open surgery, might remove the scars and restore the passage through the tubes.

FIBROID TUMORS

Between a quarter and a half of women between the ages of 30 and 50 develop fibroids. These benign tumors grow in the muscular wall of the uterus. They are usually multiple growths in several locations. Fibroids can be of three types. Those that protrude to the outside of the uterus into the pelvic cavity are called *subserosal* fibroids. *Intramural* fibroids sit entirely within the uterine wall and *submucous* fibroids protrude inside into the uterine lumen. Fibroids can also cause pain between menstrual periods, and sometimes pelvic heaviness and frequency of urination. They can cause pain and excessive bleeding. Fibroids are estrogen-responsive, that is, they grow larger with a higher estrogen level.

The majority of women with fibroids have no symptoms at all, and the tumors are discovered in routine pelvic examinations. Most often, they are diagnosed in women in their thirties and forties. In younger women, they might be discovered in a routine ultrasound examination. Fibroids grow slowly until menopause. Then they stop growing or shrink to a small size not easily detected in a pelvic exam.

It is extremely rare for a fibroid tumor to become cancerous—less than 3 per 1,000 women—but they can cause anemia if they bleed excessively. Women without symptoms need no treatment. Those with bleeding and pain have a variety of options for treatment. Medical treatment with hormones such as progestins, natural progesterone and GnRH analogs can modify the bleeding, and pain medication can alleviate the pain symptoms. Herbs such as black cohosh and dong quai are also said to decrease the bleeding. None of these substances can effectively shrink the fibroids but can tide over the symptons until menopause.

Fibroids are the most common reason for hysterectomies—removal of the uterus—because fibroids have a tendency to regrow if the uterus is left in place. If surgery is called for (as it often is), a hysterectomy would remove the uterus and thus the fibroids. But not so fast. There are many things to consider before you let anyone remove your uterus. The most important things to consider are your age, whether or not you want children, and how close to menopause you are, for when estrogen diminishes on its own, the fibroids usually shrink away anyway.

Myomectomy, another surgical procedure, would remove the tumors only and leave the uterus intact. With this procedure, the fibroids return in about 25 percent of women. However, myomectomy could scar the uterus. There are also laparoscopic surgery techniques that remove the fibroids while leaving the uterus in place.

Non-surgical Treatment

Current research is focused on medical treatment of fibroids to replace surgery because if fibroids can be successfully treated until menopause, they will go away on their own once estrogen levels decrease. A new non-surgical treatment for shrinking fibroids that bleed severely was being used successfully by gynecological teams at some hospitals. This procedure is uterine artery embolization.

A catheter is inserted through arteries in the thigh to reach the artery in the uterus. A radio contrast material is injected through the catheter to allow an X-ray to show correct placement of the catheter. Then polyvinyl alcohol, an inert plastic substance, or a gelatin-like material (gel foam) is injected to block the bleeding arteries. This has been a standard procedure for gastrointestinal bleeding for a long time. Now the procedure is being used to interrupt the blood supply to the fibroids so that they will shrink.

This is a one-day outpatient procedure, but may involve an overnight stay in some cases. Cramps may follow the procedure but the bleeding should subside in a few days and menstrual periods return to normal.

In cases of severely bleeding fibroids, uterine artery embolization can be an alternative to a myomectomy that may result in infertility. The uterine artery embolization is less likely to result in infertility.

OVARIAN CYSTS

Because ovaries have so many types of cells, including cells that can manufacture all other types of cells, a variety of tumor types can form on an ovary. The most common is the benign cyst that contains the ovum but has a thicker wall and does not rupture at the right time during the ovulatory cycle to release the egg. When this cyst ruptures, it might cause pain or bleeding or both.

Cysts that are common in younger women are *dermoid* cysts, those appearing on the surface of the ovary. These contain particles of hair, fatty tissue, and even teeth, and are believed to be remnants of embryos present before birth. They are usually benign, but should be removed or watched.

A cyst on an ovary can grow large enough to eventually cause a feeling of fullness and pressure on the lower abdomen. Such cysts are fluid-filled, rather than solid like cancerous tumors, and are diagnosable with ultrasound (sonography). By placing the transducer on the lower abdomen or inside the vagina, ovarian cysts can be visualized. For the best delineation of the tumor both techniques are used. Ovarian cysts should be watched carefully, because, in some cases, they are a sign of early ovarian cancer. They do not always have to be removed, however. If a doctor suggests removing an ovarian cyst, get a second opinion.

Ovarian cancer is the most malignant of all reproductive tumors because it is rarely completely removable at the time of the first symptoms. It usually occurs in older women except when it is familial. Women in these families should be surveilled and screened periodically as young adults. For more details, read on in this chapter.

Polycystic Ovary (PCO) Syndrome

The PCO syndrome, a condition of unknown cause, is associated with multiple cysts in the ovary, amenorrhea with infertility, obesity, elevated levels of male hormone, and mild hirsutism (presence of hair on the lip and chin). In a common variant, a tough membrane surrounds the ovary so that no egg can free itself, and no ovulation occurs. In this condition, many cysts compress normal follicles and interfere with their maturation.

PCO syndrome affects about 5 percent of women. In the past, an operation on the ovary called *wedge resection* usually restored the function of the ovary. Wedge resection is rarely done anymore, but in some cases laparoscopic removal of the thickened ovarian capsule restores menses and function. A number of medications are effective for the other manifestations of polycystic ovary syndrome.

In 1997, the *New England Journal of Medicine* reported successful treatment of PCO syndrome in twenty-five women with *troglitazone* (Rezulin), a new medication recently developed for use in adult-type diabetes.

ENDOMETRIOSIS: A COMMON CAUSE OF INFERTILITY

Endometriosis is a common cause of secondary dysmenorrhea, or menstrual cramps, and a common reason for infertility. It is a condition in

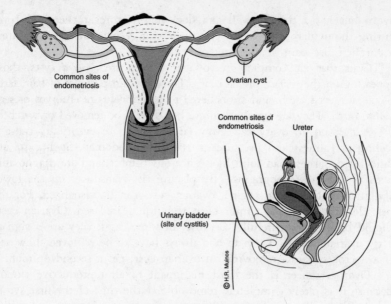

Figure 14. Endometriosis.

which cells similar to those lining the inside of the uterus, the endometrium, get implanted in various "wrong" places. The cells might attach themselves to the peritoneum, frequently behind the uterus in the deep "cul-de-sac" pocket, or to the surface of the ovaries.

Endometriosis affects about 5 million women in the United States— one woman in fifteen, or 7 percent of all women of reproductive age. About 40 percent of women suffering from endometriosis are infertile. There is a familial tendency toward endometriosis. Some women with endometriosis give a history—if asked—of severe pelvic pain and infertility in their aunts and sisters. Classically, endometriosis does not develop right after menarche but after several years of menstrual function, usually in women in their twenties, but it can occur as early as the age of 17.

When menstrual cramps do not disappear with the onset of menstrual flow, or when the pain is on one side only or in the back rather than over the entire pelvis like normal menstrual cramps, and when there is no relief with aspirin or other anti-inflammatory remedies, endometriosis is suspected. It is most painful during menses because of pressure generated by the bleeding into the pelvic and abdominal cavities. The pain characteristically stops with the end of menstrual flow, although in some women the pain of endometriosis might persist. The pain and tenderness of the mass of endometriosis can be so severe as to interfere with intercourse.

Endometriosis is a noncancerous condition that, nevertheless, is complicated to treat. The lining cells of the uterus have become displaced outside the uterus into the pelvic cavity and, being estrogen-responsive, undergo cyclical changes causing intermittent bleeding and pressure.

The mechanism of pain of endometriosis is tied up with responsiveness of the endometrium to female hormones. The lining of the uterus is sensitive to estrogen and progesterone, and grows in response to these hormones. Scattered nests of endometrial cells that might be present in abnormal locations outside the uterus, also respond to the hormones in the course of the menstrual cycle, as if they were in the uterus. Under the influence of estrogen, these nests of cells proliferate and form mounds and nodules. Under the influence of progesterone, the cells secrete mucus (just as the normal endometrium does). Both hormones stimulate the growth of blood vessels, which grow into the mounds and nodules.

When the estrogen and progesterone levels fall (as happens just before the menstrual flow), these blood vessels break and the blood escapes into the pelvis. This blood cannot escape outside as does the normal menstrual flow, so pockets of blood accumulate in the pelvis, usually near the ovaries. When the blood flow stops and the pockets of hemorrhage close off, cysts are formed. These cysts are called "chocolate cysts" because the blood in these cysts decomposes to a brown, chocolatelike color. The cysts of endometriosis frequently form on the surface of the ovaries and might also penetrate deeper into the substance of the ovaries. This severe form of disease is called "deep endometriosis" or "endometriosis with cystic ovarian disease" and is associated with very severe pain during the menstrual period.

If endometriosis becomes imbedded on the bladder wall it can cause urinary symptoms, such as the increased feeling of a need to urinate. Endometriotic tissue might also implant itself on the wall of the intestine. During successive episodes of bleeding and healing, scars form, and symptoms can include bowel movement abnormalities, intestinal pain, and even intestinal obstruction. Less frequently, endometriosis is found in the upper abdomen. When, even more rarely, endometriosis affects the chest, a woman might experience chest pain and might be spitting blood at the time of her period. The navel and any existing abdominal scars can also act as points of attachment for the errant endometriosis cells.

We don't know why these cells become implanted in the wrong place. There are theories about it but no confirmed knowledge. The dominant theory is "reverse menstruation." The cells lining the uterus, instead of being totally shed at the time of menstruation, are vacuumed up backward by the Fallopian tubes and are then propelled by the abnormal movement of the tubes ("reverse peristalsis") back through the fringed end (fimbria) out into the abdominal cavity.

Some investigators have isolated a protein that normally seals off the opening of the tube in the uterus at the time of menstruation. This protein, they hypothesize, is essential for proper implantation of the embryo into the endometrium. It was found that a number of women with endometriosis were lacking this protein. Perhaps the absence of this substance in patients with endometriosis accounts for the frequent occurrence of infertility in these women.

Another theory is that endometriosis is not a disease so much as a variant of a normal process. In most women, it is believed, some menstrual debris gets outside the reproductive tract and into the peritoneal cavity. Normally, the healthy immune cells clean up this debris by causing it to shrink and dry up. However, if the immune system fails to do this, this debris develops into endometriosis.

Symptomatic endometriosis is considered a progressive disease as long as there is estrogen to act on those cells. Once it becomes associated with pain, it gets worse with each menstrual cycle as more nodules form and interfere with the anatomy and function of the Fallopian tubes and ovaries. A 1997 study showed that even mild or moderate cases of endometriosis can be a reason for infertility, and early treatment can double a woman's chances of becoming pregnant. The author of the study suggested that women with unexplained infertility undergo a diagnostic laparoscopy.

Diagnosis of Endometriosis

Definitive diagnosis must be made by looking inside the pelvic cavity with sonography or echography and ruling out other conditions such as pelvic inflammatory disease (PID), described on page 219, which has similar symptoms.

Diagnosis can be made more definitively with a laparoscope, inserted into the pelvis through two small openings in the abdominal wall. The procedure is minimally invasive and carries relatively few risks. The physician can also insert a surgical tool through the 'scope to biopsy and destroy the lesions. (Laparoscopy allows the diagnosis and treatment of organs through two small openings in the abdomen, and laparotomy allows diagnosis and treatment through a linear incision of the abdominal wall for better visualization of the lesion.)

Medical and Surgical Treatment for Endometriosis

Endometriosis is never really cured with medical therapy alone until the source of estrogen is dried up. That happens when the ovary either spontaneously undergoes menopause or is surgically removed. While current medical treatment is ineffective in eliminating the severe disease in most women without endangering their estrogen source, and thus their fertility, it is possible to control endometriosis over several years.

Mild and moderate endometriosis can be treated, and fertility can be restored in some women through a combination of surgical and medical therapy. Treatment aims to alleviate and prevent pelvic pain and restore fertility, and the choice of treatment depends on which goal is foremost in the woman's mind. Therapy depends on age, reproductive plans, and severity of symptoms. Many gynecologists believe that fertility can be restored only when the endometriosis is fully eradicated. Others question whether infertility is directly related to the amount of endometriosis.

Medical treatment is often used as primary therapy for symptoms of endometriosis or as an adjunct to conservative surgical management of pelvic pain and/or infertility. While it is the gynecologist who confirms the diagnosis and initiates the treatment of endometriosis, it is the principal physician who should be in charge and who has the skills to continue the medical (hormonal) treatment. It is also the principal physician who should assess the patient's need and readiness for a more definitive surgical treatment.

Hormones such as danazol can suppress estrogen production and shrink the endometriosis. Hormone therapy is expensive, however, and requires periodic visits to the doctor. Danazol is a synthetic testosterone, the male hormone. It controls the pain and, as an added bonus, increases bone density. However, it adversely affects blood cholesterol and lipid metabolism. Other side effects include weight gain, muscle pain, acne, and occasionally hirsutism. With larger doses of danazol, your voice might deepen. Dark-haired women seem more susceptible to these masculinizing effects of danazol than blondes, perhaps because of the associated differences in skin structure.

GnRH analogs and antagonists are sometimes used to block the hypothalamus-pituitary-ovarian axis, stop the production of estrogen and progesterone and arrest the endometriosis. Side effects include hot flashes.

Some physicians place young women with a family history of endometriosis on a regimen of oral contraceptives; the reasoning is that these women need the medication for birth control anyway and perhaps the progestin in the contraceptive can prevent the development of endometriosis at the same time. This "preventive" maneuver should not be used indiscriminately. More research is needed to identify those women who are destined to develop endometriosis.

In recent years, laparoscopic laser microsurgery has revolutionized the treatment of endometriosis because of more complete and accurate destruction of the endometriotic tissue. This treatment cleans up the reproductive organs by freeing and emptying the pouches of cells, clearing off the surface of the ovaries, opening up the tubes, and vaporizing the endometrial implants.

A woman who does not plan to have children might prefer a radical, but more definitive, surgical cure with a thorough removal of the uterus, ovaries, tubes, and all the endometriotic implants. This treatment, *panhysterectomy*, is likely to result in a permanent cure of endometriosis as long as no endometriotic tissue is left behind. The panhysterectomy is followed by estrogen therapy for relief of the menopausal symptoms that are likely to follow the removal of the ovaries. Women who want to have children usually opt for a combination of medical and surgical procedures to ease pain and restore fertility.

ADENOMYOSIS: A VARIANT OF ENDOMETRIOSIS

Uterine adenomyosis is a benign lesion and a variant of endometriosis. The lining of the uterus invades the wall of the uterus itself and forms nests of endometrial tissue. Adenomyosis leads to abnormally heavy and prolonged menstrual flow, pain, cramps, and infertility in most cases. It is more likely to affect women in the later years of their reproductive life and around menopause.

Adenomyosis, when associated with severe bleeding and pain, is best treated with hysterectomy, unless a woman is close to menopause and chooses to wait until her estrogen level declines naturally and the lesions shrink. The symptoms are likely to vanish as long as she does not take estrogen replacement therapy. Should she plan to take estrogens after menopause because of her susceptibility to osteoporosis or coronary heart disease, or for menopausal symptoms, a hysterectomy might be a better way to treat adenomyosis.

CANCERS OF THE REPRODUCTIVE SYSTEM

Cancers of the reproductive tract—endometrium, cervix, ovary, and vulva—are discovered in about 70,000 women a year in this country, of which 22,000 die from them. Screening and early detection can prevent or cure most of these deaths. The most difficult cancer to detect early, however, is ovarian cancer.

Although diagnosis can be made by your principal physician or gynecologist, cancers of the reproductive system should be treated by a gynecological oncologist, a specialist in cancers of the reproductive tract. He or she should always be included in the discussions of treatment, and should also stand by in the operating room in case more cancer is found. If the cancer is advanced, this specialist should perform the surgery.

Once surgery is performed and lymph nodes and other tissue have been analyzed by the pathologist, treatment with radiation or chemotherapy might be called for.

Ovarian Cancer

This is the most difficult cancer to diagnose early and the most malignant. After uterine (endometrial) cancer it is the second most common gynecological cancer. It will occur in over 25,000 women and will kill 14,500 each year. One woman in seventy develops ovarian cancer in the United States. The risk of getting this cancer is apparently related to the number of ovulatory cycles in a woman's lifetime. For example, women who have never had children would have had more ovulatory cycles than women who had many pregnancies from an early age.

Delayed childbearing, and having had colon, breast, or endometrial cancer, are risk factors for this cancer. The genetic risk factor accounts for fewer than 5 percent of women diagnosed with epithelial ovarian cancer. But hereditary ovarian cancer risk means having two or more first-degree relatives—mother and sister, for example—who had ovarian cancer.

Reduced risk is associated with having used oral contraceptives for five or more years. Pregnancy, breast-feeding, and fewer ovulatory events are also believed to lower the risk.

Familial ovarian cancer is closely linked with familial breast cancer, that is, cancer; members of the families with breast cancer gene 1 and 2 (BRCA1 and BRCA2) are at high risk for ovarian cancer as well as breast cancer.

Symptoms. The reason ovarian cancer is rarely diagnosed early is because the symptoms are so vague. Women might experience a change in bowel habits or feel bloated. Pelvic discomfort might occur. The symptoms are a result of the ovarian tumor pushing on the wall of the colon. Many women think they are only gaining weight and do not seek an explanation for abdominal swelling. Fluid accumulates in the abdomen because of the cancer, and this fluid then seeps into other parts of the body, such as the chest. Often, tumor lesions from the ovaries spread to the liver, the colon, the stomach, or the abdominal wall, and can even metastasize to the lungs, before the cancer is discovered.

There is no effective mass screening for this disease, and even regular pelvic examinations cannot determine signs of this cancer. Transabdominal and transvaginal ultrasound of the ovaries can sometimes detect the difference between malignant and benign masses, but often miss a small tumor that might have already spread.

Treatment. Treatment includes surgery to remove the tumor(s), followed by a course of chemotherapy in an attempt to eradicate cancer cells throughout the body. Surgery depends upon the extent of the disease, but usually means a hysterectomy and oophorectomy (removal of the ovaries), as well as removal of any nearby organs that might be showing signs of cancer. Chemotherapy, which includes very toxic substances such as platinum and taxol that cause severe side effects, produces a remission in about a third of the patients but has only a modest effect on survival.

Prevention. Prevention of ovarian cancer is problematic because we don't know what causes it or how best to detect it early. In women with a family history of ovarian cancer and those with breast cancer, physicians might institute a close surveillance such as performing annual pelvic sonography and various blood tests (CA-125), but even they might not be successful at turning up cancer that has already spread.

Cervical Cancer

Cervical cancer is easily detectable at an early stage, and mortality is preventable through an appropriate pelvic examination and an accurately prepared and analyzed Pap smear. Nevertheless, it was diagnosed in 13,700 women and claimed 4,900 lives in 1998 despite the easy detection at a curable stage because of the failure to perform these examinations. Cervical cancer is the third most common gynecological cancer in this country, and it occurs almost twice as often in young African American women than it does in young white women. After age 65, black women are three times more likely to get this cancer than white women. The death rate is highest among American Indian women, and is also high among Asian Pacific Island Americans. It is believed that these women do not receive regular pelvic exams and Pap smears because in their cultures these tests might be considered shameful. Worldwide, cervical cancer is the most common gynecological cancer.

Having intercourse at an early age and having many sexual partners are both risk factors for cervical cancer. Smoking is also a risk factor. The risk is highest during the teenage years, when cervical cells are forming. A sexually transmitted infection, the human papilloma virus (HPV), can lead to this cancer later in life. This infection (see chapter 9) is transmitted sexually, and most often among men and women who have both had many sexual partners.

An impaired immune response system is also suspected of being a risk factor for this cancer because it strikes women who have HIV infections and who have had kidney transplants. In these individuals, cervical cancer grows fast, like a prairie fire.

Symptoms. There are no symptoms in the early stages, and this is why the Pap test is so important. Once the disease is more advanced, there might be a vaginal discharge, bleeding, or spotting after intercourse or between menstrual periods. Once the disease has spread beyond the cervix, the bleeding can be profuse, the discharge might begin to have an odor, and there might be swelling of the lower extremities and weight loss. Uremia, an endstage kidney disease associated with a toxic condition of the blood, might occur in advanced cases because the tumor spreads to the ureters, causing obstruction to the outflow of urine and shut-down of the kidneys.

Diagnosis. If cervical cells show any abnormality after a Pap test, surveillance is called for, with additional tests in three to six months. If subsequent tests are normal, then annual testing can resume. If the cells are still abnormal, then cervical tissue should be biopsied in one of several possible ways.

The extent of the disease can be determined by a series of diagnostic tests such as CT scan of the pelvis and abdomen, bone scans, chest X ray, and blood tests. If the cervical lesions are known to be large and interfere with the function of the bladder and rectum, then they need to be surgically removed.

Treatment Options. If cervical cancer is discovered and treated early, it is curable. Treatment is either surgical removal of the uterus (hysterectomy) or radiation therapy. If the cancer has progressed to a later stage, and if it involves the adjacent lymph nodes, then surgery, radiation, and possibly chemotherapy are all used in treatment.

Radical hysterectomy and lymphadenectomy, removal of the lymph nodes, is a treatment option for women with small lesions where there is no metastatic disease. These treatments are sometimes used together. It is important to talk with your doctor about which treatment would be best for you.

Cervical cancer is usually treated with radiation therapy of the entire pelvis. This continues for five days a week for four to five weeks (see an explanation of radiation in chapter 17). Side effects of this treatment can include fatigue, frequent urination, diarrhea, and nausea. Medications can help to manage these symptoms during therapy.

The cure rate is about 90 percent with one treatment and 99 percent with two. Follow-up surveillance is critical because recurrence of cervical cancer is usually found within the first two years after treatment. If the disease recurs, further surgery, radiation, or chemotherapy might be needed.

In February 1999, the National Institutes of Health alerted doctors about the results of five studies showing that chemotherapy should be added to radiation therapy as standard treatment for locally advanced or invasive cervical cancer. Chemotherapy makes the cancer cells more vulnerable to radiation and thus, treatment is more effective.

The Pap tests are continued even after a hysterectomy or menopause despite a controversy about their cost-effectiveness after hysterectomy.

Follow-up Pap tests might show abnormalities in about 10 percent of women after treatment, indicating a need for further treatment.

Endometrial Cancer

This cancer of the lining of the uterus—endometrium—will be diagnosed in 32,000 women a year, and will account for 5,600 deaths. It is the most common of the gynecological cancers in the United States, and is curable if detected early. This cancer is rare before the age of 40, but 25 percent of all endometrial cancers occur before menopause.

Mortality and complications of endometrial cancer are relatively easy to prevent because the endometrium can easily be checked for abnormal cell changes. A biopsy of cells can be done in the doctor's office by snipping a piece of tissue from the endometrium. Tissue can also be scraped away in a dilatation and curretage (D&C) without disturbing the rest of the uterus. This way, endometrial tissue can be evaluated for precancerous cell changes so that a preventive course of action can begin.

Risk Factors. Excessive amounts of estrogen appear to be the major risk factor. The estrogen causes hyperplasia of the endometrium, a condition in which the cells lining the uterus grow abnormally. The oversupply of estrogen can be caused by estrogen replacement therapy or by too many fat cells: some fat cells convert inactive adrenal hormones into estrogenlike hormones that stimulate the cells lining the uterus to grow out of control. Simply being overweight increases the risk of endometrial cancer by three times, and being obese increases the risk by ten times. Women who began menstruating early, or who go through menopause later, or who are infertile and do not have children, are at risk. Diabetes, hypertension, hypothyroidism, and gallbladder disease have all been associated with endometrial cancer.

The use of tamoxifen, a synthetic steroid used to treat breast cancer, is also a risk factor. Tamoxifen acts as an anti-estrogen in breast tissue but as a weak estrogen in the endometrium.

Symptoms. Painless postmenopausal bleeding is the most common warning sign. This can be one episode of spotting or profuse vaginal bleeding. Before or during menopause, menstrual irregularities and spotting between periods might occur. Once the disease is advanced it can cause weight loss, urinary retention, and lymphedema (swelling), especially in the legs, which are also at risk for *thrombosis*, or clogging, of the veins.

Diagnosis. An endometrial biopsy can be performed in the doctor's office during a pelvic examination. The tissue taken from the uterus lining is sent to a laboratory for analysis. Transvaginal ultrasound can also help to determine the thickness of the cells of the endometrium and detect abnormalities. In the presence of symptoms, however, this is not enough. A biopsy is also called for.

Treatment. The most common treatment is to remove the uterus, and usually the ovaries as well. Some lymph nodes will be removed also and tested for the presence of cancer cells. During surgery, the entire area will be carefully examined by the physician to see if there appears to be cancer elsewhere. Pelvic radiation and chemotherapy might also be called for.

Follow-up surveillance is critical, and because women with endometrial cancer are at greater risk for breast cancer and colon cancer, patients should be screened for those diseases on a regular basis.

Vaginal and Vulvar Cancer

Cancers of the vulva and vagina are rare. Vaginal cancer is found in women whose mothers took diethylstilbestrol (DES) in the 1950s because they were at risk of losing their pregnancies. This cancer now puts the daughters at risk of losing their pregnancies. It develops around the age of 19, and if it is identified early it is curable with hysterectomy. A registry has been established to keep track of the daughters of the women who took DES. A major lawsuit against the drug company went on for years and was settled in the 1990s.

Vulvar cancer usually strikes women during the menopausal years, and begins as a small growth or lump on one of the vaginal lips. It might itch or cause pain. It is curable if discovered early with a biopsy and removed with a partial vulvectomy, whch involves excision of the growth along with a margin of tissue around it. Lymph nodes in the groin are also removed to be checked for the presence of any cancer cells. If the cancer has spread there, then radiation treatment is necessary.

COMMON TREATMENT PROCEDURES

Many diagnostic procedures can be done in a doctor's office using endoscopic techniques. The hysteroscope is a flexible fiberoptic tube with a light (or video camera or lens) on the end that enables the physician to examine the inside of the uterus. Tiny scalpels, scissors, and other instruments can be inserted through the tube to perform a variety of functions, including taking a piece of tissue for biopsy or removing polyps. Hysteroscopy is used with gynecological procedures in the operating room as well.

Dilatation and Curettage (D&C)

The lining of the uterus is usually removed with this procedure, which can be done under local anesthesia in a hospital. With a speculum inserted through the cervix to dilate the passage, a small sharp instrument like a spoon (a curette) is used to scrape out the lining of the uterus. This is similar to a dilatation and evacuation, which is used for abortions (see page 206).

Polypectomy

Endometrial or cervical polyps can be removed with this procedure. Polyps are small, tubelike growths that project from a mucous membrane. They are commonly found in the uterus and cervix (as well as the nose and rectum), and are most often benign. Polyps in the uterus can cause excessive bleeding and sometimes sterility. Cervical polyps might bleed during intercourse. These polyps must always be removed and checked by a pathologist for the possibility of cancer. Polypectomy is like a D&C, only a hysteroscope is used to locate the polyp, and an endoscopic instrument with a snare at the end removes the polyp and cauterizes the incision.

Myomectomy

Fibroids can often be removed from the uterus with this surgical technique. This is a more difficult procedure than a hysterectomy, because the uterus must be surgically invaded but left in place. Once the fibroids are removed from the uterus, the muscle wall of the uterus is stitched back together.

HYSTERECTOMY: A TREATMENT OF LAST RESORT

In the nineteenth century, many doctors thought all female problems came from the uterus and ovaries. So when there was trouble, they took them out. This would frequently set off an acute sudden premature menopause with severe agitated depression. If a woman had in the past suffered from depression, the sudden and severe menopause led, in some cases, to commitment to an insane asylum. It was not until the later part of the twentieth century that the practice of indiscriminate hysterectomy and oophorectomy diminished.

Although the number of hysterectomies performed by surgeons in this country has decreased enormously, some believe they are still overused. It is still the second most common surgery in women of reproductive age in America. The purpose of a hysterectomy is to treat cancer, fibroids that cannot be medically controlled, or endometriosis. However, hysterectomy has often been used to treat any and all gynecological problems with the thinking "If we remove the uterus, the problems will stop."

After cesarean section, hysterectomy is the most common surgical procedure in the United States. Each year, more than half a million American women undergo this procedure. Hysterectomy is a surgical procedure, therefore it creates a fee for a surgeon (gynecologist). Many surgeons have been quick to remove the uterus from a woman at the first sign of trouble, without bothering to look any further for ways to treat. This is especially true for middle-aged women, because it was assumed their organs were of no further use. The hysterectomy is a staple of the gynecology business. By the age of 60, one in three American women will have lost her uterus to this procedure. The figures are less drastic elsewhere. In Italy it is one in six women, while in France it is one in eighteen.

Pamela became a patient of mine after she had a hysterectomy at the age of 45 that led to serious health problems as well as an inability to achieve orgasm. Pamela had had painful fibroids, and her male gynecologist had decided on hysterectomy. He had advised her that the easiest way to end her suffering was to remove the uterus, which, after all, she no longer needed at her age. After the surgery, the doctor put Pamela on estrogen, but the dosage was too high, and after her breasts swelled and became painful, she stopped taking the estrogen. Pamela became extremely unhappy, and developed disabling hot flashes, sweats, palpitations, and severe insomnia. She decided to find another doctor.

What Pamela's gynecologist had never told her was that he had removed her ovaries. He had also failed to explain that without a uterus she would also be without the uterine contractions that are a pleasurable part of orgasm. He also never bothered to find out just how much hormone replacement therapy she really needed. After a thorough history and physical examination, and careful study of her medical records, I began a program to restore Pamela's physical, emotional, and sexual good health. We started her with half the normal dosage of estrogen and some vaginal estrogen cream. Pamela also found a support group so she could talk with other women who had had unnecessary hysterectomies. Pamela sued her gynecologist and eventually won her case.

The uterus continues to be a vital part of our body's endocrine system. It continues to respond to hormones and continues to create some of its own, such as beta endorphins (our built-in painkillers) and some prostaglandins, which inhibit blood clotting. This loss might explain why women who have had a hysterectomy, even without the removal of the ovaries, are prone to cardiovascular problems such as hypertension.

Because women have begun to resist this surgery, new procedures are now under study and are being developed for treatment of fibroids and irregular bleeding, the most common reasons for hysterectomies. Endometrial ablation (cauterization with laser) is a procedure that is now being investigated as an alternative to hysterectomy.

Removing the uterus should be the treatment of last resort. Unless diseased, our reproductive organs are better left in place for all of our lives, even after menopause. The ovaries continue to produce estrogen throughout our lives, although in lesser amounts. The structure of the uterus and Fallopian tubes is stronger with the uterus kept in place.

When the entire uterus is removed, along with the cervix, it is called a total hysterectomy. Depending on the problem, it can be done in one of several ways.

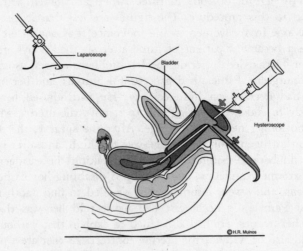

Figure 15. Hysteroscopy and laparoscopy.

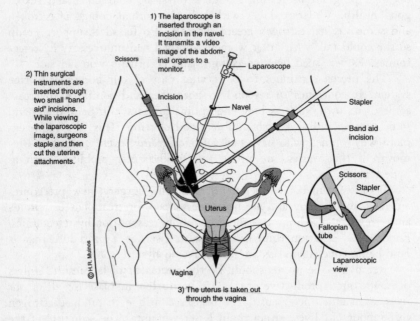

1) The laparoscope is inserted through an incision in the navel. It transmits a video image of the abdominal organs to a monitor.

2) Thin surgical instruments are inserted through two small "band aid" incisions. While viewing the laparoscopic image, surgeons staple and then cut the uterine attachments.

3) The uterus is taken out through the vagina

Figure 16. How a laparoscopic vaginal hysterectomy is performed.

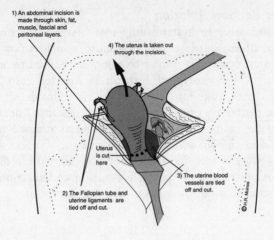

1) An abdominal incision is made through skin, fat, muscle, fascial and peritoneal layers.

4) The uterus is taken out through the incision.

Uterus is cut here

3) The uterine blood vessels are tied off and cut.

2) The Fallopian tube and uterine ligaments are tied off and cut.

Figure 17. How an abdominal hysterectomy is performed.

Subtotal hysterectomy (also called *partial* or *supracervical hysterectomy*) is the removal of the fundus and corpus of the uterus. The cervix is left behind.

Total hysterectomy is the removal of the entire uterus, including the cervix. The ovaries and Fallopian tubes are left behind.

Panhysterectomy (also called *total hysterectomy with oophorectomy*) is the removal of the uterus, the tubes, and the ovaries.

Radical hysterectomy is removal of the uterus, tubes, and ovaries, as well as the lymph nodes and support structures, such as the ligaments.

The surgery can be done through open abdominal surgery and general anesthesia or through the vagina. Side effects of hysterectomy might include premature menopause, loss of sexual sensation, inability to achieve orgasm, depression, and impaired memory.

Ovarian Surgery: Oophorectomy

The ovaries continue to produce estrogen, albeit in smaller amounts, after menopause. Yet they are routinely removed with the uterus in panhysterectomies, as if to sweep away all further problems in the now-retired reproductive organs.

If a man is faced with removal of his testes because of cancer or metastases, a huge fuss is made to assuage his ego, his manhood. Yet ovaries are routinely removed, and if a woman resists, she is patronized.

The side effects can include premature menopausal symptoms, depression, and impaired memory.

The Future: Balloon Ablation

This is an alternative to hysterectomy that destroys the uterine lining but leaves the uterus in place. The procedure, which is now being used in several clinical centers, is similar to angioplasty, used to open clogged blood vessels. A balloon-tipped catheter is inserted into the vagina, through the cervix, and into the uterus. Fluid inside the balloon is heated for a period of time, and that heat destroys the endometrial tissue. Then the balloon is deflated, the fluid is drained out through the catheter, and the whole thing is removed.

This procedure is used mostly for heavy menstrual bleeding (menor-rhagia) that is not caused by cancer, fibroids, or endometriosis. It is also used for patients in whom the D&C was not successful.

IDENTIFYING SEXUAL DYSFUNCTION

We certainly talk about sex more than ever these days, and our consciousness is constantly bombarded by television, billboards, and the admonitions of Dr. Ruth, the famous radio and television sex therapist. Some of us, perhaps, know more about the "technical" part of sexuality than the emotional part. In the past, nobody went to their doctors because they were not interested in sex or could not achieve an orgasm. Ground-breaking research on human sexual inadequacy by the famous team of Masters and Johnson in the 1950s and 1960s first described the physiology of sexual response. Today there are many sexuality clinics and medical specialists who treat sexual dysfunction.

Given the attitudes about sex in this country, it is difficult to determine if a sexual disorder comes from environmental conditioning, religious and cultural taboos, fear, disgust, medications, past sexual abuse, trauma or rape, feelings about one's sexual partner, the partner's insensitive technique, or one's own insecurities and shyness.

It is believed that about 15 percent of women, at some time in their lives, have trouble reaching orgasm. This can be caused by all of the reasons previously mentioned. Or it could be she is taking too many antihistamines. Or she is trying too hard. A woman might not be orgasmic with her partner, but she might be attracted to other men and reach orgasm through masturbation enriched with fantasy. With another partner, she might enjoy sex. Or a woman might have little general interest in sex but be able to respond sexually to her partner because of her intense feelings and interest in that person.

The good news, however, is that if a woman is not having what she perceives to be a satisfactory sex life, she can do something about it. There are many ways to determine the cause—physical and/or emo-

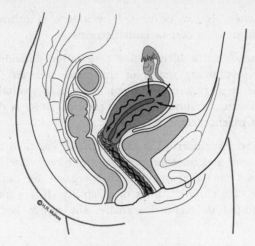

Figure 18. Arousal.

tional—and treat it with a variety of therapies that include medication, psychotherapy, and behavioral therapy.

Failure to Become Aroused
Arousal causes physical changes to the body such as vaginal swelling and lubrication. This is so automatic a response that most women do not think about it. But problems can occur in a few women after childbirth or menopause, when a change in hormonal levels impairs the normal response to sexual stimulation. Estrogen replacement plus tiny doses of testosterone, the male hormone, might restore her sexual response.

Orgasmic Disorder
Once a young woman begins to participate in sex, she might erroneously believe she should have an orgasm the first time—when, in fact, it takes a woman's body more time to adapt and respond to sex. It can take several years before she can achieve satisfactory orgasms, so it is important that women do not immediately think they are unable to enjoy sex, or that they are "frigid," a term no longer used by the medical establishment, because it is not accurate.

Studies have indicated that about a quarter of all women achieve orgasm by intercourse alone, but most need more stimulation—direct, such as touching the clitoris; or indirect, such as the warmth and encouragement of the partner.

Dyspareunia. This is pain during vaginal penetration. It might occur as soon as the vagina is penetrated, or only when it is deeply or roughly penetrated. It can be caused by a lack of lubrication or by pelvic infection, or by a cyst or endometriosis.

Vaginismus. This problem makes penetration difficult and painful because of an involuntary spasm of the pubic muscles. This can be temporary, due to a physical problem, such as a genital abscess, or because of past sexual trauma. Once no physical cause is discovered, it is treated with psychotherapy.

Medical and Psychiatric Causes. Neurological conditions that affect the spinal cord and the core of nerves and blood vessels that control the pelvic region can often interfere with orgasm. So can loss of self-esteem because of a chronic illness or disability. If a woman perceives herself as distorted or maimed sexually, she might not be able to respond.

Substance-Induced Dysfunction. Certain medications, alcohol abuse, and drug abuse can block the sexual response system. Antidepressants, antihistamines, some antihypertensives, and other drugs can have this effect.

The late Dr. Helen Singer Kaplan was one of the leading physicians involved in the treatment of sexual dysfunction; she trained generations of physicians specializing in human sexuality. She also wrote many books that are still in print, and these would be a good place for a woman to begin to look for help.

For referral to a human sexuality professional for help in sexual dysfunction, call the Cornell Human Sexuality Center at 212-821-0700, or Dr. Kaplan's old office at 212-517-9300.

broadenoma

fibroadenoma, a benign tumor that does not invade the neighboring uctures and does not metastasize (does not spread to other structures), a common tumor, far outnumbering cancerous tumors. It is usually al or round and lies deep in the breast.

In the past, the diagnosis of fibroadenoma could not be made unless biopsy was done. Now, a mammogram and ultrasound can help make e diagnosis. Excision is unnecessary unless the doctor suspects another sion underneath the fibroadenoma.

IAGNOSING BREAST CONDITIONS

ost breast lumps are benign tumors, but you cannot be sure of that nless you get a clinical examination and possibly a mammogram and urgical biopsy. Most abnormalities need more than one test. If you can el it, then it needs to be looked at with mammography or ultrasound. it feels like a cyst, then a needle aspiration can be done in the doctor's ffice. (There's more information on breast self-exam on page 246.)

ine Needle Aspiration

reast aspiration is an office procedure in which a thin needle is inserted hrough the skin into the breast lesion to draw out some cells so a iopsy can determine if the lesion is benign or malignant. This is often he first step when evaluating a lump to find out if it is fluid-filled (a yst) or solid. The contents of the syringe are inspected *grossly* (by eye) nd microscopically on a slide for presence of blood or pus and are then ent to the cytopathology lab for study under the microscope. Such esting for malignant cells is 90 to 95 percent accurate, but if it is a umor with closely packed cells, it would be more difficult to aspirate nd analyze. If no malignant cells are found this way, it does not neces-sarily mean there is no cancer.

Surgical Biopsy

Part or all of a lump can be removed surgically to determine whether or not it is malignant or benign. This is an outpatient surgical procedure done with local anesthesia and sedation.

If a tumor is small, the entire tumor will probably be removed. This is an excisional biopsy. If it is a large tumor, a sample might be removed. This is incisional biopsy. Most tumors smaller than three centimeters, about the size of a pearl, will be entirely removed.

Needle-guided Biopsy

When a tumor is extremely small, or if calcifications are discovered in a mammogram, a needle-guided biopsy might be called for. This is also

··17··

Breast Health

The female breast has been the center of great controversy for some years, ever since women decided breast cancer was not getting the atten-tion it needed from the medical establishment. Once women began to make demands, more research dollars became available, the media paid attention to the issue, breast disease specialists and breast centers sud-denly appeared, and more women began to understand the necessity for early detection of breast cancer. The battle over when women should begin getting routine mammograms seems to have been settled.

A Clinical Breast Examination (CBE) by a health professional—doctor or nurse-practitioner—should be a part of your regular health care. Every physician who plays the role of a principal doctor should do a thorough exam of the patient's breasts at least once a year. Not uncommonly, however, the doctor might be concentrating on your other, more visible symptoms and might forget the breast exam. It is appropriate for you to remind him or her of the exam. Also, ask your physician when you should start having mammograms.

The breast is made of glandular tissue, fat, and stroma. *Stroma* is the connective and fibrous tissue in between the lobules of the gland. This is what keeps the glandular tissue together and determines the shape of the breast. The glandular tissue consists of alveoli, cell-lined tiny bubbles that open up to a ductule. A group of alveoli and ductules flow together to form bunches and lead to a larger duct; this pattern repeats itself until fifteen to twenty major ducts are reached that end up as tiny openings at the nipple.

Normally, the alveolus is the major secretory portion of the breast; it is capable of secreting mucus and milk into the ducts, and eventually these secretions appear at the nipple.

The nipple is surrounded by a circular patch that is darker than the rest of the skin, called the *areola*. The nipple includes large sweat

239

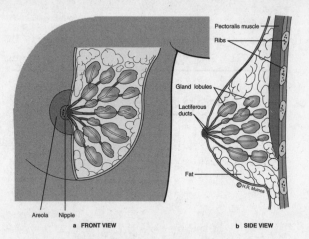

Figure 19. The female breast.

glands and sebaceous (oil-secreting) glands as well as the openings of the major breast ducts. In general, estrogen causes growth of the ducts. After ovulation, when progesterone rises, the alveoli open up and enter the secretory phase.

Before menarche, the breast is dormant, inactive, and the alveoli are collapsed. With each menstrual period, under the influence of estrogen and progesterone, the alveoli open up and branching of the ducts and ductules from which milk is secreted becomes more intricate. Most breast cancers arise from a duct.

FIBROCYSTIC BREASTS

The most common benign condition of the breast is so-called fibrocystic breasts, or *cystic mastitis*. It is characterized by patches of overgrowth of the stroma, fibrous tissue, where the alveoli expand like balloons forming cysts. It is thought by some that perhaps the overgrown stroma encircles the ductules like a tough scar that cuts off the flow of secretion from the alveoli so that the alveolus balloons out. The combination of fibrous and cystic proliferation leads to the name "fibrocystic" condition. In the past, this condition was known as "fibrocystic disease." But we have learned that it is not a disease, merely an overresponse to the rise of estrogen. The condition is common, and it might be a familial characteristic.

Others believe that the fibrocystic process begins in the alveolus, which, under the influence of estrogen, overproduces secretions. These harden, form a plug, and cut off their own exit from the alveolus. The alveolus stretches into a cyst. And the fibrous scar formation is a result

of a secondary inflammatory reaction to the pressure cyst. Whatever the primary reason for this overgro tissue plus cyst formation, the process, because of i patchiness, results in many irregular lumps—so-calle

With each menstrual cycle, under the influenc progesterone, the breast is stimulated; these normal f mone levels lead to fibrocystic changes in the predisp premenstrually that we see the effect of the sustained hormones on the breast. This is why premenstrually tender, painful, and enlarged even without the fibrocy

After the first pregnancy, the fibrocystic condition somewhat, although some soreness might recur periodi ing the premenstrual part of the cycle. The fibrocystic again cause discomfort at the time of menopause, when imbalance of hormones and different ratios of estrogen

Still, many physicians have pragmatically advised fer from premenstrual engorgement and fibrocystic lum ing coffee and tea, avoid chocolate, and abstain from A number of women are satisfied that their symptom on this regimen, but few continue to stick religiously free regimen. Some physicians have also advised their vitamin E (400 milligrams twice a day), vitamin C, an vitamin B_6 (100 milligrams three times a day) before m to prevent engorgement. Although this course of actio supported by research, many women experience relief of breast/premenstrual symptoms. Women who suffer from strual breast engorgement and fibrocystic lumpiness helped by the administration of a small-dose balanced mild tranquilizer.

There are many types of fibrocystic formations. It i that even *the most common, typical, garden variety benign fib carries somewhat increased risk of cancer.* There are, howeve less common lesions in the breast characterized by atypi (overgrowth that can be determined by biopsy) in whi developing cancer—perhaps decades later—is much great

The real problem with the fibrocystic condition is t difficult to discover a new unusual nodule when there are lumps in the breast. Most often the lump of the fibro tender; it might be painful even without palpation. It is might be multiple lumps in both breasts, which is very re multiplicity of lumps speaks for a benign process. Durin up of a patient with fibrocystic condition it is not unusua nodule to disappear and new nodules to appear in the other breast.

an outpatient surgical biopsy, but it is preceded by placement of fine needles into the breast. First, in the radiology department, and under direct mammographic visualization, the lesion is identified on the screen and the coordinates are established. With the patient under local anesthesia, a fine needle can be inserted through the skin into the lesion. Another X-ray picture is taken to ensure that the needle points exactly into the previously identified clump of calcifications. In the operating room, the surgeon, with the help of that film, removes the lesion together with the needle.

Mammotomy

A *stereotaxic* mammotomy is a minimally invasive outpatient procedure that employs a special biopsy needle and X-ray equipment that helps direct the needle accurately into the suspicious area. The local area is numbed with xylocaine. The only incision is a tiny nick in the skin, so there is no scar. The needle is inserted quickly into a breast lesion while rotating around clockwise and taking slices of tissue. At the same time, a vacuum suction removes blood and fluid from the same site. This enables sampling of more tissue from the area of interest than the standard core biopsy, and thus the results are more definitive.

When a tiny area is biopsied in this fashion, it might actually be removed by this procedure, which is why in those cases a tiny metallic clip is left in the breast at the biopsy site for future reference, in case surgery is needed.

WHEN TO GET A MAMMOGRAM

Good breast health necessitates screening for cancer. In this country, as well as most other Western countries, the incidence of breast cancer is on the rise because, as the experts believe, the disease can now be detected in its earliest, perhaps precancerous stages called *ductal carcinoma-in-situ* (DCTS). The other possible reasons are that as women live longer, the breasts are exposed to more toxins in our environment over longer periods of time.

In the United States one woman in eight will develop breast cancer by the time she is 85. While breast cancer is more common in older women, it is usually more aggressive in younger women. In older women the cancer generally grows more slowly and may metastasize less readily.

The controversy over whether or not women should begin screening with mammograms when they are 40 or 50 was settled in a dramatic 1997 capitulation by the National Cancer Institute, which agreed to agree with the American Cancer Society that the tests should begin at age 40. (Actually, high-risk women might need to begin at 35.) The previously recommended age to start mammograms was 50 since mammograms are difficult to read for women below that age. There are many false positives and false negatives, and this makes screening less cost-effective. Everyone agrees, however, that 50 is the age when all women enter the high-risk period.

The American College of Radiology, the American Medical Women's Association, and the American College of Surgery also recommend that a baseline mammography be performed between the ages of 35 and 40 and that annual or biennial mammography be done between the ages of 40 and 49. In women with a positive family history for breast cancer and in women with a suspicious lump, mammography should be done more often and as needed.

Because mammography is not perfect—there is a 15 percent margin for error—any finding needs to be supplemented by a clinical examination. At 51 Monica breathed a sigh of relief when a mammogram did not show any abnormality, even though her doctor had discovered a small lump on the lower part of her left breast, near the ribs. There was a similar lump in the same area of her right breast, but this one was larger and clearly felt like a cyst, which showed up on the mammogram. When Monica reported the mammogram results to her doctor, a woman, the doctor examined Monica's breasts again. Still not satisfied, the doctor urged Monica to have a surgical biopsy of the lump in the left breast and referred her to a breast surgeon. After some resistance from Monica, who did not want to go through any more medical procedures for what was probably benign, the biopsy was done. Monica did indeed have breast cancer, but it was detected early enough to be cured. Monica was eternally grateful for her doctor's insistence that she follow up until the lump was explained.

As Monica's case illustrated, women often will have a cancer that will be missed by mammography. More often it is missed in younger women because their breasts are more dense. Films of younger breasts, with more dense tissue, can be more difficult to read.

Nobody knows for sure how long after the age of 50 screening should continue. Because a breast tumor is more likely to grow slowly the older a woman is, some clinicians feel that after the age of 70 women need a mammogram every two years. Women who take estrogen replacement therapy, however, should continue to have a mammogram every year for the rest of their lives.

Even though nearly 85 percent of cases occur in women over 50 and 30 percent of these deaths can be reduced by mammography in women 50 and older, in 1990 only 40 percent of women over 50 had ever had a mammogram. And the performance of breast self-exam (BSE) had actually declined. Only 40 percent of the estimated 60 million women at risk are referred by their physicians for screening mammography. Failure by the doctor to order a mammogram has already led to malpractice suits.

Women are about eight times more likely to have a mammogram if the physicians talk to them about it during an office visit.

Medicare pays for mammography screening, and at least forty states require insurance companies to pay for mammography as this book is being written.

What to Know About Mammograms

As of 1994, all mammography facilities were required to be accredited by the American College of Radiology. The accreditation seeks to standardize mammography and achieve the highest level of accuracy possible. This means the equipment must be up-to-date and the staff properly trained in breast mammography. Some diagnostic centers do all kinds of X rays, and they are not necessarily proficient at mammography. The newer technology has reduced the radiation exposure drastically and made mammography safer. Standard testing involves taking pictures of both breasts from two angles: from above and from the side. The skill of the technician is necessary to get the proper compression of your breast between the metal or plastic plates while it is being photographed.

Reading a mammogram is not an exact science. Both benign and malignant tumors can show up as masses, calcifications, or densities, so it is critical to have an experienced radiologist—a physician specializing in diagnostic radiology—read your films. If you have previous mammography films, the doctor should compare your new films with those.

Periodic mammograms, clinical breast examinations by trained health professionals, and breast self-examinations form the triple base of screening for breast cancer. Screening is sometimes called the "secondary prevention." In this setting, the secondary prevention identifies early localized disease and prevents complications of spreading cancer. The hope of many women is to be able to exercise primary prevention, which means preventing breast cancer from happening in the first place. Primary prevention is problematic at present. For the effect of diet on breast cancer prevention see below (page 252). The use of tamoxifen and raloxifene for primary prevention is also discussed later in this chapter (page 252).

Other Breast-imaging Techniques

Sometimes, if a mass is unclear on a mammogram, an ultrasound can gather more evidence, especially in younger women with dense breasts. An ultrasound will determine if the mass is filled with fluid, and is therefore a cyst, or if it is a solid lesion, and possibly cancerous. CT scans and MRI are sometimes used to look at the lymph nodes near the collarbone, as well as the chest wall, and are generally done to try to rule out any metastasis of breast cancer.

Scintimammography is a technique employing a radioactive contrast agent (mostly a substance called *technetium-99m sestamibi*) that is injected into the arm vein. From there the contrast agent flows into the breast where it visualizes the highly vascular tumor and its spread, if there is any. A gamma camera picks up the gamma rays emitted by the contrast material and permits the surgeon to focus on the residual tumor. This technique is being tested in several clinical centers as a follow-up of mammogram.

Sentinel node biopsy is another technique being tested during breast cancer surgery as a substitute to removing as many as 20 armpit lymph nodes to ascertain if the tumor has spread. Sentinel node is the first node to which cancer migrates from the breast. A blue dye is injected around the tumor; as the dye flows to the axilla the first blue-stained sentinel node is identified and biopsied. If the node is free of tumor there is no need to remove the remaining lymph nodes under the arm. A new modification of this procedure by doctors from the University of Vermont on 443 patients involves using a radioactive marker instead of a blue dye. The sentinel node is identified through the detection of radioactivity and excised. Both techniques allow surgeons to reduce the number of lymph nodes removed at breast cancer surgery, sparing women pain and the damage to lymph ducts and nerves that often occurs with the standard axillary-node biopsy and that causes chronic fluid accumulation (*lymphedema*) and loss of function in the upper arm. Both procedures are in the experimental stage at present.

BREAST SELF-EXAM (BSE)

Doctors examine many breasts during the course of a year, and even when very accurate records are kept in the chart, it is difficult for the doctor to recognize a change. On the other hand, if you become familiar with your own breasts it will give you the advantage of recognizing anything unusual, like a new lump or a change in the shape of the breast or the nipple. Perform BSE every month at the same time, ideally within the first ten days of your menstrual cycle. If your breasts are large and dense, it will be more difficult to find any abnormalities. Smaller breasts, naturally, are easier to examine.

Breasts need to be examined in two positions—standing and lying down (see Figure 3, page 45). This way you can do a thorough job of it. While you are standing, it is easier to examine the top portion, and when lying down, the middle and underneath portion. Before you examine your breasts, look at them in the mirror. The more you do this, the easier it will be to spot something unusual, such as new puckering, a "valley" or a swelling in the outline of the breast, or a changed position of the nipple.

Stand in a well-lighted place with your hands on your hips. Press your hands against your hips or push your palms together or raise your arms and lock them behind your head. All three maneuvers tense your pectoral muscles and help you visualize abnormalities. Then with your arms over your head see if there is any swelling or puckering anywhere. Raising your arms pulls on the ligaments and might bring out skin changes over masses that are fixed either to the skin or to the ligament. Lower you arm and squeeze your nipple gently to check for any fluid escaping, milky or otherwise.

Lying down on a bed is the best place to do the rest of the BSE. When lying on your back, elevate your shoulder with a pillow and raise that arm above your head. This allows the breast to spread evenly over the chest and makes it easier to detect lumps. Examine your breast with the fingers of your opposite hand. Use your finger flats, not the finger-tips, which would distort the tissue and limit the area of palpation.

I prefer the daisy pattern in the palpation of the breast because it is the most thorough. Think of your breast as the face of a clock—a daisy clock. Place the flats of your fingers at the periphery of the opposite breast at ten o'clock. Press gently on the breast and guide your fingers toward the center of the nipple, along what would have been the minute hand of the clock. Having arrived at the nipple, reverse the direction and move your finger toward what would be eleven o'clock all the way to the periphery and into the armpit. Move on in this clockwise fashion all around the breast. Peel the petals of the daisy until you come back to ten o'clock.

Palpate the outer upper quadrant of the breast twice since this is the most common area for lesions to start. About 60 percent of breast cancers occur in this area. You might inscribe small circles with your fingers as you move them along the radius of the breast. Vary the depth of the palpation so that you can feel the superficial and deeper-lying structures. Use starch powder to prevent sticking of the fingers to the normally moist skin.

Examine your underarms separately. Reach up with the opposite hand high into the armpit and then press down and feel all the structures in the walls of the armpit, the front, the inner, outer, and back walls.

BREAST CANCER STATISTICS

It is estimated that 178,799 new invasive cases of breast cancer will be diagnosed in women in the United States during 1998. Between 1973 and 1990 there was a significant increase in the incidence of breast cancer.

In the 1970s,	1 woman in 20 developed breast cancer in the United States.
In 1983,	1 woman in 13.
In 1989,	1 woman in 10.

In 1991,   1 woman in 9.
In 1994,   1 woman in 8.

Since 1994 breast cancer incidence has leveled off, according to figures released in March 1998 jointly by the American Cancer Society (ACS), the National Cancer Institute (NCI), and the Centers for Disease Control and Prevention.

About 43,500 American women will die of breast cancer, according to the above estimates. Death rates declined significantly since 1990, probably because of general improvement in lifestyles, earlier detection, and better treatment.

In contrast, the incidence of a very early breast cancer and precancerous breast lesion ductal carcinoma in situ (DCIS) has dramatically risen since 1973 when it was 2.2 and 1.7 for every 100,000 white and black women, respectively. The figures increased to 15.5 and 14 per 100,000 for white and black women. This rise was especially steep among women older than 50; from incidence of 6 it went up to almost 50 per 100,000. The increased use of mammography has meant more breast cancer is detected in the very early, precancerous stage and cured before it has a chance to metastasize.

Out of 100 women with a localized breast cancer 92 will survive for at least five years, and some of them will be cured altogether. This is up from 78 percent in 1940, primarily because breast cancer is detected and treated earlier now. When a breast cancer has metastasized to regional lymph nodes, the survival rate is 71 percent. If the cancer spreads to other parts of the body, such as the bones or lungs, only 18 women out of 100 will live five years after the diagnosis.

The growth rates of breast cancer cells vary and so do patterns of metastases. The slow-growing tumors with long preclinical phases offer us an advantage of possible early discovery, either through clinical breast exams by a doctor, or through periodic self-examinations by the patient, or through periodic screening with mammography. When discovered early, the disease has a better prognosis than when it has grown large enough to be discovered accidentally by the patient.

Risk Factors for Breast Cancer

The connection between estrogen and breast cancer is intriguing. Women who start menstruating early and undergo menopause late are at higher risk for breast cancer. By the same token, women who have their ovaries removed before the age of 37, and therefore produce no more estrogen, have less risk of breast cancer.

Nulliparity, having no children, increases the risk threefold, because the exposure to estrogen has lasted longer. There is a high incidence of breast cancer in nuns, for example. Having the first baby after the age of 35 increases the risk four times.

Several studies document an increased risk of breast cancer in women who smoke and in women who consume excessive alcohol.

Many women ask if oral contraceptives and postmenopausal hormone replacement therapy increase their risk of breast cancer. The old-time oral contraceptives that contained a high-estrogen dose were associated with an increased risk, especially in younger women. Some studies suggest that present-day doses of oral contraceptives do not affect breast cancer risk. Oral contraceptives, in fact, decrease the incidence of cervical and ovarian cancer. Several studies have demonstrated, however, that women who develop breast cancer early, before the age of 45, tend to have histories of using oral contraceptives (presumably of present low dose). (See chapter 8 for more on oral contraceptives.)

There is continuing controversy about the breast cancer risks associated with hormone replacement therapy in women after menopause. Short-term use, up to five years, apparently does not change the risk, but long-term treatment, for more than six years, raises the risk slightly, the relative risk being about 1.5 percent. Combined with a positive family history of breast cancer, the risk goes up to 2.5 percent.

Family History

If your mother or sister had breast cancer before menopause or in both breasts (bilaterally), your risk of getting breast cancer rises nine times. Not all women with a positive family history have a familial cancer. After all, with the high frequency of breast cancer in our society there is a good chance of having family members with this disease. We suspect familial breast cancer if there are two or more first-degree relatives with this disease. To prove the cancer is familial and genetic requires the identification of a mutation in the DNA of the women involved, a mutation that is missing from the family members who do not have and will not develop the familial breast cancer.

In the 1990s two breast cancer genes were identified: BRCA 1, responsible for 40 percent of heritable breast cancers, BRCA 2, responsible for 30 percent of heritable breast cancers. Together, these two genes account for about 70 percent of heritable breast cancer. BRCA 1 and 2 are dominant genes, and women in such a family have a 50 percent chance of having inherited the gene and have an 87 percent lifetime risk of breast cancer. A man has a 50 percent risk of being a carrier and of having offspring with that same chance of being carriers.

Race and Ethnicity Factors

The breast cancer gene occurs in 1 percent of Jewish women of Eastern and Central European origin—or one in fifty Ashkenazi Jews. Most American Jewish women are in this group. A controversial study reported in the *New England Journal of Medicine* in 1997 found that the risk to Jewish women with the mutated gene was less than originally thought.

The study, by Dr. Jeffrey Streuwing, a genetic epidemiologist, was done at the National Cancer Institute. The investigators found that mutations in the two breast cancer genes meant the women had a 56 percent chance of breast cancer and a 16 percent chance of ovarian cancer by the time they were 70 years old, regardless of family history. Previous estimates were 85 percent for breast cancer and 60 percent for ovarian cancer.

What made the study controversial, however, was the way it was done. The research team recruited over 5,000 Jewish women and men in the Washington, D.C., area and set up stations at community centers and synagogues. They took blood samples and asked the volunteers for family histories. Critics complain that few people—especially men—would have accurate memories of why a grandmother died, for example. This goes back to an era when few people talked about disease, especially one in a reproductive organ. The test subjects were not informed if they had the genetic mutation until the statistics were compiled.

Many studies are continuing in the Jewish population, and regardless of the amount of risk, it is clear to all that there is high risk. As many as a million Jewish women in this country and in Europe have one of these gene mutations. A Columbia University study reported in the January 1999 issue of the *Journal of Clinical Oncology* suggested that genetic screening for BRCA1 and BRCA2 mutations is beneficial and cost-effective for Ashkenazi women.

The National Cancer Institute reported that *death* from breast cancer has declined among white women in the United States, probably because of earlier detection, but no such decline has shown up for black women under the age of 50. Continuing research should help us understand why there is such a high mortality rate from breast cancer in minority women, especially African Americans. We need more information about race-specific risk and potential differences in tumor biology. Breast cancer in black women, although less common than in whites, is more likely to occur at a younger age and be more lethal. Whether it is more lethal because of late diagnosis or there is a biological reason, we don't know. At Harlem Hospital, in a predominantly black neighborhood of New York City, half of all breast cancers were incurable on admission and only 5 percent were in the first stage; that is, small and contained within the breast (see "The Stages of Breast Cancer" later in this section). The National Cancer Institute's previous decision to forgo screening below the age of 50 would have affected black women disproportionately because breast cancer tends to strike them at an earlier age.

Environmental Factors

The female population of Suffolk County on Long Island has the highest national prevalence of breast cancer. These women banded together and formed one of the most powerful lobbying groups in the breast cancer movement. Their contention was that contaminated groundwater put them at risk, but this was never proven. Some women point to the mass spraying of entire neighborhoods with DDT when they were children in the 1950s and 1960s. There is still no direct proof, although many studies are in progress. A recent study showed no correlation between breast cancer and levels of DDT residuals in the tissues.

Many chemicals are now known to have carcinogenic effects. They include pesticides such as DDT and its relatives; industrial pollutants such as PCB (polychlorinated biphenyls), breakdown products of many plastics, and DES (diethylstilbesterol). Pesticides live in our stored body fat. This is the same as it is for animals and fish. Often, fish and other water life are washed up on the beaches deformed from toxic pollutants in the ocean.

Other Risk Factors
The following substances and conditions have also been found to increase a woman's risk of getting breast cancer.

• Obesity, diabetes, hypertension, smoking tobacco, and uncorrected hypothyroidism all increase the risk; but once corrected, hypothyroidism does not. While Japanese women have lower rates of both breast cancer and obesity, the heaviest postmenopausal Japanese women were at more than double the risk of developing breast cancer when compared with the thinnest, according to the study reported in the January 1999 issue of the *International Journal of Cancer*.

• Immunosuppressive drugs, like corticosteroids, cyclosporine (used in transplantation), methotrexate, and cytoxan (used in chemotherapy), are associated with an increased incidence of many tumors, including breast cancer.

• A history of cancers of the endometrium, colon, ovary, and salivary gland; lymphoma; and leukemia increases the risk of developing breast cancer.

• Women who received radiation and survived Hodgkin's disease are seventy-five times more likely to develop breast cancer than women in the general population. (Older age at the time of radiotherapy and higher radiation dose were associated with significantly increased risk of breast cancer.)

• Having had two or more biopsies for benign breast disease.

• Women with 75 percent or more dense breast tissue, which makes reading mammograms difficult.

• The less common atypical type of fibrocystic breasts increases the risk of cancer two to three times. This difference between the typical and atypical fibrocystic breasts can be established on a biopsy only.

• Cancer in one breast increases the risk of a second primary tumor in the other breast fivefold.

• High bone density, which points to increased lifetime exposure to estrogen, has been associated with increased risk in menopausal women. This is another piece of circumstantial evidence tying estrogen to breast cancer.

All above listed risks account for less than 20 percent of breast cancer. Increasing age is the most significant risk factor.

The Effect of Diet on Risk and Prevention of Breast Cancer

There have been many studies about the effect of animal fat on breast cancer, and there were years of debate, with a great deal of belief that diets high in animal (saturated) fats were a high risk factor. So far, however, there has been no definitive implication for breast cancer as there has been for others such as colon cancer. A recently reported study points to olive oil (*monounsaturated* fat), but not to vegetable oil (*polyunsaturated* fat), as offering protection from breast cancer. Polyunsaturated fats (vegetable fat) offer protection from heart disease.

We do know that high-fat, low-fiber diets are bad for health. Fat clogs the arteries and causes heart disease. Lack of fiber creates digestive problems and leads to colon polyps. It follows that eating well-balanced meals with plenty of fresh fruits and vegetables, and less fats, will keep a person healthier and at less risk for any disease.

However, there are some studies that are looking at particular foods that might be protective. In addition to the olive oil studies, scientists have been studying cruciferous vegetables for some time because they are believed to shift estrogen oxidation toward a "benign" pathway. Cruciferous vegetables are mostly in the cabbage family: Brussels sprouts, broccoli, and all cabbages. Because women who live in countries with high consumption of cabbage had less breast cancer, research was led in this direction.

Some vegetables also contain special estrogenlike substances. These are *phytoestrogens,* and they are found in many vegetables, including soybeans and yams, and also in green tea. Women in the Far East—Japan, China, and Korea—consume large quantities of soybeans in various forms, including tofu and miso soup, and have lower rates of breast cancer. (The men there also have much lower rates of prostate cancer.)

Medications and Prevention of Breast Cancer

Ingestion of aspirin and NSAIDs (non-steroidal antiinflammatory drugs) seems to decrease the risk of breast cancer as it does colon and other cancers. In women at high risk for breast cancer *tamoxifen* (a drug previously used in women *with* breast cancer) was found to prevent breast cancer, the spokesman for the National Cancer Institute announced in 1998. However, tamoxifen use is associated with an increased risk of endometrial cancer and cannot be taken for a lengthy period of time by women with an intact uterus. Preliminary results of a trial indicate protection from breast cancer by the use of *raloxifene*, a new estrogen agonist/antagonist that is not associated with endometrial cancer.

The Stages of Breast Cancer

Once the diagnostic testing and biopsies have been performed, breast cancer is "staged" so you and your doctors will have an idea of how widespread it is and how best to treat it. Staging is based on the clinical examination (clinical stage) and the pathologic findings (pathologic stage). There is a rather elaborate system that takes into account all of the variables of the particular disease to arrive at a stage. Most breast cancer is staged in grades from 1 to 4, and these stages are often broken down into subcategories such as Stage IA or 1B. This is augmented by the TNM system—tumor, nodes, metastasis—to more finely tune the diagnosis. In general the stages break down like this:

Stage I means the tumor is two centimeters or less, with or without fixation to the underlying chest wall; there is no sign of metastasis or lymph node involvement.

Stage II is a breast tumor of more than two, but less than five, centimeters, with or without fixation to underlying fascia, and no sign of metastasis. Lymph nodes might or might not be involved.

Stage III means the disease is locally advanced; that is, it has spread to the nearby lymph nodes but has not metastasized elsewhere. The tumor might be greater than five centimeters, with or without fixation to the underlying fascia.

Stage IV applies to tumors that have spread to other organs far away from the breast, such as the bone, lung, liver, or brain; that is, thus have *"distant metastases."*

TREATMENT FOR BREAST CANCER

In the last several years breast cancer treatment has improved greatly due to more sophisticated diagnostic and surgical techniques, more medical specialists with better experience, better insurance coverage, better reconstructive surgery, and more involvement of the well-informed patient.

Breast conservation, or lumpectomy plus radiation, is becoming the standard treatment for most women with early breast cancer. A study concluded in the 1980s showed there was no difference in survival of women who had undergone lumpectomy (removal of only the lump) and radiation and those who had a modified radical mastectomy (complete removal of the breast). In the past, surgeons preferred to remove the entire breast to be sure they got all the cancer cells—and also because there had been little progress or research in surgical techniques in this woman's disease.

While most (71 percent) of these tumors were treated inappropriately with total mastectomy in 1973, the proportion of those treated with lumpectomy and radiation increased. Still the proportion of cases treated with mastectomy is inappropriately high, particularly in some areas of the country lacking sophisticated treatment facilities and staff. Studies have proved that lumpectomy, followed by radiation and chemotherapy, is just as effective as mastectomy, but often doctors are afraid to risk the chance of leaving a microscopic cancer cell behind.

In the past it was assumed—by male doctors—that older women would not care if their breast was removed, but this discriminatory practice has been corrected. A woman of any age can choose to have her breast removed in order to feel certain that the entire tumor has also been removed. And a woman of any age also has the option of reconstructive surgery, so that her breast can be rebuilt.

Breast conservation is also possible for women with relatively large tumors as long as they have not metastasized. (About 20,000 to 30,000 women fall into this category.) Chemotherapy is used before surgery to shrink the tumor, so that lumpectomy can be performed and the breast saved. Thus, breasts can be saved in an additional 40 percent of women. Chemotherapy used this way is called *neoadjuvant* therapy. Surgery is then followed by additional chemotherapy, known as *adjuvant* therapy. In one study at Georgetown University, 56 percent of women survived and were disease-free five years after a mastectomy. Among women who had preoperative chemotherapy and lumpectomy, 77 percent survived and were disease-free after five years. This procedure holds out hope for breast conservation for many of these patients. However, we cannot ever know if a microscopic cancer has already moved along to some other part of the body, so the question of proper treatment remains controversial.

Surgical Procedures

Following is a brief description of the various surgical procedures in use for breast cancer. Some of these have already been mentioned, but we list them here so you can easily compare them.

• **Lumpectomy** is removal of the tumor and a margin of tissue surrounding it. Five-year survival rates of women with Stage I breast cancer are no different with a lumpectomy followed by breast irradiation than they are after a mastectomy. Whenever possible, the least-mutilating procedure is preferable, but it is not appropriate for all breast cancers.

- **Quadrantectomy** is removal of that quadrant, or quarter, of the breast involved with cancer.

- **Simple mastectomy** is removal of the breast but not all the mammary tissue.

- **Modified radical mastectomy** is total removal of the breast and all axillary lymph nodes, while preserving the pectoralis muscles, to facilitate reconstructive surgery. Modified radical mastectomy was first devised by Dr. Halstead, a breast surgeon, and it has been a standard for treatment of breast cancer since early this century.

- **Radical mastectomy** is complete removal of the breast, pectoralis major and minor muscles, and axillary lymph nodes.

- **Bilateral prophylactic mastectomy** is the removal of both breasts, sometimes performed in women at high risk of breast cancer, such as carriers of BRCA1 or BRCA2 mutations. It can significantly reduce the incidence of breast cancer, although it does not completely get rid of all breast tissue.

Lymphadenectomy

Removal of lymph nodes under the arm (axillary nodes) on the same side as the affected breast is necessary in order to find out whether the tumor has metastasized, as this influences subsequent treatment. Removing these nodes is usually done while the lumpectomy or mastectomy is performed in surgery.

New techniques of diagnosing the lymph nodes are being developed that will allow for testing the nodes under the arm without surgery. This involves injecting a dye and radioactive sulfur into the pathway the tumor would take to reach the first, or sentinel, lymph node. A probe like a Geiger counter is then used to track the dye. If it produces beeps, the single node is then removed in a simple surgical procedure. If that first node is cancer-free, then it is highly likely the others will also be cancer-free. If the node is positive for cancer, then the remaining underarm nodes would be removed with the traditional surgical technique.

If lymph nodes are positive for cancer, adjuvant treatment with chemotherapy or tamoxifen, or both, might be prescribed.

Reconstructive Breast Surgery

Many women who have had a mastectomy choose to have their breasts reconstructed by a plastic surgeon as soon as possible, and this procedure is always planned in advance and is often begun at the same time as the mastectomy. Some women choose to have their other breast removed

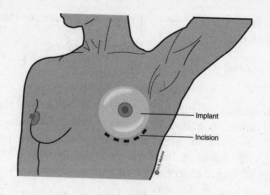

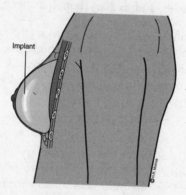

Figure 20. Reconstructive breast surgery.

as well, not only to reduce the risk of another primary cancer but so that reconstruction can give them two perfectly matched breasts.

Most surgeons feel that the reconstruction after a mastectomy should be delayed so that the skin being approximated will have a chance to stretch and adjust before the prosthesis is introduced. When reconstruction is done simultaneously, the tightness of skin might be painful and conducive to the formation of a fibrous capsule around the implant. There is also the psychological aspect of delaying the reconstruction to consider. Women see the immense improvement after a delayed reconstruction and are more satisfied.

The initial stage of surgery is the implant, a saline-filled plastic bag or the patient's own fat tissue from the abdominal wall. After this surgery heals, a nipple and areola are fashioned out of the patient's groin skin. Only salt water and the patient's own fat implants are used. Silicone had been used since 1962 for breast augmentation and for breast reconstruction. Since 1992, the question of whether silicone-gel-filled breast implants cause connective tissue disease and symptoms has been a focus of controversy. In 1992, the FDA banned the use of silicone-gel-filled breast implants except in clinical trials. There is overwhelming evidence, however, from many epidemiological studies that there is no increase in the incidence rate of presumed "collagen disease" symptoms among women who had the silicon gel breast implant over controls.

If reconstructive breast surgery is not done skillfully, there could be complications, such as infection and tight scar tissue around the implant, which would be difficult to fix. Also, if you are going to have chemotherapy, you need to consider immediate reconstruction after surgery, or else you will have to wait until the course of chemotherapy— perhaps several months—is completed.

If you choose reconstructive surgery, it is very important to be well informed and do considerable research before making up your mind. Ask your doctor, or check your library, for the latest studies about breast implants and reconstructive surgery following breast cancer. Ask your doctor, or check with a breast cancer support group, for the name of a woman who has recently had reconstructive surgery. Talk with her about her experience and ask if you can see her breasts, so you will know what to expect.

Radiation Therapy

Radiation therapy usually begins soon after the surgical scar is healed, and its goal is to kill any remaining cancer cells in the area of the surgery. This is meant to mimic what a mastectomy would do. Studies have shown lumpectomy and radiation to be as effective as mastectomy in similar cases.

Find a radiation center that treats lots of breast cancer patients, and where the technology is up-to-date. Modern radiation treatment is vastly improved, and the exposure to radiation is safer than in the past. You want to be treated in a center where your radiation oncologist works with a physicist and a docimetrist who use computers to confine the radiation to the precise area of the breast that needs to be treated. Technicians will measure and calculate, then mark your breast with tiny tattoos to indicate the field for the radiation beam. Then you will be fitted for a cradle that will hold your body in place on the table so that each day when you come for a treatment, the beam will reach the exact same treatment area on your breast.

Treatments are given five days a week, usually for about five weeks. The treatments are painless, and the usual side effects might be a feeling of fatigue and some redness of the skin. Report these to your doctor, who will probably prescribe a gentle cream to soothe the skin on your breast and advise you to take a nap during the day or to go to bed earlier. Most women continue with their normal work and family schedules during this treatment.

Lumpectomy plus radiation has a cosmetic advantage: The general shape of the breast is not changed. The redness from radiation disappears within a few months, although occasionally some pigmentation persists. So cosmetically it is a better result. The disadvantage is that radiation treatments require daily trips to the treatment center over the following five to seven weeks.

Chemotherapy

Chemotherapy is the use of "chemicals" to treat a disease. What we know as chemotherapy for cancer involves the use of cytotoxic drugs—drugs that kill cells. This means the medications kill the cancer cells as well as many of your other cells. The normal cells grow back, but it is hoped that the cancer cells die forever. The cytotoxic drugs have a predilection for aggressive cells. This is why cancer cells, which multiply rapidly, are killed preferentially. Because of this cell death, the side effects can be severe, which is why there is loss of hair, nausea, and vomiting.

If breast tumors metastasize to the axillary lymph nodes, chemotherapy is needed, because it is a systemic treatment that can kill all cancer cells anywhere in the body. It is not known if chemotherapy in women with node-positive tumors truly cures them of cancer or simply postpones the appearance of metastatic disease. Some workers in the field believe, however, that adjuvant chemotherapy actually helps eradicate microscopic clusters of malignant disease elsewhere in the body and is, therefore, curative.

A course of chemotherapy for breast cancer can take several months, depending upon the extent of the disease, the medications used, and the stage of the disease. There will still be side effects such as nausea and loss of hair, but these conditions are much less potent than they used to be. Medications have been developed to combat the nausea, and creative hair styling, and even wigs, can be used if your hair gets thin or falls out.

Chemotherapy is usually given in the office of the oncologist by intravenous injection. The side effects might be strong for the day or two right after treatment, but they generally subside. Treatments might be weekly or every three weeks, depending on your particular treatment.

Most women are able to continue their lives by adjusting their schedules to accommodate the treatments. For example, having a treatment on Friday would mean you have the weekend to recover before going back to work on Monday.

Recent development of Herceptin targeted against an "oncogen"— a cancer virus that becomes part of the cancer cell DNA—has raised hopes of eventually controlling even widespread breast cancer. This treatment is still experimental.

Hormone Therapy

Women who have lumpectomies might follow that surgery with five years of hormonal therapy with tamoxifen. Tamoxifen is a synthetic substance that acts as an anti-estrogen (estrogen antagonist) on the breast tissue and is associated with longer survival of patients with breast cancer. Tamoxifen acts like estrogen on other tissues. Like estrogen, it prevents bone loss and lowers cholesterol, thus protecting you from coronary heart disease. Unfortunately, tamoxifen also acts like estrogen on the lining of the uterus. It can cause overgrowth, polyps, and occasionally endometrial cancer. It is not unusual for women who take tamoxifen to develop abnormal vaginal bleeding or polyps on the endometrium. This might require a hysteroscopy or D&C. Periodic surveillance is required while taking tamoxifen, such as transvaginal sonograms to carefully monitor the endometrium.

Occasional nausea, gastrointestinal discomfort, and mild hot flashes might be present when beginning the therapy, but they usually disappear.

In general, estrogen-receptor-positive tumors have a better prognosis and respond well to either tamoxifen or chemotherapy. In some younger patients, both therapies are used simultaneously. In general, but not always, younger women do better on chemotherapy; postmenopausal women do better on hormonal therapy.

Some physicians believe that if the tamoxifen protects against breast cancer recurrence it should be continued indefinitely. Others believe that the risk of endometrial cancer is too great with prolonged use. In a 1997 issue of the *Journal of the National Cancer Institute*, the results of one study indicated that there was no appreciable benefit to taking tamoxifen for more than five years. Women who took the drug for ten years did not survive any longer than those taking it for five years. At present, most physicians prescribe tamoxifen for five years.

Pharmaceutical companies are developing new estrogen antagonists that do not have an agonistic effect on the endometrium. One of these is raloxifene, produced by the Eli Lilly Company and approved by the FDA as Evista.

YOU CAN BEAT BREAST CANCER

Ethel's mother had two mastectomies, at ages 45 and 55; her sister at 42; and her maternal aunt at 48. This kind of family history was consistent with a genetic mutation, either breast cancer gene 1 (BRCA-1) or breast cancer gene 2 (BRCA-2). Ethel began monthly breast self exams at age 30, and biennial mammograms at 40. She was 48 when she first saw me. An accomplished artist and the happily married mother of two daughters, she was enjoying tennis and hiking. Her menstrual periods had been waning for the last two years.

Her mammogram visualized an abnormal cluster of calcifications in her left breast. And excisional biopsy with axillary lymph node sampling revealed an eight-millimeter (less than a third of an inch) tumor that was estrogen-receptor-positive, and no involvement of any of the lymph nodes. Because of the small size of the tumor and the negative nodes, Ethel was an ideal candidate for lumpectomy with radiation. But because of her family history she was worried about other areas in her left breast and decided on modified radical mastectomy. At the time of the mastectomy, a skillful plastic surgeon fashioned an implant from the skin and fat of her abdomen and inserted it into her left mastectomy area. Subsequent examination of the excised breast revealed multiple precancerous lesions (*cancer-in-situ*). Ethel decided then to undergo the simple mastectomy of her opposite breast. With simple, the breast tissue is removed but all muscles and ligaments are left intact. That right breast tissue was negative for any tumor or precancerous lesions.

Ethel healed fast. Because of the small size of the tumor that was estrogen-receptor-positive, she was placed on tamoxifen for five years and not chemotherapy. She resumed all her activities, won a number of amateur tennis contests, and walked the Appalachian trail. I saw her last fifteen years after her surgery, and no disease was present. She was happy, planning for her husband's retirement from the publishing business. Her two daughters have been pursuing the same breast surveillance that has been so successful in their mother.

Because of her ominous family history Ethel chose at the time modified radical mastectomy. However, many women choose lumpectomy with equally successful outcome on long follow-up. As long as the axillary nodes are not involved the prognosis nowadays is good provided the woman had followed the mammogram surveillance prior to the discovery of the cancer. Even having positive lymph nodes is not a death warrant these days. Several of my patients have survived many years after the surgery and adjuvant therapy for breast cancer with positive nodes. Some of them are still alive and some died of unrelated causes.

WHO TREATS BREAST DISEASE?

Breast cancer was traditionally discovered by gynecologists, and mastectomies were then done by general surgeons.

Today there are specialized breast treatment centers in most major hospitals, and surgeons who do only breast surgery. It is very important to get treatment, and certainly surgery, by a specialist who sees and treats many cases of breast cancer and who is up on all the latest information and treatment techniques. If you can, try to get treatment at such a place, often associated with teaching hospitals in the larger metropolitan areas. Ask your principal physician to refer you to such a center if you have breast disease.

Treatment for breast cancer includes a team of a surgeon, a chemotherapist, and a radiation oncologist. Your principal physician will also be involved in your care if you have other conditions that need to be monitored.

There is a great deal of good information available now about breast cancer treatment. There are many books and Internet web sites where you can find out more about your options. Some of these are listed in Appendix 1.

There are also many support groups, which is where many women go after being diagnosed to find out what other women in the same situation did. It has been shown that women who participate in support groups for breast cancer live longer than those who do not.

Follow-up Care

Once your breast cancer has been treated, lifelong surveillance is necessary because you are at greater risk for recurrence. However, most women who had their cancers detected and treated early survive into old age. You will need a mammogram every six months for the first two years following surgery, and then annually. And checking your own breasts monthly should be as normal now as brushing your teeth. Refer back to page 246 for information about how to do this.

·· 18 ··

The Female Immune System

The immune system is our own personal National Guard. Units of troops have very specific assignments as they protect us from foreign invaders such as bacteria, fungi, viruses and internal invaders such as altered cancerous cells. It is a complex system of thousands of interactions, hundreds of obscure cellular networks, and dozens of cell types responsible for encoding our response to disease, determining when or if we get sick, and deciding how long we stay sick.

The immune system is unlike any other human system in its need for absolute synchronization. Immune cells are everywhere. They are in the thymus, in the brain, the lymph channels and nodes, the spleen, and the liver. When something upsets the body's equilibrium, such as disease or stress, the system is called upon to defend us. In certain circumstances, however, this defense system can be rendered helpless.

When we are children, we catch colds from one another easily because our immune systems are still developing and are not strong enough to protect us. In old age, the immune system weakens and once again leaves us more vulnerable to infections. If you were born without a functional immune system because of a genetic defect, you would need to live in a totally germ-free environment to survive, like the "boy in the bubble" stories we read about in *Life* magazine many years ago. An immune system deficiency can occur after the system itself is attacked by an infection or virus or disease. The HIV virus, for example, destroys the important cells of the immune system so that there is no protection from other infections.

Allergies are caused by a certain malfunction of the immune system. And when the immune system misguidedly attacks the cells of the body itself, it causes autoimmune diseases such as lupus or rheumatoid arthritis.

The immune system will attack a transplanted organ such as a heart

262

or a kidney because the immune system recognizes this invader as foreign and mounts an attack-and-destroy action. Medications are used to override the immune system and prevent this.

The female body, however, has the special ability to modulate the immune system during pregnancy to prevent rejection of the fetus, which, in a sense, is a partially foreign invader because it contains DNA from another person. This special ability to protect the fetus implies a system that is more complex and elaborate than that of a man. On the other hand, women suffer more autoimmune disorders than men, which may be due to the enhancing action of estrogen.

HOW YOUR BODY PLAYS "DEFENSE" AND "OFFENSE"

Our skin is our first immune system line of defense, then the mucous membranes, tonsils, and adenoids. If we inhale bacteria, viruses, or fungi, the macrophages in the nasal mucous membranes, and the sweeping action of the cilia in the bronchial tubes, go into defensive action. If these fail to protect us from offending germs inhaled or ingested, the lymphatic system takes over. This is a system consisting of lymph nodes, spleen, and lymphatic vessels—like the cardiovascular system consists of blood vessels. In fact, the lymph system works in concert with our veins as it drains most of the organs. At strategic points along the route of lymphatic drainage from the organs there are lymph nodes, which are like filters that drain the system and catch the garbage. The nodes contain lymphocytes, special types of white blood cells that kill germs.

The way the immune system responds to threats is by encounter, recognition, activation, deployment, discrimination, and replication. It encounters the invader, recognizes the invader for what it is, activates relevant fighting cells, deploys them at the site of invasion, discriminates between the invader and the innocent bystanders, and produces lethal weapons (antibodies). Units of cells and networks scattered around the body have diverse functions.

T cells, from the thymus gland, have a variety of jobs. Some direct and manage the immune responses, and others attack cells that are infected or cancerous. These are the killer T cells. Once an antigen (invader) has been recognized as foreign by the memory T cells, the killer T cells destroy it. Then the T-helper cell stimulates antibody production by the B-cells and the suppressor T cells modulate and stop the response once the danger is over, while the memory T cells keep the memory of the response and activate it if the invasion recurs. T cells must get close to the invader in order to destroy it. They are unlike the B cells in this way.

B cells come from the bone marrow. Each B cell makes a specific

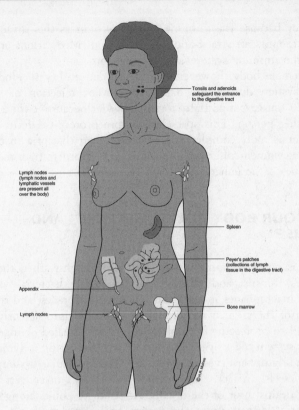

Tonsils and adenoids
safeguard the entrance
to the digestive tract

Lymph nodes
(lymph nodes and
lymphatic vessels
are present all
over the body)

Spleen

Peyer's patches
(collections of lymph
tissue in the digestive tract)

Appendix

Bone marrow

Lymph nodes

Figure 21. The immune system.

antibody against a new antigen in order to render the antigen powerless. These antibodies can interact only with the antigen for which they were designed. The B cell is activated by the T-helper cell.

Lymphokines are substances that are released by the various cells of the immune system to target other cells in the system. Lymphokines are the telephone lines that facilitate their communication, interaction, and networking.

Macrophages are reconnaissance cells, the first to spot an invader. They are the metal detectors in the airport, screening every piece of baggage and every person who comes along. The macrophage will engulf and digest the foreign invader, then push its digested components to the surface like a flag and present it to the T cells, either the "naive" T cells if this is a new attack, or to the memory T cells if it is a recurrence. Macrophages are our first line of defense. They encounter, signal, and activate the immune system, but without the T cells and B cells, macrophages would be unable to fight off invaders.

Antibodies are proteins manufactured by the activated B cells that have a perfect fit for the invader. They hook onto the antigen, immobilizing it, making the whole complex digestible by still another group of cells, the scavengers in the spleen, liver, and lymph nodes. Antibodies frequently persist after the first attack, and their response is more efficient with a recurrent invasion. Antibodies give us short- or long-term protection. For example, we get mumps only once and are protected ever after. When we breast-feed our babies, we pass along our antibodies, which give their immune systems more protection.

Cellular Memory

Whenever an antigen appears again, the memory cells activate the entire response, including the antibody response, more quickly than with the first attack. This is the principle of immunization. Immunization is not always perfect; sometimes a foreign invader is down but not out. Chicken pox, for instance, is caused by a virus that can remain after the illness, dormant in the body, and might even emerge as shingles (Herpes zoster) years later in adulthood. The herpes simplex virus can also stay in the body forever and flare up now and then.

ALLERGIC ASTHMA

Allergies can cause us to get a rash, a runny nose, or a full-blown attack of asthma—or, if they are severe, we can go into shock. This happens when someone is stung by a bee or gets a shot of penicillin without knowing she is allergic to the drug, which is made from mold, a common allergen.

An allergen is an antigen that provokes the allergic response. If you breathe in cat dander or dust mites, for example, your immune system sees it as a threat and goes into action—or overkill—which causes a great deal of discomfort. The antibody response to an allergen frequently involves an increase in a special group of antibodies known as the immunoglobulin E (IgE) rather than the usual antibodies, known as immunoglobulins M and G (IgM and IgG). Allergy is a misguided hyperactive response of the immune system when it recognizes a minor threat, such as a speck of dander or a mold spore, as a deadly enemy.

Histamine and other more potent irritants such as leukotrienes are released by the union of the allergen with its corresponding IgE. This provokes an inflammatory response that causes the bronchioles to constrict (as in the case of asthma) or the blood vessels to dilate, and might cause a runny nose and watery eyes. More than 40 million people in this country suffer from hay fever, or allergic rhinitis and conjunctivitis. Such allergies might begin in childhood or during the adult years up to about 45, then decrease with age.

Asthma, on the other hand, might not go away. Asthma is most commonly caused by a reaction to an allergen, but it can be caused by exercise as well (see page 76). Asthma is a condition that causes the airways to become inflamed and narrowed. It can be chronic or occasional. It is currently thought that inflammation of the bronchioles plays a major role. This has led to treatment with anti-inflammatory drugs that also counteract the immune system responses. In general, more boys suffer from asthma in childhood than girls, but women are more likely than men to develop asthma in adulthood, middle age, and old age. Nearly twice as many women than men die from asthma.

The American Lung Association reports that there are 15 million asthmatics in this country, and one third are children under 18. The number of cases has risen by two thirds since 1980, with a disproportionate increase in lower-income Hispanic Americans and African Americans. The death rate in the United States from 1989 to 1991 was approximately 1.3 men per 100,000 population. This number jumped to 2.7 for women. The reason for the difference is unknown.

Asthma is affected by the waxing and waning of hormones, and often strikes during puberty. Some believe asthma attacks in women are precipitated by a drop in estrogen levels before menstruation, but studies have not backed this up. There is no real difference in this except during pregnancy with some asthmatic women. As many as 4 percent of pregnancies are complicated by asthma. (For more information about this, refer back to page 203.)

Asthma can be caused by any number of allergens, including dust, mold spores, animal dander, ragweed, pollen, and even certain foods such as shellfish or nuts. A recent study pinpointed cockroach droppings as a major cause of the increasing incidence of asthma in children of the inner cities.

Medical Treatment for Asthma

Avoidance of the allergens is part of the treatment, but this is not always possible or enough. There are airborne allergens, for example, such as pollen, that we cannot always avoid. Treatment by a physician—internist or pulmonary specialist—is necessary to monitor asthma, and to prescribe effective drugs. Because asthma can be a chronic disease, comprehensive asthma treatment should include periodic lung function tests in order to assess the extent of lung dysfunction.

The classes of drugs used in asthma are anti-inflammatory, bronchodilators, and antibiotics. Many of these drugs are usually inhaled, so they cause fewer side effects in the rest of the body. Steroids (cortisone analogs) such as prednisone are used to combat inflammation in severe cases. Inhaled steroid preparations are used to prevent or to keep inflammation at a minimum, but these have recently become controversial because of their implication in the formation of cataracts in some children as well as adults after long-term use. Bronchodilators that relax the surrounding muscles, and widen the airways, are commonly used to relieve symptoms of an attack. A new group of drugs for asthma has recently been cleared by the FDA. These are *anti-leukotrienes,* which work against the potent irritants that are released from the cells as a result of the exposure to allergens.

AUTOIMMUNE DISORDERS: A WOMAN'S PROBLEM?

Autoimmune diseases are the result of some unknown stimulus causing the immune system to attack itself. The body mistakenly creates antibodies and sends killer cells after its own organ tissue, cells, or membranes that it believes are foreign invaders. Nobody knows what provokes the body to start producing autoantibodies. The current thinking is that a genetic predisposition leaves a person susceptible to the development of an autoimmune disease such as lupus, multiple sclerosis, scleroderma, rheumatoid arthritis, juvenile diabetes, and Crohn's disease.

Recent studies are leading investigators to what they see as "molecular mimicry." This is when one of the body's own structures has a similar biochemical structure to some of the invaders that the immune system has learned to attack. A mishap might occur when the immune system makes a mistake and regards as foreign the body's own proteins and antigens. Thus, the immune system attacks itself. The 1996 Nobel Prize for medicine went to Peter Doherty and Rolf Zinkernagel for their discovery of how the immune system recognizes virus-infected cells. It is hoped this new knowledge will help us understand how the immune system also recognizes invading foreign cells like cancer and the body's own molecules that cause inflammatory diseases such as rheumatoid arthritis, lupus, and other auto-immune diseases.

But the big question is: Why does this happen more often in women? Perhaps estrogen stimulates the T cells, which then go on their rampages against foreign bodies—and themselves as well. Autoimmune disorders are more common in female Scandinavians than African women, but in this country white and black women have about the same rate of incidence.

SYSTEMIC LUPUS ERYTHEMATOSUS (SLE)

The classical example of an autoimmune disorder is systemic lupus erythematosus (SLE), which affects primarily young adult women and children of both sexes.

There is a strong familial component in many lupus cases, and affected members of the family might also suffer from other autoimmune disorders. If one identical twin develops lupus the other twin has a 58 percent chance of developing lupus or a related autoimmune disorder.

An abnormal gene that predisposes someone to lupus is not enough to produce the disease. An infection of some sort, or exposure to a chemical or a physical agent such as sunlight or a drug, is needed to trigger production of the autoantibodies.

The lupus autoantibodies, directed at many cells and organs, can show up in two or more body systems. Joint pains (*arthralgias*) might occur alone or with skin lesions, inflammation of the heart (*myocarditis*), and inflammation of the heart's covering membrane (*pericarditis*). Pleurisy and/or pneumonia with cough, chest pain, and shortness of breath are also symptoms. Neuropsychiatric symptoms, such as seizures, periodic muscular weakness, and mood changes, can occur in about two thirds of lupus patients and lead to misdiagnosis of multiple sclerosis or a neurosis. Lupus symptoms can come and go in cycles. It is difficult to predict what might precipitate a bout of lupus, and impossible to be certain in retrospect that something did. This is another reason it is often misdiagnosed.

Sunlight or sun exposure has been known to precipitate a lupus attack in a susceptible person. A 17-year-old patient of mine with fair skin and freckles had always been warned by her mother to avoid too much sun, but she went to the beach one day with her friends. Two days later, Alice had a rash across her nose and cheeks in the shape of a butterfly. She assumed it was sunburn even though it did not fade for three weeks. During that time she did not feel well, but she ascribed it to having caught a chill sitting around in a wet bathing suit. Eventually, she was well again and forgot the episode until ten years later, when she was immunized for rubella as part of a public health campaign for employees in the hospital where she worked as a secretary. Alice submitted to the rubella immunization gladly since she planned to marry soon and start a family. A few weeks after the vaccination, she developed severe pain in her hands, wrists, knees, and ankles. Even the joints in her jaw hurt. The hospital doctor told her to take Motrin, which helped somewhat, but soon Alice was running a low-grade fever and feeling sluggish.

When she came to see me I noticed a faint pinkish rash on her face and asked if she had ever had such a rash before. This is when she recalled the long-ago "sunburn" after her day at the beach. That rash, like this one, was shaped like a butterfly with the body of the insect over the nose and the wings spreading across the cheeks. This butterfly rash is characteristic of lupus. In all probability, Alice had lupus. I concentrated on questioning her about possible exposures to substances that elicit immune antibody response. Except for the remote sunburn and the measles vaccination, there had been none.

Alice's brother had Crohn's disease, an inflammatory bowel disease, and her maternal aunt had hypothyroidism, both indicative of immune system malfunctions. Alice's blood tests revealed anemia, a mild decrease in white blood cells, and an elevated sedimentation rate, which is frequently associated with immune response. Another blood test, the antinuclear antibody test (ANA), was positive for lupus. Antinuclear antibodies are usually present in large amounts in women with lupus, although smaller amounts can be found in people with other autoimmune disorders and even in a small proportion of completely normal individuals. Urine (and blood) is analyzed for kidney malfunction, which could be a life-threatening complication of lupus.

Lupus can cause arthritis that appears much like rheumatoid arthritis. However, the arthritis of lupus is not destructive and seldom results in joint deformities. Until the use of steroids, lupus was almost uniformly fatal. Fortunately, therapy has changed significantly the natural history of that disease

Treatment for Lupus

Treatment for lupus depends on the severity of the disease and which part of the body is involved. Nonsteroidal anti-inflammatory drugs (NSAIDs) such as Motrin are used for mild cases of muscle and joint pains, and fever. Antimalarials are also used for mild and moderate cases. Corticosteroids, cortisonelike chemicals, are the mainstay of therapy for moderate to serious cases, but must be carefully controlled by an expert in treating lupus. Cytotoxic drugs (drugs that kill cells) are used for very severe cases, especially if the kidneys are involved.

A rheumatologist is usually called in to treat lupus. This is an internist with advanced training and certification in autoimmune diseases such as lupus, rheumatoid arthritis, and scleroderma, as well as other nonautoimmune conditions involving the musculoskeletal system such as osteoarthritis and osteoporosis. Together with a rheumatology consultant, I treated Alice with an antimalarial medication used for early lupus in mild-to-moderate cases. Alice began to feel better. Joint pains ceased, the rash faded away completely, and her fever subsided. We monitored Alice carefully for any side effects to the medication such as eye involvement and rash. Such surveillance was especially important when she became pregnant because lupus flare-ups are common then. During pregnancy lupus frequently becomes more severe because antibodies that are directed at various components of cell membranes might cause generalized clotting throughout the body—at which point the prognosis is grave, even if the pregnancy is terminated.

After eight months the medication dosage was tapered off until it could be stopped. It is important to monitor for resurgence of lupus and its symptoms. Fortunately, Alice's lupus never progressed beyond the first presentation. After a while even her ANA test became negative.

Once diagnosed with lupus, it is important to avoid excessive sun exposure as well as any injections containing "foreign protein" such as allergy shots and most vaccinations. These foreign proteins can perhaps act as antigens stimulating the production of antibodies. Blood transfusions, especially, must be avoided since they are replete with foreign antigens.

RHEUMATOID ARTHRITIS

The term *arthritis* refers to inflammation of a joint or joints. *Arthros* means "joint" or "articulation," and *itis* means "inflammation." Therefore, arthritis does not refer to bones or to muscles, but rather to the connection between the bones. A pain in your forearm does not mean arthritis, but a pain in the shoulder, elbow, wrist, or finger joints could. If there is no inflammation in the joints, it may be defined as *arthralgia*, or pain in the joints. If there are signs of inflammation such as swelling, heat, pain, and redness, then the process is arthritis. Rheumatoid arthritis is a serious, painful, crippling, systemic, and usually progressive disease that shortens a woman's life span. While a few men get rheumatoid arthritis, it is overwhelmingly a woman's disease. Rheumatoid arthritis, unlike osteoarthritis, affects younger women between 30 and 50.

Although the cause of rheumatoid arthritis is not known, most researchers consider this chronic, polyarthritic (involving many joints), symmetrical systemic disease to be caused by an autoimmune process. Autoantibodies form in the blood and attack the synovial cells, the lining of the joints, causing inflammation, swelling, pain, and erosion of contiguous bones. The lining of the joints, cartilage, then bone, becomes inflamed.

This disease affects 2 percent of the population and increases with menopause. The activity of the disease is higher when estrogen is low. Pregnancy causes improvement, but the condition flares up six to eight weeks postpartum. So, while there is a respite during pregnancy, there is also a higher rate of spontaneous abortions and death of the baby before or after birth. The disease can be sporadic or progressive until it immobilizes.

Women with rheumatoid arthritis are subject to premature heart disease and osteoporosis, both of which might be caused by long-term treatment of the disease with corticosteroids. The most ominous complication of rheumatoid arthritis is not the pain—which may be considerable—and not the swelling, fatigue, or weight loss. It is the development of joint deformities that result in disability and immobility. These deformities interfere with getting around, going to work, even with getting dressed.

Rheumatoid arthritis is different from *osteoarthritis* (see page 409), which is not a systemic disease. Osteoarthritis is the common wear-and-tear, traumatic variety of arthritis affecting middle-aged and elderly individuals. Osteoarthritis is usually asymmetric and targets joints that are more frequently used. The morning stiffness of osteoarthritis usually disappears within an hour and responds more promptly to external heat. The pain of osteoarthritis is felt when moving the joint but rarely persists at rest the way the pain of rheumatoid arthritis does. With osteoarthritis there is frequently deformity and mild swelling, some pain and tenderness during the active phase, but rarely any redness and almost never any fever.

The cause of rheumatoid arthritis seems to be both genetic and environmental, especially when it is so severe it requires hospitalization. There is three to four times more incidence of the disease in women who have a mother or sister with the disease. Chromosome 6 contains genes that ensure that every person is different, and those with a special DR4 and DR1 gene on chromosome 6 are more likely to have rheumatoid arthritis. There is a theory of interplay between a genetic predisposition and an environmental factor, perhaps a microbial infection. This combination could be the initial stimulus. Stress, we believe, makes it worse, but this is a clinical impression, not yet backed up by long-term studies.

How Rheumatoid Arthritis Affects the Joints

Rheumatoid arthritis characteristically involves hands and the proximal (near) finger joints, but it can affect many joints of upper and lower extremities (hands and hips). Several hand joints can be affected by rheumatoid arthritis and it is critical to diagnose the distribution of the involvement correctly. The wrist—carpus—consists of a series of relatively small bones (carpal bones) that are located at the end of the long bones of the forearm. The many joints among the carpal bones ensure flexibility at the wrist. From the wrist spring five longer (metacarpal) bones, which constitute the hand. All fingers except the thumb have three joints. The thumb has two.

In medical terminology, *proximal* means "closer to the center of the body," and *distal* means "farther from the center of the body." So your fingertips are distal, and your knuckles are proximal. The tips of your fingers are connected to the middle segments by the so-called dip (distal interphalangeal) joints; the joints between the middle segments of your fingers and the proximal segments of your fingers are called pip (proximal interphalangeal) joints. Rheumatoid arthritis usually involves the pip joints, which are swollen, painful, and can be discolored and warm to the touch. The pain persists even at rest. Other joints frequently involved are also on the periphery of the body—feet, ankles, neck, shoulders, and elbows. Rheumatoid arthritis causes deformity of the joints, and muscles atrophy because it becomes too painful to move them. When the disease progresses, it spreads to the shoulders, elbows, and hips.

Diagnosing Rheumatoid Arthritis

In retrospect, Janice recalled that two or three weeks before her joints began to ache she had a brief head cold with a sore throat and low-grade fever. One morning she woke up with stiff, aching, and puffy hands and wrists. The symptoms lasted for half an hour or so, but in the rush of getting ready to go to work, she soon forgot the stiffness. But it recurred every morning and lasted for hours. At first she thought it was from her tennis game the previous weekend. Her husband, who suffered from tennis elbow, agreed. After a while, however, she began to have difficulty holding even her toothbrush, and at breakfast, the knife felt unwieldy when she buttered her toast. In addition, she worried about similar symptoms on her left side. She was right-handed, but did use her left occasionally in tennis for a backhand swing.

At work Janice found it painful to type and frequently had to rest her wrists at the computer. Her symptoms fluctuated up and down the next few months. With the help of Advil and occasional aspirin, she was able to function. It did occur to Janice that her symptoms might be arthritis, but she reasoned she was too young—only 35. Her grandmother had it, but she was past 75. Janice decided she had strained her hands with too much typing.

When her hands became swollen and painful to touch, despite the over-the-counter painkillers, Janice came to see me. I could almost make the diagnosis when I saw her hands. I avoided gripping her hand for fear of causing pain, but merely touched it to greet her.

Although the appearance of Janice's hands suggested rheumatoid arthritis at first glance, it was important to perform a complete workup to rule out any other conditions. A thorough history of Janice's family satisfied me that her condition did not seem to be familial. Her 75-year-old grandmother had the more common osteoarthritis, involving mostly the distal finger joints.

Symptoms of rheumatoid arthritis can also look like the arthritis caused by Lyme disease, but Janice said she had not been in any outdoor areas frequented by deer and had not noted any ticks on her body. She did not own a dog or cat that could carry a tick into the home. Lyme disease arthritis can involve any of the joints and can mimic both osteoarthritis and rheumatoid arthritis. Even though Lyme disease was unlikely, I tested her blood for it anyway. It would be a pity to miss a potentially curable condition. A series of tests were needed to rule out all other possibilities before properly diagnosing rheumatoid arthritis.

• An elevated white blood cell count might indicate the presence of a hidden infection someplace in the body; occasionally an abscessed tooth or an abscess deep in the abdomen might become a cause of distant joint pains. This is called "reactive arthritis" or "focus-of-infection arthritis."

• Anemia often accompanies rheumatoid arthritis, especially in the later stages, but does not usually accompany osteoarthritis.

• Rheumatoid arthritis is frequently associated with an elevated sedimentation (sed) rate, while osteoarthritis is not. Janice exhibited a moderately elevated sed rate. This is defined by the height of blood column that settles down in one hour. In women, anything above twenty-five millimeters in one hour is defined as elevated, above thirty as significantly elevated.

• Latex fixation tests can show the so-called rheumatoid factor, a substance present in the blood of about 80 percent of people with the disease and considered characteristic for this disease. About 20 to 30 percent of people with rheumatoid arthritis do not have the substance in their blood, and it can be present in a number of other conditions, including lupus.

• An X ray of the joints can look for any signs of erosion, which can guide us on treatment. The presence of erosion indicates the need for aggressive treatment targeted at the modification of the disease process, not just pain relief.

Medical Insurance Limitations

Sometimes, early recognition and diagnosis of rhematoid arthritis and aggressive treatment combined with physiotherapy can arrest the disease and prevent deformities. Yet, health insurance rules often limit patients to diagnostic tests of a certain type or a certain number. Because there are many tests needed for a careful and correct diagnosis not only of rheumatoid arthritis itself but for the stage in which the disease exists, you might need to talk with your physician and your health insurer to be sure you can get all the tests you need.

Many women are enrolled in plans that would not allow all of the tests I gave Janice. Additionally, if you cannot go to another physician, or one you choose because of reputation, you might not be able to afford the best diagnosis or even a second opinion. Without proper diagnosis, you are less likely to get the proper care. Studies have shown that poor women do not respond as well to treatment because they have less access to comprehensive health care. They often do not get treatment soon enough. Higher education is actually associated with lower prevalence of rheumatoid arthritis in women, but not in men.

Treatment for Rheumatoid Arthritis

In recent years, the treatment of rheumatoid arthritis has undergone a drastic change. It has now been established that in the first year or two after diagnosis there is a window of opportunity to modify the disease process, to slow it down or even stop or reverse it. New disease-modifying drugs, together with physical and occupational therapy, are used to accomplish this.

In the past, therapy of rheumatoid arthritis was targeted at the symptoms, primarily the relief of pain. Tylenol, which is a pain medication, anti-inflammatory agents including NSAIDs, corticosteroids, and even narcotics have been used, even though the use of narcotics is not wise in such a chronic condition because they can become addictive.

Disease-modifying Drugs (DMDs)

Disease-modifying drugs (DMDs) include the antimalarial medications (chloroquine and hydroxychloroquine), intramuscular gold injections, penicillamine, and methotrexate. This type of medication actually suppresses the primary autoimmune process responsible for destroying the lining of the joints. The anti-inflammatory drugs suppress the inflammation, the secondary process, while the painkillers only help the pain. Some women are unable to tolerate the DMDs or their disease process becomes refractory, meaning they no longer respond to the drug.

• **Methotrexate** is the most immunosuppressive medication of the three. Recently, another such drug, Cytoxan, has been investigated for use in rheumatoid arthritis. Methotrexate and Cytoxan are commonly used for cancer treatment. They destroy a number of cells in the body, especially those that multiply fast, such as tumor cells, and also the T and B lymphocytes involved in autoimmune response.

• **Antimalarial drugs** are only partially immunosuppressive and are used in mild early cases.

• **Gold injections** are given intramuscularly, at first weekly, then biweekly, finally one a month. Nobody knows exactly how gold therapy works, but after the gold reaches a certain level, about a month or three after therapy begins, it relieves the pain and even helps correct the deformities.

Treatment must be closely monitored with frequent urine and blood testing. It is difficult sometimes to maintain an effective dosage of medication while avoiding toxic side effects. Renal toxicity might develop while on gold therapy, and severe bone marrow suppression can occur from treatment with methotrexate.

• **Penicillamide** absorbs abnormal proteins, including the autoantibodies and excretes them in urine.

If treatment with DMDs is unsuccessful or impossible, alleviation of pain is the only thing left other than physical and occupational therapy.

Anti-inflammatory Drugs

Of the anti-inflammatory medications, NSAIDs and aspirin are the least toxic, although they can cause gastrointestinal or kidney effects and stomach ulcers. Corticosteroids are also in this class of drugs. Their continued use can cause side effects such as osteoporosis, accelerated atherosclerosis, hypertension, diabetes, and steroid myopathy with severe muscle weakness. Corticosteroids are the treatment of last resort. Continued use of steroids is discouraged because of the serious side effects. The side effects of steroids must be counteracted whenever possible. For instance, when treating with long-term steroids a woman who is either menopausal or has other evidence of deficient or disrupted ovarian function, it is important to replace her estrogen unless the hormone is seriously contraindicated. Estrogen and progestins must be added if the woman has an intact uterus, and also vitamin D and calcium to prevent osteoporosis.

In Janice's case, we had a window of opportunity to approach the disease aggressively with DMDs to prevent erosion and deformity of her joints. In consultation with a rheumatologist, we treated her with gold therapy. Antimalarials were too weak since she already had some erosion of the joints. If the gold failed we would have to treat her with Cytoxan. She got weekly injections of gold, combined with an intensive rehabilitation of physical and occupational therapy. Janice was monitored with periodic urine and blood serum counts to calibrate the dosage of gold. It took several months before Janice began to feel relief from her symptoms.

Physical and Occupational Therapy
Physical therapy is the mainstay of treatment for rheumatoid arthritis. The goal of physical therapy is to strengthen muscles, increase the range of motion around the joint, increase mobility, and prevent deformities of the joints. It also improves flexibility, gait, and posture. Exercises are aerobic, weight-bearing, resistance, balance, and workout of a particular limb or the upper body or neck. Women are not always eager to engage in physical therapy because of the pain, but those who get past the discomfort and think of getting better are more successful with treatment.

Occupational therapy is directed at improving the activities of daily living and working, thus the name. This therapy devises better ways of functioning despite pain and other limitations. For instance, getting out of bed, getting dressed, picking up objects from the floor, placing objects up on shelves, eating with utensils (sometimes especially designed for a particular disability), opening doors, navigating in a small space at home and outside, typing, writing, getting on a bus, or entering a car.

Learning how to use the wrists differently is a good example of adapting to rheumatoid arthritis. More damage is done to the wrist joints on the outside of the wrist, the side with the pinkie finger. This makes it difficult to turn a doorknob to the left with the left hand, for example. This is called *ulnar deviation*. Janice balked at first, but learned to overcome this tendency of her hands to deviate to the outside. She learned to open doors by turning the knob counterclockwise when using her right hand, and vice versa with her left.

There has been no significant progression in Janice's disease, and she feels well and is working full-time. Not everyone is as lucky. Failure to get treatment early enough, before erosion and joint destruction have already begun, means any treatment might be too late, even with DMDs. Also, if you are unable to pursue vigorous and persistent physical therapy, the joints might freeze or lock in place and cut down on mobility and agility.

Joint-replacement surgery is sometimes indicated to correct the deformities that can freeze a joint in a nonfunctional position.

New Treatment of Promise Etanercept, a soluble substance that intercepts the action of the "tumor necrosis factor"—one of the culprits in rheumatoid arthritis—at its receptor, has recently been found to be beneficial in combination with methotrexate when methotrexate alone no longer works.

SCLERODERMA

This is a progressive systemic disease of unknown origin that attacks the skin and internal organs. The body makes excessive collagen, which causes the skin to thicken, and internal organs can become incapacitated.

There are four to twelve cases of scleroderma per million women in this country, but incidence has increased in the last three decades. It is equally distributed in all geographic and racial groups, with modest increases in young black women. It is three to four times more common in women than men and most commonly begins in the forties or fifties. There is no accepted treatment of this disease and few experimental protocols.

RAYNAUD'S SYNDROME AND RAYNAUD'S DISEASE

Raynaud's is a circulatory condition that is called Raynaud's disease when it happens by itself, but when it develops along with an underlying disorder such as scleroderma, lupus, or rheumatoid arthritis, it is called Raynaud's syndrome. We mention it here because it is often associated with these autoimmune diseases.

Women have Raynaud's syndrome about twenty times more frequently than men, and usually experience the first episode as young adults. Raynaud was the French physician who first described this condition, which is a problem for about 10 to 20 percent of the population. For some reason, the body's circulation has an exaggerated response to cold. The small blood vessels in the skin get their signals mixed and send blood from the skin to the internal organs to protect them against the cold, leaving the skin of the extremities to fend for itself. Fingers and toes become like icicles, and sometimes the nose is affected, too.

There is no known cause, but Raynaud's is associated with a sudden drop in body temperature, spending time in an over-air-conditioned space, going out without gloves in cold weather, and even being in a stressful situation. The resultant disturbance in control of the vascular responses causes the release of chemical messengers that constrict the blood vessels and keep them that way. These areas then get no oxygen, and blood pools in the surrounding tissue, causing the bluish and purplish skin color. Numbness and pain develop. Something else unexplainable triggers a return to normal.

MULTIPLE SCLEROSIS (MS)

Women are two to three times more prone to the most common neurological disorder, multiple sclerosis, which is believed to be caused by an abnormal immune system response to the myelin that covers the nerve fibers. MS affects about 300,000 young adults in the United States. It occurs rarely in childhood, and rarely after the age of 50. When it becomes chronic, it leads to disability.

The cause of MS is unknown, but there is evidence that myelin is attacked by T cells in this disease, causing "demyelination"—loss of myelin around the nerve fibers. We do know that various factors, such as viral infections, genetics, and where you live, play a role. For example, the disease is much less common in the countries around the equator, and more common in the colder areas. It has been suggested that a virus, pregnancy, or trauma precedes the autoimmunity, but this has not been proven. Also yet to be explained is why it is so much more common in women, although it is thought to be related to the hormonal factors.

Symptoms are related to the area of the brain that is affected. If the optic nerve is inflamed, then loss of vision occurs. In fact, the occurrence of *optic neuritis,* or inflammation of the optic nerve, might be the first symptom of MS, with other symptoms to follow within five years. Double vision, slurred speech, tingling, or weakness can be symptoms. If the nerves affected are in the pelvic area, then bladder, bowel, and sexual dysfunction can result. Tremor, spasticity, and sphincter dysfunction can also be symptoms of MS, as can impaired memory. There have been cases, discovered on autopsy, where the patient never had symptoms and never knew she had the disease. MS symptoms can be abrupt and then go away, and then come back again in several weeks.

The disease does not appear to reduce fertility in women, although it does seem to affect the ability to achieve orgasm. Both sexes suffer loss of libido with MS. The disease has little effect on the outcome of pregnancy, such as causing miscarriage, premature birth, or birth defects. In fact, the disease seems less aggressive during pregnancy, but after pregnancy it seems to return with more force. Long-term disability from the disease, however, seems no different in women who had children while they had the disease and in those who did not.

Diagnosis of MS

Because symptoms are often confused with other conditions, it is difficult to diagnose MS correctly. There have been cases of women having been told they had MS when, in fact, they had chronic fatigue syndrome. Other women have suffered the symptoms of MS for years and were never diagnosed correctly, and therefore became progressively worse over the years.

A variety of tests are needed for correct diagnosis: neurological examination, and a combination of clinical and laboratory exams, a lumbar puncture to test the spinal fluid for an abnormal protein pattern that could be a clue. MRI scans of the brain or spinal cord, or possibly both, are used to identify the demyelinated white matter plaques of MS. There are also tests to calculate the speed of nerve impulse transmission, which is often changed by the loss of the protective coating myelin.

Treatment and Management of MS

Steroids, either by pill or injection, are the most prescribed treatment for MS. Other immunosuppressive drugs like Cytoxan and Imuran are used, as are two types of interferon called Betaseron and Avonex. Interferon medications are very expensive. Pain is treated with other drugs.

In 1997, a drug called Copaxone (*glatiramer acetate*) was approved by the FDA for treatment of relapsing MS. This drug could replace the interferons. Copaxone is a synthetic form of naturally occurring myelin proteins that bind to the T cells, diverting them from attacking the body's myelin. Tests have shown that Copaxone modulates the immune system's effect on the myelin and reduces the number of flares of MS. In clinical trials, patients had fewer relapses, although the drug did not seem to make getting around any easier, and it had no apparent effect on the disease progression. This drug worked better with early cases of MS and had little effect on patients with chronic progressive MS.

The glatiramer is given by injection under the skin and can cause side effects such as pain at the injection site, flushing of the skin, tightness in the chest, and anxiety. Depression and flulike symptoms caused by interferon are no more common with the copaxone. Additionally, clinical trials have shown no toxicity in the blood or liver, but whether it is safe for pregnant women, or if it is excreted in breast milk, is unknown.

Zanaflex (*tizanidine*) is used to treat the spastic symptoms of MS. This drug has been avalable for a dozen years in Japan and Europe, where it is used as a short-term muscle relaxant. Other drugs have been used to treat the increased muscle tone and painful muscle spasms of MS. These include Lioresal (baclofen) and others that, taken orally, are ineffective in the long term. They also cause weakness, sedation, and if withdrawn suddenly can cause seizures or hallucinations. Some patients only benefit from these drugs with continuous dosage with an implanted pump, but this can lead to overdosage or infection.

Zanaflex, is fast-acting, especially if taken with food so that it is completely absorbed. The effects of the drug reach a peak an hour or two after taken and then disappear within six hours. Clinical trials have shown the drug effective in decreasing daytime muscle spasms and reducing the number of times the patients awake during the night with painful spasms. In trials in England, the tizanidine medication was about as effective as baclofen in patients with MS.

Adverse effects might include sedation, dry mouth, dizziness, and in rare cases visual hallucinations. Zanaflex also interacts with other drugs and alcohol, and might cause problems, especially with oral contraceptives, antidepressants, and drugs for hypertension. Tizanidine is usually taken at bedtime, and the dosage is increased gradually while blood pressure is constantly monitored.

At the Université Pierre et Marie Curie, researchers have used a substance (eliprodil) that enhances myelination of nerve fibers in a tissue culture. While promising, the drug has not been tried in humans yet.

MS is a long-term, chronic disease that requires a great deal of coordinated treatment and management by a principal physician and a neurologist. The disease, which can lead to disability and mobility only by wheelchair, is managed with supportive services and physical therapy. Diet, rest, and avoiding temperature extremes—especially heat—are important.

··19··

Disorders of the Endocrine System

Our hormones are like a city's bicycle messengers, or the FedEx delivery trucks, carrying vital information from one part of the body to another. The word *hormone* itself means "to spur on." Each hormone is a complex chemical produced and secreted to our bloodstream by an endocrine gland. Some hormones are secreted by special cells in some organs, such as parts of the digestive tract or the heart. The actions of hormones metabolize other chemicals and nutrients entering the body. They balance the supply of minerals and water, modulate our reaction to stress in response to the central nervous system, and of course, have a great deal to do with our sexual development.

The hormones are controlled by a system of feedbacks that lets a gland know when it can stop producing a particular hormone for the time being. Some glands are controlled by the *pituitary,* the master gland, near the base of the brain. The pituitary, in turn, is controlled by the *hypothalamus,* which is part of the brain. If a gland fails to produce for any reason, we sometimes can replace the missing hormone with a medication that mimics the action, such as the use of insulin injections by a diabetic when the pancreas stops producing insulin for the regulation of the body's sugars.

THE TWO TYPES OF DIABETES

There are two types of diabetes; both are chronic conditions that require long-term care and management. Type I diabetes, sometimes called "juvenile onset" diabetes, is an autoimmune disease that begins in childhood or adolescence and affects both men and women almost equally. It accounts for less than 10 percent of the diabetics in this country. The more common Type II diabetes, or "adult onset," strikes mostly women and is caused by multiple factors, including genetic predisposition, obesity, and a sedentary lifestyle. The risk increases with age. Women of color are more susceptible to Type II diabetes than Caucasians. This type of diabetes is the fourth leading cause of death for black, Hispanic, and Native American women. Worldwide, it is more frequent among urbanized populations than rural communities.

It is estimated that about 16 million Americans have diabetes. Half of them know it and the other half do not. About 1 million of them have Type I, which is managed by closely monitoring blood sugar levels and taking daily insulin injections. This type is also known as insulin-dependent diabetes mellitus (IDDM) (*mellitus* means "sweet").

The other 15 million have Type II, non-insulin-dependent (NIDDM). The body produces sufficient insulin at first but develops a resistance to its actions. Blood sugar levels rise, and if uncontrolled, this can lead to blindness, kidney failure, circulation problems, and other complications. In many cases of Type II diabetes, weight loss can bring the disease under control and dietary changes and regular exercise can then keep it under control. In 10 to 20 percent of patients, however, this does not work, so they need either oral medications that stimulate insulin production and lower their levels of glucose, or insulin itself.

How Sugar Is Metabolized

Diabetes develops because of a problem with insulin and glucose. Insulin is essential for the body's ability to use glucose. Glucose is the body's most important fuel. Insulin facilitates the entry of glucose into cells, where it is "burned"—oxidized—to provide energy for the cell's function. Glucose is the preferred fuel used by all tissues of the body. This fuel allows the organs to perform their work, grow, and stay viable. When we eat foods that contain carbohydrates, either concentrated sweets such as candy or cake, or complex carbohydrates such as grains, vegetables, and fruits, our digestive system breaks down the food into ever smaller components (see chapter 26 for more about the digestive system). The basic unit of which all carbohydrates are composed is glucose. Glucose is absorbed from the intestine into the bloodstream and is carried first to the liver and then to other tissues of the body.

Our cells need glucose to stay healthy and perform their designated functions—to contract muscles, produce glandular secretions, make our brains function, and cause our hair and nails to grow. If glucose is unavailable, a cell is likely to cannibalize itself; that is, burn its own fat and protein. This is especially true of the fatty tissue cell (the *adipocyte*), which shrinks or self-destructs in the absence of the fuel. The liver, a very resourceful repository of various body fuels, intervenes when glucose is scarce. Having stored a portion of every meal as glycogen, a complex carbohydrate, the liver transforms some of the glycogen stores into glucose and releases it into the bloodstream. Muscles can also store a limited amount of glycogen to be burned as glucose in an emergency.

However, glucose needs help to break through the membrane of the cells, and the hormone that makes this possible is *insulin,* which is produced by the pancreas, an oblong organ that sits behind the stomach and supplies digestive juices to the intestinal tract. The digestive (*exocrine*) function of the pancreas has little to do with its *endocrine* (hormone-insulin) function. The insulin-producing cells form patches or islands (*insulae,* in Latin) in the pancreas called the islets of Langerhans, after the German anatomist who first described them. Insulin, the product of the islets, is secreted into the blood and carried to virtually all tissues in the body. In the absence of insulin, glucose is unable to breach the cell membrane, so it accumulates in the blood until it is excreted into the urine, thus starving the body of necessary fuel. Large amounts of glucose in the blood and urine cause an excessive amount of urination.

A study at Harvard published in 1997 in *Journal of the American Medical Association* showed that people who eat too much starch as a way of eating less fat might be setting themselves up for later diabetes. Participants in the study ate lots of potatoes, white bread, and white rice, all of which have almost no fiber. They drank a lot of soft drinks. They had two and a half times the rate of diabetes found in women who ate less of these foods and more fiber, specifically from whole-grain cereals. The high-starch diet increased risk factors for diabetes.

Carbohydrates in refined foods like white bread and white rice are quickly absorbed by the body, causing a big surge in blood sugar, which in turn causes the pancreas to secrete high levels of insulin. These foods, ounce for ounce, increase glucose levels more than eating sugar itself. Potatoes, which have always been a staple of the diets of poor countries, have prevented starvation. However, in a sedentary civilization like ours, excessive amounts of them are harmful. While carbohydrates represent the largest portion of foods we should eat each day, they must contain fiber and nutrients.

Left undiagnosed and untreated for years, diabetes causes irreversible damage to the health. In the long run, women with diabetes—type I and II—are more likely to have high blood pressure and suffer a heart attack, stroke, and kidney failure. There is also lowered resistance to infections, sepsis, and gangrene, leading to amputation of the limbs. Diabetes vies with glaucoma as the leading cause of blindness in our country. As many as 24,000 people go blind every year from diabetic retinopathy. Damage to the nerves and blood vessels causes 54,000 amputations a year, according to the American Diabetes Association. All told, there are 178,000 deaths from complications of diabetes each year in this country.

Because of the difficulty of regulating glucose levels in the blood, high glucose can damage nerves over time. This is called *neuropathy.* It decreases your ability to feel pain and other sensations, especially in the feet. Neuropathy also reduces perspiration, which can lead to cracked, dry skin. It might shorten tendons and weaken muscles. The shortened tendons can actually change the shape of the foot. Obstructions to the arteries are more likely to occur in diabetics, and thus, poor blood flow interferes with healing. Once an ulcer or infection takes over, gangrene can occur, and this means removal of the affected toe, foot, or even the entire leg.

Type I Diabetes

Type I diabetes is less common and usually more severe than Type II. It begins in childhood or adolescence. The body for some reason has created antibodies that attack the insulin-producing cells of the pancreas. This type is associated with certain genetic variants represented on the human chromosome 6. The presence of these genetic variants does not predict diabetes; it only causes a predisposition to diabetes. Both genetic predisposition and outside environmental factors play a role, but we do not know if it is a physical or chemical injury. Most researchers believe the precipitating event is an infection from a virus that stimulates an immune response of antibody production. The antibodies neutralize and destroy the invading virus.

However, because of an accidental but uncanny structural similarity between that virus and a structural component of the insulin-producing cells of the pancreas, the antibodies start destroying the islet cells in the pancreas. Such anti-islet antibodies are sometimes detected in the blood of Type I diabetics early in the disease process. Once all insulin-producing cells are destroyed, the autoimmune process burns out and the anti-islet antibodies disappear from the blood. By the time the person develops full-blown diabetes it is usually too late to detect any of the anti-islet antibodies.

As a result, there is severe deficiency of insulin, and the burning of fats eventually results in production of large amounts of fatty acids that turn the internal environment of the body acidic (sour). The human body requires a delicately balanced, slightly alkaline (sweet) internal environment to function efficiently.

When the blood turns acid, we call it *acidosis*. With acidosis, many enzymes stop working, and eventually all living processes stop. The brain is acutely sensitive to the effect of acidosis, and it makes the diabetic stuporous, as if she were drugged, and then comatose. In acidosis of Type I diabetes, fatty acids are further burned to produce ketones. Overproduction of ketones is detected in the breath, which smells like nail polish (which is made of acetone). Ketoacidotic coma is an extreme complication of diabetes Type I, and very rarely occurs with Type II.

Type II Diabetes

While Type I diabetes means there is an absolute deficiency of insulin, in type II diabetes, there is a combination of resistance to insulin and relative deficiency. The pancreas, in a sense, gets tired of producing enough insulin to keep up with the overabundance of glucose. The level of insulin might be high, but it is still insufficient to do the job because the body is resisting the insulin action, so it is a relative deficiency.

When a person is obese there is a decrease in the number of insulin receptors on the membranes of cells so that insulin cannot get attached to the cell membrane to get the glucose into the cell. The glucose stays in the blood and levels rise. The islet cells of the pancreas are stimulated by the high blood sugar level and respond by pouring more insulin out, but that insulin again encounters resistance at the cellular level. The absolute level of insulin might be high, but it cannot overcome the resistance. With time, the islets will become exhausted and then absolute insulin deficiency might intervene. When this happens, a Type II diabetic would need to take insulin.

Type II is more likely than Type I to run in families, and it involves a combination of many genes in some complex fashion not yet understood. There is a degree of "social" inheritance; that is, people grow up following their parents' eating habits and sedentary lifestyle. Type II diabetes calls for weight loss, adjustment of diet to lower the carbohydrate burden, and exercise, as well as quitting smoking. Nicotine raises blood sugar levels on its own.

Type II diabetes tends to be mild initially, causing few symptoms. In fact, it sometimes exists without the person's being aware of it. Half of the 15 million Americans who have diabetes have not yet been diagnosed. The patient might be brought to the physician for unrelated reasons and diabetes is discovered through the testing of the urine or of the blood.

The risk for Type II diabetes increases with age, as the body's ability to produce enough insulin for the overwhelming amount of food wears down. The risk doubles every ten years after age 40, and if you are overweight the risk is higher.

Latinas have more diabetes than blacks or whites, yet Cuban Americans have only half the rate of other Americans. More than 11 percent of black women have diabetes, and 5.8 percent of white women. The Pima Indians of the Southwest have especially high rates of diabetes and obesity. About 40 percent of Pima Indian women have Type II diabetes. Genetics plays an important role in Type II diabetes; there are probably multiple genes involved.

The known risk factors are these:

• Being overweight and sedentary is the major risk factor.

• Being a member of a high-risk minority—African Americans, Hispanics, and American Indians—or having a relative with diabetes.

• Having delivered a baby weighing more than nine pounds, or having been diagnosed with gestational diabetes.

• Having impaired glucose tolerance or fasting glucose levels.

Warning Signals for Diabetes

Type I diabetes is usually discovered in a young person because of excessive urination, excessive thirst, hunger, and often some weight loss.

Type II diabetes is often discovered accidentally when a patient comes to a doctor for a checkup, or for some other condition, and a blood or urine test reveals high glucose levels. Symptoms of diabetes per se may be absent. Frequently, diabetes is not discovered until the complications begin.

There is evidence that diabetes exerts greater negative impact on the health of women than on men: In two comparable groups of long-term Type II diabetics, almost 40 percent of women and fewer than 20 percent of men developed eye complications, 35 percent of women and only 15 percent of men wound up with diabetic kidney disease, and 45 percent of women and 28 percent of men suffered from neurologic complications.

These complications can be avoided with early detection and treatment. There are some warning signs of Type II diabetes; if you notice any, see your doctor.

• More frequent urination, especially at night

• Increased thirst, dry mouth

• Excessive hunger

• Blurred vision or a change in vision

• Weight loss might or might not be present; the person might have actually *gained* weight prior to the development of diabetes

• Chronic fatigue

• Tingling or loss of feeling in hands or feet

• Infections that recur or will not heal

Screening Guidelines for Diabetes

Blood sugar levels once considered normal were deemed to be too high in new guidelines issued in 1997 by the American Diabetes Association. The guidelines were also endorsed by federal health authorities. Diabetes, either type, is diagnosed when two readings on two different days reach 126 milligrams per deciliter or higher on a blood test known as fasting plasma glucose or fasting blood sugar. The cutoff used to be

140 or higher. The normal rate is below 110. The danger zone is from 110 to 125.

The new guidelines call for all healthy people 45 and older to be tested every three years. This is about 77 million Americans, and such screening is expected to detect 2 million new cases of diabetes. People at higher risk should be tested more often.

Emotional Side Effects of Diabetes

Having diabetes is always traumatic to the patient as well as her family. The emotional reaction to Type I is especially overwhelming, because it usually comes at the time of major biological and psychological transitions of adolescence. The diagnosis of diabetes, a chronic disorder that she will carry with her for the rest of her life, might sound like a death sentence to a teenager. There is frequently denial of the diagnosis and the child or adolescent might skip her insulin through forgetfulness or on purpose, as if trying to bring the diagnosis into question. Other diabetic children are aware of the frightening effect of their illness on their parents and might exploit it by rendering themselves "a little sick"—either by skipping a dose or by taking an excessively large dose and inducing hypoglycemia. Some of the so-called labile or difficult-to-control diabetic cases are due to a child who is willfully manipulating her insulin doses. It is a cry for attention from a child who feels overwhelmed by her illness.

Julia had Type I diabetes. At 12 she began to wet her bed. She tried to get out of bed each time but she could not always hold her urine and still wet the bed. She was losing weight, was constantly thirsty and drinking an abundance of fluids, yet her mouth felt parched. She felt light-headed, and her mother took her to the pediatrician, who diagnosed Type I diabetes.

Julia had a temper tantrum at first, and then became morose, refusing to have anything to do with insulin and self-care. Then she encountered a wonderful nurse in a specialist's office. Read on page 287 how Julia began to manage her diabetes.

With Type II diabetes, which usually occurs in adulthood, the emotional problems center around the frustration and depression of changing the habits of a lifetime. The difficulty of complying with the prescribed regimen is familiar to anyone who has ever tried unsuccessfully to lose weight and change her lifestyle. The frustration, depression, and sometimes resignation are not uncommon. Instituting an oral pill regimen might signify to some patients that their illness can be taken care of with "medicines" and that no effort at modifying the diet is necessary. This is not true, of course, because weight loss and exercise are essential parts of the treatment of diabetes.

MANAGING TYPE I DIABETES

Diabetics can lead normal lives when their disease is managed well. They can do whatever anyone else does—have children, work, compete in sports—as long as they understand how to control two basic reactions to their disease.

Low Blood Sugar (Hypoglycemia)

If a meal is skipped, or too much insulin is used, or there was more exercise than usual, low blood sugar will develop. This is *hypoglycemia*, which causes irritability, nervousness, clammy skin, and a tingling on the tongue. The remedy is to immediately eat sugar, such as a piece of candy, or drink a glass of orange juice to bring sugar levels up as quickly as possible.

High Blood Sugar (Hyperglycemia)

When there is too much sugar in the blood because there was not enough insulin or there was too much food for the amount of insulin, and the patient did not do her normal exercise, *hyperglycemia* can occur. Hyperglycemia plus acidosis (see page 283 for information about ketones) can lead to a coma. The skin becomes hot and dry, breathing might become labored, abdominal pain might be present, and sleepiness will set in.

Diabetic coma and hypoglycemia can usually be avoided by regular urine testing, so that insulin, diet, and exercise can be adjusted accordingly. However, to be safe, a diabetic should carry a few lumps of sugar or a candy bar around, and should wear a bracelet or carry a card identifying her as a diabetic.

Urine Testing

The simplest way to monitor glucose levels is to test the amount in the urine. This is generally done twice a day—morning and evening—but it is done more often with difficult-to-control diabetes, or during pregnancy, when levels can fluctuate more. Urine is tested for the presence of glucose by using a sugar-testing paper. When the paper is immersed in the urine, resulting yellow, red, and brown colors mean there is too much sugar in the urine, indicating that the insulin dose needs to be increased. Blue and greenish colors mean there is little or no sugar present and the insulin dose need not be increased.

Insulin Injections

Diabetics need to give themselves injections, usually in the thigh or abdomen. The nurse taught Julia how to monitor urine and blood glucose levels using an instrument called a glucometer and how to practice the self-injection technique using a large orange. She also taught her to use combinations of regular (fast-acting) and NPH (longer acting) insulin three times a day with her meals. Occasionally she needed additional insulin before going to sleep if there was too much sugar in her urine at that time. Her excessive thirst and frequent urination abated. Insulin used to be made from beef or pork insulin, but now we have human recombinant insulin, which gives rise to fewer allergic reactions. Recently a very fast-acting recombinant human insulin has become available.

Exercise Therapy

Regular exercise is an important part of managing diabetes. Vigorous exercise acts like insulin, so it lowers the need for injectable insulin. If a diabetic exercises and does not adjust the injected insulin, however, the resulting hypoglycemia interferes with the nutrition of her brain and other vital organs. This low blood sugar can make her faint or black out. In Julia's case, she had such episodes of hypoglycemia on the evenings she played basketball at school. Julia was eventually placed on an insulin pump and was able to regulate her blood sugar adequately. She became a good partner in her health care by asking questions of her doctor and reading up on diabetes. Encouraged by her endocrinologist, she eventually went to medical school and specialized in diabetes, helping other people overcome their afflictions.

MANAGING TYPE II DIABETES

Helen G. had been chubby since childhood. With her first pregnancy, however, she added 50 pounds to her usual 140 and, after delivery, was able to lose only ten of those. Her second pregnancy produced twins, and Helen ate "for three." When she got on a scale that spring she topped 210 and became panicky about her wardrobe and ("Forget it") bathing suits. The weight was slow to come off. Attending to her twins and the toddler kept her busy at home, and she had to forgo her workouts and jogging.

Undressing one evening she noticed a pimple under a skin fold on her lower abdomen. She wiped it with witch hazel, but the pimple did not heal. When it got as big as a quarter, she consulted her family doctor, who prescribed hot soaks and antibiotics. The pimple shrank with the treatment but, after a few weeks, started to grow again and soon oozed pus. New pimples appeared. She also found smaller ones in her groin, her armpits, and under her right breast. Then she noticed large pimples (*furuncles*) of varied sizes scattered over her body. Her blood pressure was moderately elevated, too.

Helen had diabetes; she had had it for some time, and it was out of control. Her brother had diabetes and had to have a toe amputated because of an infection resulting from circulatory problems. It was hard for her to accept the diagnosis, even though she saw firsthand the effect of the disease on her brother's toe infection. Diabetes lowers the resistance of the body to infections, especially to those initiated by the *staphylococcus*, a bacterium that is commonly present even on healthy skin. Staphylococcus thrives in an environment high in sugar. The moist skin between body folds, the so-called kissing surfaces, provides a natural point of entry for the bacterium, which is resistant to normal hygiene and standard antibiotics. This is not an uncommon first manifestation of diabetes.

After a thorough workup that ruled out thyroid disease, we devised, with the help of a dietitian, a diet that was low in concentrated sweets, moderately low in calories, and high in fiber—vegetables, fruits, and grains. Topical treatment consisted of daily showers with a mild antiseptic (Phisohex, in her case) applied over the infected areas. Then the skin is rinsed carefully and patted dry. I advised Helen to wear cotton underwear to absorb body moisture. Her furuncles soon began to shrink and dry up.

With an exercise program and diet Helen's blood sugar normalized, and she did not need insulin. She gradually lost weight but required vigilant monitoring, periodic visits to the dietitian, and some help from a psychiatrist to continue this difficult lifelong assignment. The memory of her brother's suffering added to her resolve, and so did the worry that her daughters might inherit her disease.

Treatment of Type II Diabetes with Oral Medications

In the 10 to 20 percent of patients whose diabetes cannot be controlled with diet and exercise, oral medications can either stimulate the production of insulin (a group of old drugs called *sulfonylureas* like Glucotrol, Micronase, Diabinese, and DiaBeta tablets, all now available for many years), or slow down the absorption of sugars in the intestine (new drug Precose), or lower the body's resistance to insulin (Rezulin). All these mechanisms result in lower glucose levels. These oral drugs are designed to offer some diabetics an alternative to daily insulin injections.

A new drug, Rezulin, part of a new class of drugs intended to attack the underlying cause of the disease—the resistance to insulin—was approved by the FDA in 1997. Known chemically as troglitazone, it is one of a class of drugs known as insulin sensitizers. In other words, it helps make better use of the insulin already produced by the body. It is recommended for use by patients with Type II diabetes who are not helped by the normal treatment modes of lifestyle changes and weight loss. Troglitazone is not recommended for women who are pregnant or for women with heart or liver disease. Another insulin sensitizer drug, Avandia, is awaiting review by the Food and Drug Administration.

Another new medication, *acarbose* (Precose), delays the absorption of sugars in the intestine, thus preventing high peaks in blood glucose levels.

Understandably, many patients with Type II diabetes whose blood sugar cannot be controlled with diet and oral medications resist bitterly the necessity to start insulin injections. Yet, it is not unusual for some patients to realize how much better they feel once insulin therapy has been started.

Protecting Feet from Diabetic Neuropathy

Because diabetes causes circulatory problems, about 15 percent of patients develop sores on their feet or legs at some time. If these persist and are not immediately treated, amputation of the foot might become necessary. About 54,000 amputations a year are related to diabetes.

A new screening tool can help identify any nerve damage in the foot that might lead to ulcers. This is a nylon fiber attached to a handle. A doctor pushes the filament against several areas of the bottom of the foot and notices when you feel pressure. Regular screening with this device can help prevent 50 to 90 percent of amputations caused by diabetes, according to the U.S. Health Resources and Services Administration.

Any foot injury needs to be attended to so an ulcer does not form. This means your shoes must fit well and anything such as an ingrown toenail or a a blister—any minor irritation—must be treated before it causes irreversible damage. Some ways to prevent damage include:

• Wear shoes made of natural, soft leather with wide toes. Synthetic materials do not allow your feet to breathe, and wearing them all day can make your feet sweat, leaving moisture between your toes. Avoid too-high heels and shoes with thin straps, especially thongs between the toes.

• Stretch the muscles in your foot by rolling a bottle with your toes. If the feet remain flexible, this will prevent stiffness that can lead to deformities and irritation.

• Moisturize your feet with a lotion or cold cream, but do not use it between the toes.

• Keep your toenails short, but before trimming them, soak your feet in warm water for about ten minutes. This is the only time soaking of the feet is recommended, but it makes the nails more pliable to trimming. Cut them straight across with a toenail clipper and file the sharp edges so the adjacent toes will not be irritated.

• Inspect your feet every day. Look for redness, blisters, calluses, corns, warts, and athlete's foot. When you wash your feet, do not use overly hot water. Gently pat your skin dry, and make sure no moisture remains between the toes.

• See your doctor immediately if you get any type of foot ulcer. It might be necessary to X-ray your foot to look for bone damage, and to test your blood to rule out infection. The wound can be cleaned with a saline solution and dressed. Ulcers won't heal with continued pressure, so you will likely have to stay off your feet. Special shoes, insoles, or crutches will give you some mobility. If an ulcer does not respond to treatment, you might need to be hospitalized.

Where to Get Information
• American Diabetes Association. Check their web site, www.diabetes.org, to find your local chapter.

• National Diabetes Outreach Program, 800-438-5383

THYROID DISEASE

All abnormalities in thyroid activity—both excesses and deficiencies—are much more common in women than in men. The incidence of benign and most malignant thyroid nodules (small lumps) is also higher. It is not well understood why the female thyroid is so much more easily perturbed, but we suspect the thyroid is more sensitive to changing body needs in women because the progression of pregnancy and delivery require rapid adjustments in the metabolism. If this is so, women pay a price for this adjustability by succumbing to a greater risk of thyroid ailments throughout their lifetime.

The thyroid gland, in the neck, controls the metabolism of every cell and organ in the body. It dictates the rate at which fuels are burned and how fast or slow each organ functions. It does this by producing two hormones: thyroxin (T4); and the triiodothyronine (T3).

Hypothyroidism and Hyperthyroidism
It has been known for over a century that the excess activity of the thyroid—hyperthyroidism—causes many organs to overact. The heart rate accelerates and might become irregular, or fibrillate. It can cause nervousness, excess perspiration, shaky hands, diarrhea, and weight loss. The classical form of hyperthyroidism, called Graves' disease in America and England and Basedow's disease in Europe, causes the eyes to become prominent and protrude from the sockets, and the enlarged thyroid forms a sometimes visible goiter in the neck. (Barbara Bush had Graves' disease and was treated with iodine 131. Interestingly, her husband, the former president, also got a form of hyperthyroidism that led to abnor-

mal heart rhythms while he was in office. The Bushes' dog developed a thyroid condition, too.)

On the other hand, when the thyroid is sluggish, you become tired and the heart rate is slow. Skin is frequently dry and thick, and sometimes it becomes yellow and itchy. Everything slows down, even the bowels, and constipation might ensue. Cold intolerance, lethargy and sleepiness, facial puffiness, and menstrual disturbances (such as heavy and frequent menses) might be combined with other more non-descript symptoms such as joint aching, decreased perspiration, hair changes, muscle cramps, weight gain, decreased memory, and mental impairment. Some of the symptoms of hypothyroidism are easily recognized by doctors, but more subtle ones, like muscle spasm and pain, are not.

The most common cause of hypothyroidism is *Hashimoto thyroiditis,* which occurs when autoantibodies invade the thyroid gland. While the first stage is infiltration of the thyroid by lymphocytes, the destruction of the organ is characterized by scarring. This autoimmune process is the most common cause of hypothyroidism in women.

The treatment of hypothyroidism consists of replacing the missing hormone with a synthetic L-thyroxine.

Both types of thyroid dysfunction—hyperthyroidism and hypothyroidism—are much more common in women than in men.

FIBROMYALGIA

In the face of thyroid deficiency, muscles are more susceptible to cramping up as a reaction to a minimal, and often unnoticed, exertion. When Abby was 15, her hypothyroidism was diagnosed and blamed for her excessive menstrual bleeding and I prescribed regular thyroid treatment. Over the years, we routinely checked her and adjusted the medication. She graduated from college, began her career, married, and had two children, all without incident.

When Abby was 34, her husband's company joined an HMO, and they decided they would both be covered by this insurance plan, which meant Abby would be cared for by another doctor. During a physical exam, the new doctor asked Abby why she was taking thyroid medication when her thyroid function tests were all normal. The new doctor explained that the drugs could not be covered under this medical coverage because the tests showed she did not need it. Abby decided to comply, after all, she felt well enough—and she had been taking thyroid medication for years.

Abby's mistake here was not asking the new doctor to call me and not showing the new doctor her medical records. After ten days without the medication, Abby could barely get out of bed. Her entire body ached, her shoulders and back were stiff, and her muscles were tender to the touch. A hot shower helped a bit, and she was able to get to work. In her high-pressure job as a financial executive, Abby worked hard that day, and the stiffness lightened up a little. However, the next morning the muscle aching was overwhelming, and she had to stay home from work.

Her husband took her to the HMO clinic, and the doctor took blood tests for muscle function and autoimmunity. The tests were negative, and the doctor diagnosed arthritis and prescribed NSAIDs, nonsteroidal anti-inflammatory drugs.

Anti-inflammatories helped the pain a little, but the stiffness and tenderness persisted. Abby felt pain with the slightest movement—even fastening her bra was excruciating. She tried to work at home, but memory ebbed away. She actually tried shaking her head to clear the fog, but a headache nearly blinded her. She was unable to rest or sleep because no matter what position she lay down in, her body ached.

Abby's husband continued to call the HMO office to find out what could be done. They assured him that a wait-and-see posture was all that was required because the tests were all negative. If the symptoms persisted, they said they would do a surgical biopsy of her muscles and skin to search further for the reason.

That brought Abby back to me. The very acuteness of her symptoms spoke of a drug reaction or an infection. She held her head stiffly, obviously unable to move her neck. She could not raise her arms above her shoulders, as if she had bursitis, an inflammation of the *bursa*, fluid-filled sacs that protect the joints. Her back was so stiff she could not bend forward or to the side without grimacing. When I touched the muscles of her neck and shoulders, she felt a painful spasm.

What Abby had was *fibromyalgia,* which means "painful muscles," a common condition provoked, among other causes, by thyroid deficiency. Although many women outgrow hypothyroidism, it was wrong to assume that a "normal" test result meant she no longer required medication.

When hypothyroidism affects the muscles, the symptoms are frequently unrecognized. The muscle cell uses glucose as its usual fuel to burn for energy. When incomplete combustion occurs, such as after vigorous exercise when there might not be enough oxygen, the burning of sugar is incomplete and lactic acid is formed. The acid can be irritating to the nerve endings within the muscles and cause pain. The muscle contracts, but might lose its ability to relax. Continued contraction of the muscles can generate a painful spasm, which we call fibromyalgia. A woman experiencing such pain is likely to "freeze" her muscles in a position of least pain, but this only perpetuates the spasm and causes more pain. A hot shower can help the blood remove and dissipate the lactic acid. Resting the extremity helps more complete oxidation of the lactic acid to carbon dioxide and water, and gentle exercise also increases the removal of the residual lactic acid and helps relax muscles.

Fibromyalgia is actually a basket diagnosis of a number of conditions that can have a number of causes, many of them not fully understood. Common circumstances before the disease is diagnosed include an awkward position of the body, repetitive strenuous movements of a group of muscles, the first effort at an exercise, such as the first ski trip of the season, or the first tennis game. Also, moving heavy furniture can bring on pain and spasm of a group of muscles.

Treatment for Fibromyalgia

Small doses of thyroid medication—synthetic thyroid hormones—were used to treat Abby. Doses must be small at first so the body is not shocked. Gentle limbering exercises, heat treatment, and moderate doses of vitamins, including vitamin C, are introduced to overcome the long-standing effect of thyroid deficiency on the muscle.

Fibromyalgia usually responds to this treatment after a few weeks. Thyroid medication might need to be continued for life, but the requirements change throughout life. During pregnancy, thyroid requirements can increase. A nursing mother might have to switch to a medication that does not pass through the breast to appear in milk. As a woman ages, she might require less thyroid medication. The most reliable indicator of the status of the thyroid is the periodic checking of the thyroid stimulating hormone (TSH) level in the blood.

Abby's story is not uncommon. Because thyroid medication is frequently overprescribed by some doctors without a valid indication, like candy, many other doctors suspect that in each case it was unnecessary. The HMO doctor's error was that he did not get in touch with the doctor who had prescribed the medication in the first place or ask Abby for her medical records.

··20··

Mental and Physical Stress

The young adult woman, as the balancer of many demanding roles, is the most stressed woman in the population. Home, family, job, and school take a great deal of energy and organization. When it becomes overwhelming, it leads to physical and mental breakdown in a variety of ways, including minor or temporary illness, temporary bouts of depression, chronic colds, and a pervasive feeling of being run-down. If it continues indefinitely, this kind of stress can lead to long-term illness such as chronic fatigue syndrome, or clinical depression.

CHRONIC FATIGUE SYNDROME (CFS): THE YUPPIE FLU

When chronic fatigue syndrome (CFS) first appeared it was labeled the "yuppie flu" because it has been associated with people balancing high-powered careers and households with children. It was said to be all in their heads, a neurosis of the age. We now know it is an infection, but we do not yet know the invader nor the organ target of the infection.

The cause of CFS is still unknown, but a number of studies indicate that it is a physical illness involving the brain and the immune system. It is estimated that from 100,000 to 250,000 people in the United States suffer from CFS. Seventy percent are women, mostly young and well educated. Anywhere from half to 70 percent of them have a history of allergies. Children can be affected if there is a presence of symptoms in other family members, a recent ingestion of raw milk, or history of allergy or asthma. Exposure to chemicals, a noxious work environment, and poor ventilation have also been suspected of playing a role.

About 2 million women a year go to their physicians with symptoms of CFS. These include muscle and joint pain, memory loss, insom-

295

nia, and disabling fatigue. In a recent study, the Centers for Disease Control and Prevention showed the disease might be more widespread than previously thought, because women with symptoms have been given short shrift by doctors who do not take them seriously or who are not informed about CFS. Current estimates in a Harvard Medical College study of more than 3,000 people indicates as many as 267 people per 100,000 might have CFS. Previous estimates were between 4 and 10 persons per 100,000.

CFS is a chronic disabling fatigue that lasts at least six months. It begins with cold or flulike symptoms—or in a few cases, women reported they felt fine and all of a sudden they were sick. It is frequently associated with intermittent low-grade fever. It was given the name chronic fatigue syndrome by the Centers for Disease Control in 1987, but similar syndromes had other names before. In the eighteenth century, a similar syndrome of low-grade fever and great lassitude and weariness was known as "febricula." In the nineteenth century it was "neurasthenia" and "daCosta syndrome," or simply "the vapors."

CFS is manifested as a flulike illness, a debilitating fatigue, with persistent unexplained relapses. In addition to the low-grade fever, muscle pain, and fatigue, short-term memory and concentration are often impaired.

A famous doctor was asked to speak at a very prestigious meeting in another part of the country. This doctor was an activist, and had a busy private practice, as well as responsibilities at the hospital and at home. When she got up to the podium, she could not deliver her talk. She had become mentally discombobulated. At this point, she decided to go home and see her own physician and find out what was wrong. She felt chronically depleted. She was diagnosed with mononucleosis, yet after weeks of rest she did not feel any better. She came to me a few months later, and I discovered she had a low-grade infection. Her chronic fatigue was due to the infection.

Some cases of chronic fatigue are due to menopause, to hypothyroidism, and to depression. When no cause is found, chronic fatigue syndrome (CFS) is diagnosed.

More recently it has been speculated that CFS might be due to hypoglycemia, multiple allergy syndrome, chronic candidiasis (see page 216), and chronic mononucleosis. It has also been associated with the *Epstein-Barr virus infection,* but in most cases there is no hard evidence of this infection. We suspect it is some kind of infection, but it has not been identified yet. CFS is also sometimes associated with fibromyalgia, or pain in the muscles. Chronic fatigue syndrome can persist for months or years, but usually becomes less bothersome with time.

Diagnosing CFS

There is no distinct diagnostic test for chronic fatigue syndrome, even though some immunologic abnormalities have been found in many of these patients. The only way to diagnose CFS is to exclude all other possible causes of the symptoms, such as thyroid or adrenal diseases, or other abnormalities and lingering infections.

Blood tests will help identify infectious agents in your body. Your doctor might palpate the lymph nodes, which might be tender. A tilt table test can identify falling blood pressure characteristic of CFS. The Romberg test for imbalance, a frequent symptom in CFS, is often administered: You are asked to stand still with your eyes closed; patients with CFS tend to fall forward. The tandem walk is placing the heel of one foot just in front of the toes of the other and walk in a straight line, very difficult to do when the sense of balance is impaired. Blood pressure can be low with CFS and it falls even further on standing still.

Laboratory tests will reveal immunologic abnormalities, such as impaired killer T cell activity, when CFS is present. There might be an increase in the number of B cells, and certain of the B cells and the IgG levels might suggest chronic viral reactivation. Other abnormalities might be circulating immune complexes, electrolyte imbalance, and elevated alkaline phosphatase.

Treatment for CFS
Medications might include an adrenal steroid to get the electrolytes back to normal, more salt intake to increase blood volume, and support stockings for blood pressure and to prevent pooling of the blood in the legs. Many patients improve over time, but often the condition never completely goes away.

CLINICAL DEPRESSION

Mental health is a prime example of how the challenges to a woman's health vary with her life phase and of how the stresses depend on responses to changing roles and conflicting societal demands. The most common mental disorders of women during this life phase are anxiety, clinical depression, panic attacks, and sleep disorders.

Untreated depression can lead to suicide, which is the third leading cause of death of teenagers and the fifth leading cause of death in adults from 25 to 64. Suicide is not a single act, but a dynamic process of conditions and events that intensify over time. Depression can present a different picture in each life phase.

The adolescent girl might be especially concerned about having a perfect body modeled on popular media advertisements. Her eating disorders grow out of such fixations, and her depression might be due to her inability to meet her own unrealistic expectations and those of her parents and peers.

In adult women, the stresses of reconciling domestic roles with those of outside work are frequent causes of depression. Difficulty in getting home chores done; meeting the needs of husband, children, and of aging parents; getting ahead at work; and being a superwoman are all circumstances tugging at women simultaneously. This may lead to acute exhaustion and physical symptoms that will call for a clinical workup in an internist's office.

A menopausal woman might suffer from fear of aging in a society that worships youth. She might suffer the "empty nest syndrome" when her grown children leave home, or perhaps the opposite, if they return to roost again in a household no longer able to sustain them. At the same time she might also be caring for aging parents herself, and feel caught in the bind of being everybody's mother.

An elderly woman mourns the loss of her peers, friends, and family members who have departed. She is acutely affected by the loss of her own capability to see well, to hear well, and to be able to walk, run, or dance without losing her balance. She resents being dependent on others for support, meals, and getting around. She might feel alien in a world of new values, new music, new attitudes. She might become suspicious that her children, or her caretakers, are cheating or neglecting her. (Sometimes, she might be right, as elder abuse is an increasing problem in this country.) She might feel discouraged from exerting effort to adjust to the new, seemingly hostile environment. She might feel that she ought to give up and move on to leave the world to the younger.

All these situations and responses to different circumstances can lead to depression, which is far more common in women than in men. Depression or emotional problems in men are more likely to show up as substance abuse. In 1996, a panel of the National Depressive and Manic-Depressive Association estimated that 24 percent of women and 15 percent of men suffer from clinical depression at some time in their lives, at an annual cost in absenteeism, medical expense, and lost production of $43 billion annually.

Depression is a public health problem in our society. Suicides, especially among young, intelligent people, are the extreme outcome of this highly prevalent illness. The dollars spent on medications alone should tell us something. The global market for the antidepressant medications Prozac, Zoloft, and Paxil and the newest psychotropic drug, Celexa, is estimated at $6 billion a year. Nevertheless, depression is still underdiagnosed and undertreated.

Our attitude is part of the problem. Some people believe being sad or unhappy is part of their personality. Primary care physicians often fail to recognize depression, or they call the symptoms hypochondria— a false belief that we are sick—especially in women. There is a need to reduce the stigma attached to any kind of psychotherapy or mental or emotional disorder, and to educate doctors as well as patients. More patients are treated by their principal physicians for depression than are treated by the mental health sector. Yet principal doctors fail to diagnose 50 to 75 percent of common mental disorders.

Insurance coverage is another barrier to treatment, because not all carriers will cover psychotherapy, and many HMOs will not pay for psychiatric medications, which tend to be very expensive.

There is evidence that depression needs long-term treatment in order to prevent relapse.

Rose is a 40-year-old housewife with two children living at home. She is from a traditional background and, unlike most women today, does not work outside the home even though she has always had a fantasy about being a travel tour director. She complains of chronic fatigue, total exhaustion, overall weakness, and dizziness. Such common and vague symptoms are difficult to define and quantify, and are most difficult to diagnose, as I discovered with Rose. (This has also been a reason for physicians' failure to take them seriously.)

"How long have you been feeling weak?"

"All my life."

"Really? When you were a child, a teenager?"

"Oh, no, not then."

"How about when you were an adolescent?"

"Yes, even then, ever since I started to menstruate."

With some prodding Rose mapped out the times when she was extremely weak: at exam times in high school, in the first year of college, after the birth of her first child, after a severe cold, after the death of her best friend, and when she caught her husband cheating on her. The weakness did not affect any one part of her body differently than the other; it was not localized.

"I wake up very early, at three or four A.M. The world is black and I feel gray inside. I cannot get back to sleep but have no strength to get up out of bed and no reason. I feel dizzy most of the time and so weak. If I do anything half strenuous I feel exhausted."

"Has your dizziness caused you to fall to one side? Do you feel nauseated with the effort to get moving?"

"Not really. Just dizzy and weak."

The early-morning insomnia might point to depression, but the weakness, fatigue, and dizziness call for a comprehensive clinical evaluation to rule out anemia, disorders of the inner ear (labyrinthitis), hormonal abnormalities such as thyroid deficiency, and ovarian, adrenal, and pituitary insufficiency—also diabetes, chronic infection, immune disorders, and cardiac and renal disease. For Rose, all the tests turned out to be normal.

Still, Rose had multiple physical complaints and what is commonly called by doctors a "positive system review." That is, she answered "Yes" to questions about every system of the body. Yes to a question about shortness of breath (cardiovascular system), yes to nausea (gastrointestinal system), yes to a question about "the room swirling around her" (inner ear or central nervous system involvement), yes to urinating a lot (urinary tract or endocrine system). Patients with such diffuse involvement of every system are more likely to have a psychiatric disorder that is manifested in physical (somatic) complaints.

When we can rule out all else, including chronic fatigue syndrome, Rose's history of lifelong recurrence of symptoms points to the diagnosis of depression. Its recurrence is triggered by her home and family situation and by the death of her close friend. Rose is deeply unhappy. Her husband is chronically unfaithful, her 17-year-old daughter might be using drugs, her 20-year-old son has dropped out of college and lolls around in bed all day watching television. Rose's mother, 65, has vascular impairment of her legs that keeps her housebound and dependent upon Rose, and Rose's 85-year-old grandmother has Alzheimer's disease.

Rose has allowed herself to become a doormat. She has swallowed her own anger and is so depressed now that she is unable to see how she can possibly change her life. She is overwhelmed and worried that her own health is failing her. She feels that there is nothing to look forward to, just more suffering, reacting to the ills in her family, trying to deal with them. Her support systems are failing. Rose seeks solace in food and has gained an inordinate amount of weight. She feels unattractive and undesirable. She sees no solution and thinks about suicide every day.

Feeling sad from time to time is common in life. There are stresses everywhere. Dealing successfully with these stresses might help you prevent the development of a profound clinical paralyzing depression. To succeed in the complex world of today you must have inner discipline and control over your life. If you feel overwhelmed, excessively fatigued, and inordinately sad, get treatment and set in motion a plan to get better.

Common Symptoms of Clinical Depression

It is important to distinguish between a passing feeling of "the blues," or sadness, and the symptoms of a major or clinical depression. Here are some indicators of clinical depression.

- Loss of interest or pleasure, depressed mood accompanied by four or more other symptoms that have lasted *at least two weeks*.

- A noticeable weight change—either loss or gain.

- Insomnia or sleeping too much.

- Restlessness, fidgeting, or slow movements, lethargy.

- Loss of energy, fatigue.

- Feelings of guilt and worthlessness.

- Inability to concentrate or make decisions.

- Recurrent thoughts of death and suicide.

- Change in appearance (haggard, untidy, "not there").

Depression leads to suicide in roughly one of six cases. It is estimated that 180 women per 100,000 commit suicide as a result of major depression.

Risk Factors for Depression

There are a variety of risk factors for depression, both physical and emotional. For example, it could be caused by hormonal fluctuation, such as after childbirth or during menopause. It could be familial if there are first-degree relatives with the condition. It can be caused, in some cases, by the "learned helplessness" of women who believe they are unable to take charge of their own lives. Being stuck in the house with small children can also lead to depression, and poverty is a very big factor in the incidence of depression. A tragic event, such as a death in the family, divorce, or loss of a job can lead to long-term depression in cases where there has been a failure to express grief and mourn for the loss.

TREATMENT OF CLINICAL DEPRESSION

Your principal physician can check your health to be sure there is no physical cause for your depression, and can also prescribe drugs that can help you overcome the symptoms. However, such drugs should not be used without accompanying psychiatric or psychological therapy and counseling to enable you to change your life. The depression might also be related to a particular life phase and hormonal levels, and this needs to be considered before prescribing antidepressants, or mood elevators.

Primary care physicians are most often the ones who are treating depression; they are also the ones who most often fail to diagnose depression. If you suspect that your symptoms are due to depression, ask your physician to refer you to a competent psychiatrist.

Psychotropic Drugs

Entire books have been written about the effect Prozac has had on our society. Millions of Americans take this or a similar drug to combat depression. It has been the subject of a great deal of debate, most of which is still unsettled. However, the goal of using such drugs for depression is short term. They are meant to give you a jump start on the road to pulling yourself out of depression. Although these drugs can be prescribed by your principal physician, they should be used only in conjunction with valid psychological counseling and a comprehensive plan to get control of your life and yourself.

There are many medications available to treat symptoms of depression. Antidepressants are helpful in the treatment of panic disorders and phobias. The newer selective serotonin re-uptake inhibitors (SSRI), such as Prozac, Zoloft, and Paxil, seem to have fewer side effects than the older antidepressants, called tricyclics because of their chemical formula, which consists of three ringlike structures.

It is essential that you follow the doctor's instructions and do not attempt to self-medicate with psychotropic drugs. A thorough physical examination must be performed first, as well as an evaluation of your hormone levels and any other medications you might be taking simultaneously.

Professional Psychotherapy

There are many types of short- and long-term psychotherapy and counseling available in almost any part of the country, from in-depth psychoanalysis, to group therapy, to behavioral therapy, and a variety of newer techniques.

Psychotherapy takes place between you and the psychotherapist (psychiatrist or psychologist) and is designed to make you feel better about yourself and your surroundings. As you share your experiences with the therapist you gain insight into your own "bag" of preconceived ideas, habits, and misconceptions. While traditional therapists are nondirective—that is, they do not suggest to you how to handle your problems—under subtle questioning by the therapists you might yourself arrive at the best ways of handling the situations.

Psychoanalysis is a long-term, intensive treatment that explores your experiences as far back as your childhood, your early relationships, and your conscious and subconscious thoughts. By understanding yourself you might be able to understand how you get into difficult situations and avoid repeating your mistakes.

Behavioral therapy, frequently used by psychologists, is based on reinforcement of a desired behavior by a series of rewards and punishments. It might consist of manipulation of the environment toward one conducive to a desired behavior. Behavioral therapy might help you stop smoking, or overeating, to get into and persist with a good fitness program.

Here's an overview of the professionals involved in mental health:

Psychiatrists are certified medical doctors who specialize in the mental health field. Being able to understand the interactions between physical health and emotions, they take a complete physical and psychological history. They can treat you with a variety of therapies, including drug therapy as well as psychotherapy. They are the only psychotherapists legally allowed to prescribe drugs.

Psychologists have doctoral degrees in the field of psychology. They are not medical doctors, and they cannot prescribe drugs, but they do use psychotherapy. If psychotherapy needs to be supplemented with medications, psychologists refer you to a psychiatrist or have you consult with your principal physician.

Psychiatric social workers have degrees in social work with training in psychotherapy. They might make good counselors but lack the depth of formal psychological training that psychologists and psychiatrists have.

Other specialists are available to help you deal with special causes of depression, such as long-term domestic violence or substance abuse. These are people especially trained to help you deal with the cause of the problem and change the situation. For example, a marriage counselor is not trained to deal with domestic violence or drug or alcohol abuse. Eating disorders need the attention of a psychotherapist as well as an internist, but alcoholism and drug abuse require special programs such as Alcoholics Anonymous and a clinical rehabilitation program. The addiction needs to be treated separately before the depression can be addressed.

If you are depressed because of a chronic illness, you can find support from medical associations that operate support groups and self-help programs for those who have cancer, kidney disease, diabetes, or arthritis. Almost every illness has an organization that can give you information and support. If you are the principal caregiver to a chronically ill spouse, you can find a great deal of help and support from groups such as the Well Spouse Foundation, which are very knowledgeable about the depression that comes from this situation.

EIGHT WAYS TO TAKE CONTROL OF YOURSELF AND YOUR LIFE

The most difficult part of getting better is deciding you want to get better and take that first step toward change. I believe very strongly that you should seek medical advice to help treat depression. And while you are doing that, I have developed my own "homespun" ideas, which I'll share with you, to help women overcome depression.

Develop an Action Plan

To change your life you need a plan with very specific objectives. Write down your stresses; list them in the order of how they affect you. Include the reasons for the stress and how you would like to have it resolved. For instance, Rose planned to have a talk with her daughter and get her into a drug rehab program, and possibly into a Tough Love program that helps teenagers and parents learn how to communicate. She planned to give her freeloader son an ultimatum about finishing school or getting a job and his own apartment. She planned to take her mother to a doctor for comprehensive medical care so she would be able to get around on her own, and possibly employ a home health worker to tend to her needs until then. The grandmother would be put into a nursing home.

Rose also had to confront her feelings about her husband. Did she want to tolerate his infidelity? Did she want to divorce him and live alone? This was a tough decision, but she planned to let him know, and show him, that she was not a doormat.

Once the list is made, get all the information, names and phone numbers, of any people needed to carry out the plans. When a course of action is decided, the timetable needs to be set. Be specific, set dates, then proceed. Imagine where you want to be in a week, a month, and a year. Visualize yourself achieving these goals. Rose had been so busy that she had not given herself time to deal with her depression and the problems that caused it. She knew she could not solve these problems overnight, but she outlined realistic time schedules for all she wanted to accomplish.

Rose planned to find some way to begin working in the travel industry and started to research it. She also planned to join Weight Watchers to get control of her weight. She knew if she did she would be on a balanced and sensible diet and have the support of others in the program.

Get a Comprehensive Physical Checkup

Be sure to have your own physical examination to rule out anemia, thyroid abnormality, hypoglycemia, diabetes, or anything that could be affecting your mood. Determine to follow a program of preventive care to remain healthy. Ask your doctor for referrals for appropriate therapy for your depression. Just the simple act of taking your health seriously is a step on the road to recovery.

Eat Properly

Three modest meals a day can help in weight control and maintaining overall health and well-being. Eat plenty of fruits, vegetables, and grains; establish a diet low in fat and meats. Skipping breakfast is the most common dieter's mistake. Having breakfast cranks the engine up and helps burn the calories. (For more complete information about nutrition and weight control, refer back to chapter 10.)

Get Regular Exercise

Vigorous exercise not only has a beneficial effect on your physical well-being but is a perfect psychological tranquilizer. When you feel mad at someone, don't bash him over the head or sit there in a snit. Instead, get out and run, do some laps in a pool, or walk fast around a block or two. This does not solve the original problem, but as your body releases its own feel-good hormones, the endorphins, you might think more rationally and come up with a more effective way to deal with the situation. Plan at least half an hour each day of recreational flexing of your muscles: run, jog, swim, bicycle, play tennis or basketball (refer to chapter 5).

Keep Busy

Being involved with and enjoying what you do, at home and work, might chase your blues away. If your work is a source of your anxiety and depression, reevaluate what you want to accomplish at work and whether your job is worth the pain it causes. Learn to say no to excessive demands at work, at home, to friends and colleagues. Find time for relaxing activities, hobbies, and learning new skills. Try to combine necessary activities like watching the children or preparing a meal with pleasant circumstances such as listening to music. Perhaps you can find private time to practice meditation, yoga, relaxation, or biofeedback.

Talk About It

If you have close friends you might wish to confide your stresses to them. Sometimes good advice from a real friend can help you perform a "reality check" on your complaints. Rose also got involved in support groups for relatives of drug abusers, which helped her understand what her daughter was going through and how they both could help resolve the problem. All in all, depend on your principal physician to direct your strategies to prevent severe depression and to encourage professional psychotherapy when it is necessary.

Get Away from It All

Although taking a vacation is not a cure-all for depression, a vacation and a change of scene might provide an opportunity for you to take stock of the situation and plan more substantive strategies. With some distance, you might see things more clearly.

Enjoy What You Have

No matter how sad or frustrating you feel your situation is, try to remember what gifts you do have. You still have two arms and two legs and a roof over your head. These are assets that someone else might be missing. List your assets and think about them; about how much sadder you would be if you did not have them. The sun might not be shining today, but perhaps it will tomorrow.

Keep in mind that, although you might be balancing many demanding roles, you are also exposed to myriad opportunities during this phase of life when you are most strong.

··21··

Domestic Violence:
A Public Health Hazard
for Women

Violence by an intimate partner is the leading cause of injury to women, and in New York City it is the leading cause of death among women. One in four women in America is the victim of domestic violence at least once, and it accounts for more than a third of emergency room visits by women of all ages. The degree of injury from domestic violence is severe. Of 218 women coming to one metropolitan emergency department with injuries, 28 percent required admission to the hospital, and 13 percent required major medical treatment, such as surgery. Almost half of the women had been there before.

Because of the devastating toll it takes on women, domestic violence was declared a public health hazard in 1988 by the American Medical Women's Association and in 1992 by the American Medical Association. In 1994 it was declared a federal crime. Since then, the police, the courts, and the medical establishment have been trying to learn better ways of helping women.

From a medical perspective, domestic violence appears as a systematic or recognizable syndrome, with symptoms in the victim similar to those of posttraumatic stress disorder, a condition characterized by recurring and debilitating symptoms of anxiety and depression. In a 1995 study by the Commonwealth Fund Commission on Women's Health, researchers established that a person's response to an acute violent event is remarkably the same whether it's from war trauma, concentration camp experience, or domestic assault. Survivors of violent acts have common reactions, such as paralyzing terror, anxiety bordering on panic, loss of control, and the sudden realization of their own vulnerability. Stress reactions are acute and lead to nightmares, insomnia, poor concentration, amnesia, hypervigilance, and hypersensitivity to any sudden noise even remotely connected with violence, such as a door slamming.

CRISIS INTERVENTION

Some hospitals have an immediate crisis intervention *team* to help you work through the violent event—they also help prevent posttraumatic stress disorders. The team helps you ventilate your intense feelings in a safe environment with supportive listeners. The goal of crisis intervention is to help bring you back to a normal emotional and physical state.

A few hospitals now have a domestic violence advocate on staff, and a few provide state-of-the-art care for women in abusive relationships. Some hospitals work closely with crisis centers in their communities to provide lasting help for women who are physically abused.

To be effective, crisis intervention should include helping you plan for safety and a way to leave the violent relationship. It should also refer you to a women's shelter and link you up to the social service and legal systems, as well as to advocates who can walk you through the systems so you can make progress. Without intervention and assistance into a support system, you are less likely to get help.

Signs of Abuse

The fight-or-flight response is our normal reaction to stress. Our adrenaline pumps up so we are ready for either response. However, women in violent relationships are stuck in overdrive. They continue to feel the stress. This wear and tear on the body and the emotions leads to many long-term health problems, among them:

- Migraine headaches
- Hypertension
- Loss of hearing or vision
- Gastrointestinal problems
- Malnutrition
- Miscarriage and other dangers to pregnancy
- Depression
- Substance abuse
- Suicide and murder

Doctors and nurses now routinely look for signs of domestic violence as part of the initial screening in emergency rooms. The American Medical Association, which acknowledges that its members have failed to identify domestic violence in as many as 98 percent of cases, has produced a learning manual for its members to help them deal with the injuries and illnesses resulting from domestic violence.

As early as 1988, the American Medical Women's Association established the Task Force on Violence Against Women, and it has developed a curriculum on how to teach doctors to recognize, diagnose, and manage domestic violence. Some of our members hold courses on domestic violence with local police forces so that they become more sensitive to the issue.

While the AMA and AMWA are both urging doctors to recognize and treat domestic violence (something most doctors neglected in the past), the Joint Commission on Accreditation of Healthcare Organizations, the national regulatory board for hospitals, has instructed its members to improve care to those coming into hospitals with symptoms related to domestic violence—or lose their accreditation.

When you arrive in an emergency room in any accredited, publicly supported, or private hospital, you must receive medical care whether or not you have insurance. In Quincy, Massachusetts, women leaving abusive relationships are given free medical care.

If you came into a hospital with a heart attack, doctors would ask about your health history from diet to whether or not you smoke—all the risk factors for heart disease. Today doctors are required to do the same thing for domestic violence. If they suspect abuse they might ask you if your partner has hurt or frightened you at any time.

Even if you have no visible bruises or broken bones after a violent incident, you might be sufficiently traumatized to be in shock and in need of medical attention. Have police or a friend or neighbor take you to the nearest emergency room for a thorough checkup and possibly X rays.

Even in a busy urban hospital emergency room, the guard at the door will have been trained to be on the lookout for an abusive man who might be trying to control an injured woman he is with. All emergency room personnel—from the guards to the receptionists to the medical staff—are trained to respond to domestic violence. The guard will report this activity to the staff inside. If your abusive partner will not leave your side because he is so "concerned," this in itself will tip off the doctor. It is a common behavior pattern of abusive men. If you feel the hospital staff will protect you from further violence, answer their questions as candidly as you can. An alert doctor or nurse will understand your reluctance to be forthcoming about domestic violence and might try to coax more information from you. Most women are relieved to finally talk about it. But you should not feel pressured or intimidated. If you are not ready to tell anyone, just say that.

No matter how you describe what happened to you, the physician will look for the following things:

• Common domestic violence assault injuries such as contusions, abrasions, and minor lacerations, as well as fractures or sprains.

• Injuries to your head, neck, chest, breasts, and abdomen—especially the latter two if you are pregnant.

• Numerous injuries on many parts of your body, which signals either an auto accident, a natural disaster, or a beating.

• Defensive injuries like fractures or bruises on your forearm that would suggest you were trying to fend off blows to your face or chest.

• In addition to physical injuries, they will look for depression, anxiety, and the psychological and emotional symptoms of stress disorders

When you talk with the emergency department doctor or nurse, if they think your story of what happened to you does not match the extent of your injuries, this is also a tip-off. Women commonly invent stories to cover up what really happened. If you say you fell down the stairs because your abusive partner brought you in and warned you not to say what really happened, try to find some way to let the physician know that it is not safe for you to talk unless the hospital can promise to protect you. The security staff can also be summoned to accompany you to different areas of the hospital, such as the X-ray room. You are entitled to be safe in a hospital.

Sadly, you are especially at risk for domestic violence if you are pregnant—as many as half of all abused women are abused when they are pregnant. And 24 percent of the pregnant women seen in clinics and hospitals have been assaulted by a violent partner. More babies are born with birth defects as a result of violence against the mothers than a combination of all diseases and illnesses for which we now immunize pregnant women.

The physical effects of violence during pregnancy are especially profound. You are twice as likely to miscarry and four times more likely to have a low birth weight baby if you have been beaten up during this time. You are at risk for a ruptured uterus, detached placenta, hemorrhage, miscarriage, and early labor. Your baby could be malformed, permanently disabled, or killed before it is born.

Ask the hospital to help you, so you do not have to return to the abusive man (see chapter 14).

Talking with Your Doctor

Many women do not go to the emergency room or hospital when they are hurt, but try to wait until their abusive partner is gone. Perhaps they wait until the next morning, when he goes to work. Others fear that if they use the same doctor who treats the abuser, the doctor will betray their confidence and the abuser will find out.

What if the doctor knows your family? If you don't feel you can share your story with the family doctor who also treats your abuser, then find another doctor. Try to find a doctor who respects women and will not treat you like a child, one who understands the problems of domestic violence or who seems well informed about new health care response. Ask a domestic violence advocate where you can find the kind of doctor you need. Call your local health network, women's organizations, the local chapter of the American Medical Women's Association. You can call a local health network, or a hospital, and ask them to recommend a family doctor, or whatever type of doctor you believe you need.

Don't let yourself be pressured or judged. You will know when you are ready for intervention, when it is safe. And each time you visit a medical setting and seek help, you are one step closer to taking the next step toward freedom.

Helen had been abused for years but had never reported it. Before marriage she had a dynamic job on Wall Street. When the children came—three of them—she became a full-time homemaker. Helen came to see me many times with chronic ailments such as headaches and gastrointestinal problems, but she was careful never to reveal the real cause of her distress.

Helen had been having severe headaches ever since her third child was born. Life began to seem like a big blur. That last child, now past the terrible twos, was not a problem. The middle child was in kindergarten, and the oldest was a sweet and "perfect" child. Helen's husband worked hard despite his fear of being downsized. But he made enough money for Helen to stay home with the children, and the house was maintained in good order. Helen assumed her malaise was her own fault.

In the park one day, watching her youngest children play, she told her friend that she woke up with headaches and they lasted all day. She could not think clearly, and her memory was faulty. "My gynecologist said all new mothers have headaches," she told her friend. "But I am hardly a new mother anymore." Her friend sent her to me for a thorough checkup.

Her history and examination was unremarkable except for anemia. She had lost weight because she was not eating properly. An MRI and a thorough neurological examination with a specialist were negative.

Helen is well organized and systematic in her daily schedule. Her children are well attended to, and the husband's dinner is on the table the minute he walks in. The three children come up with constant minor problems that she keeps solving logically and effectively. When I suggested that she could afford to get some help with the house, she said she and her husband were "private people." They did not want a stranger underfoot. Suddenly a lightbulb went on in my mind. Sometimes this kind of talk means that the husband has a problem with control, and a common characteristic of controlling men is the attempt to keep their wives isolated.

Helen had come to see me for another one of her migraine headaches, but with new insight and suspicions, I began to look for other telltale signs. A fading bruise over her temple and scalp, almost within her hairline, was camouflaged by her slightly odd hairstyle.

"How did you get this?" After staring at me for a moment, she said, "I fell." I disregarded her answer and pushed on.

"Did someone hurt you?" That's all it took: Helen dissolved in tears. Michael had been bashing her all over the head, calling her stupid and ignorant.

I gave Helen the name of a domestic violence counselor at a women's crisis center because I know that in cases of violence a marriage or family counselor is not appropriate treatment. I gave her the local and federal domestic violence hot line numbers. Michael needed to be held responsible, be punished for his crime, and get battering therapy. I urged Helen to report the incident to the police. She refused all avenues of help, afraid that Michael would punish her even more for "spilling the beans." Sadly, I knew this was true, too. The majority of abused women who are killed are killed when they attempt to leave the abuser, and thus deprive him of control.

Once again, before she left, I asked her if she wanted to go to a safe place, but she said no, her children were home with a baby-sitter and she could not leave them. I urged her to follow up with the phone numbers and find out what she could do. I urged her to talk with other women who have been through the same experience. She promised to do that but did not show up for a return appointment. When I called she whispered back that her husband had been very sweet these last weeks but forbade her to see me again. Yes, she would report to the police if violence recurred. She hung up, and I did not hear from her again. Years later a mutual acquaintance told me that Helen had left her husband. She and her children moved to the Midwest, where Helen lived with her family until she was able to get a job and her own home with her children. Thank God, I thought.

Perhaps the greatest misconception about domestic violence is that it is solely the domain of the poor and uneducated. In fact, it crosses all economic, social, cultural, and educational lines. And it is not your fault. It is the fault of the man with the problem, and his actions are against the law. In some cultures it is more difficult for women to seek help, especially where women are raised to be modest, patient, and self-deprecating.

GETTING TREATMENT FOR ABUSE

If you are being physically abused by a partner, you might feel embarrassed, and the doctor might feel embarrassed for you, but you will be sorry later if you do not get your story on the record. Tell the doctor what happened as accurately as possible and also describe any past history of violence or abuse. If you are timid with medical authority, take a friend who can do some of the talking for you and provide moral support.

Your physician should let you know exactly what kind of treatment you need, ask you if you will be able to follow up with the necessary care, and see if you need help to do this. If your physical injuries do not require that you stay overnight in the hospital, but you are afraid to go home, doctors can arrange for a safe place for you to go. They can also take you out of the hospital under guard and into protection of a shelter or the police. If you need to be transported for treatment, the hospital must see that you get there safely, without being hurt again by the man who caused your injuries.

It is important for you to receive treatment for symptoms of abuse, just as you would receive treatment for any health condition that could lead to disability and an early death without treatment. Talk with the doctors about how this can be accomplished whether you go home or not. You might not be ready to leave your abusive partner yet, but you must get medical care.

If any medication, such as a painkiller, is prescribed, ask about side effects. If the painkiller will make you drowsy, your abusive partner could take advantage of your lowered resistance to become violent again. Avoid tranquilizers or sleeping pills, because you must be as alert as possible. You cannot be walking around in a fog when your life is in danger. Discuss alternatives with the doctor.

Keeping Medical Records as Evidence

If your abusive partner broke a lamp over your head you could have glass or wood fragments embedded in your skull. These should be saved after they are removed. If you came into the hospital with blood all over your clothing, or with clothing that was torn because of obvious violence, the doctor should remove this clothing and lock it away in a sealed and labeled bag as evidence. This material can be locked up until it is needed by police, prosecutors, or your own lawyer. Evidence needs to be carefully preserved, labeled, and documented in order to be used in court.

Most hospitals have still cameras and videos for imaging injuries. With your consent they will photograph your injuries from all angles, close up and full body, including your face. Two pictures of each trauma area should be labeled with your name, the date, and the location of the injury, as well as the names of the witness and photographer. One set of pictures will be part of your medical record and the other will be locked away for later use by you or the police. The police and prosecutors might also want to photograph or videotape your injuries while you are in the hospital if criminal charges are filed against your abusive partner.

Physicians are required to document your condition and treatment and report any suspicions about partner abuse or domestic violence syndrome. Careful documentation is important because you can use it in court if you are seeking an order of protection, a divorce, or child custody. In addition to your name and address, and the time, date, and location of the injury, here is what your medical report should include.

- Medical history, including diseases, injuries, and pregnancies.

- Chief complaint and description of the abusive event described by you.

- A detailed description of your injuries, possible causes, and explanations given. The location and nature of the injuries might also be illustrated on a body chart.

- Color photographs and imaging studies of your injuries. (You might have to sign a consent for a physician to take photographs of you showing your injuries.)

- The physician's opinion on whether the injuries were adequately explained by you. If not, documentation of how the injuries occurred.

- The physician's note that he or she did ask you about domestic violence and your response to the inquiry.

- Results of all pertinent laboratory and diagnostic procedures.

- If the police are called, the name, badge number, and phone number of the investigating officer and any actions taken.

- Name of the physicians and nurses who treated you.

- Name and address of anyone who is with you.

Pay attention to the details of your medical report. Because several people might be making entries onto your medical records, there can frequently be errors. Ask to read the report before you leave, or have someone read it to you if you are unable to read it because of your injuries. Ask for copies of your medical record when you leave the hospital or doctor's office if you think you will need it right away to apply for a protective order or to file a criminal complaint with the police.

Physicians who treat women for injuries inflicted by their intimate partners are often called on to testify in court about what they saw, the extent of your injuries, and how they treated you. They can also become involved as expert witnesses, who give medical testimony about the nature of the injury or condition, as well as any reasons to suspect abuse. This could include, for example, giving an opinion as to whether an explanation given by a patient for a particular injury is consistent with medically recognized abuse.

Doctors are usually required to report to police any gunshot or stab wounds or any other injuries that they suspect are a result of felonious assault. If your injuries are less drastic, they still might report them in some states.

Doctors might ask if you want them to report the violence. If you agree to allow the police to be called, or if the hospital is required to call them because of the nature of your injuries, then a social worker or domestic violence advocate should also be present with you during this meeting.

Protecting Your Confidentiality

If the hospital has your address already on file—from previous visits or from your medical insurance card—ask them to change this in the computer and show a separate "mailing" address. Women have often refused to get proper medical treatment for conditions caused by abuse because they are covered on their abusive partner's insurance coverage and fear he would find out they were getting medical treatment. If this is your case, explain this to the physician caring for you.

The health care system generates lots of paperwork. Many things might be sent to your home after you leave a hospital or clinic, such as lab test results and billing statements. If you do not want reports or bills sent home, do not give them your real address. Tell doctors and staff you might not be at that address, or that your partner will see the medical reports and destroy them. He knows they are evidence. Have your reports sent to your job, or to a friend or family member you can trust.

Nobody with a life-threatening injury or disease would be allowed to leave the hospital. Naturally, they cannot lock you in the hospital, but if they advise you not to leave and you insist on leaving anyway, you will probably have to sign a statement that you left "against medical advice."

An accredited medical facility cannot let you go home without finding out if you have or need a safety plan, if you have someplace to go, and if you need a domestic violence advocate. They cannot let you go until they assess the risk that you might commit suicide or be killed by the violent man after you leave the hospital.

The national domestic violence hot line number is 800-799-SAFE (7233). For the hearing impaired the number is 800-787-3224 TDD.

PHASE III

THE PERIMENOPAUSAL YEARS

AGES 45–65

....

INTRODUCTION:
THE SANDWICH GENERATION

At the beginning of the twentieth century, when the average life expectancy of an American woman was barely 50, menopause, which begins anywhere between 35 and 58, was considered a taboo topic even among grandmothers who had survived the perils of childbirth. Today, a woman's life expectancy is 76. Most of us will spend *at least* a third of our lives without the benefit of the full complement of estrogen produced by our ovaries.

When life expectancy was nearer 50 few women survived beyond menopause. Those who did were seldom accepted by the Western civilization as full-fledged citizens. In the Middle Ages and in Salem, Massachusetts, in the seventeenth century, mature single or widowed but active women were feared—and some were burned as witches. Today, women are taking charge of their own destinies and writing books about menopause to put to rest the myths that have been handed down over the generations.

We continue to be parents, workers, and lovers. We might also be caught in the middle of a generational gap as well. Because we are all living longer, this time of life poses the added condition of being sandwiched between two generations. Not only are we parents to our children, many of us become caretakers to our parents as well. While we are coming close to achieving many of our life's goals, and perhaps more time for ourselves, we are also taking on more responsibility at a time when our bodies are beginning another hormonal transition that will toss us onto that cyclical choppy sea again.

Menopause, the so-called change of life, is a normal phase of every woman's life, and not necessarily the last one. In the past, women dreaded menopause, which was viewed by society as the *end* of a woman's useful (read "reproductive") life. Fifty years ago a woman of 45 was considered over the hill. She had little to expect

319

after wearing out her reproductive function, except perhaps to clean house for her husband and work at a dull and unfulfilling job. No more babies, hence no more sex, no role in the world.

The dominant youth-worshipping ideology in our society makes many women feel that if they look their age after menopause, they are less attractive. This is not true. Good health, good nutrition (including appropriate vitamin intake), proper balance of exercise and rest, satisfying work, and relationships contribute enormously to a mature woman's good looks.

Thank goodness attitudes are changing. However, despite our strength and youthfulness well into advanced age, some women still fear this perimenopausal phase, the years from approximately 45 to 65, believing they will lose their attractiveness, grow hairs on their chins, and lose interest in sex. And worse, their husbands will lose interest in having sex with them, or will run off with a younger woman. And if a woman is still single at 45, surely she will never get a man!

At best, men know very little about menopause and what to expect during this change in a woman's life, but it is apparently not true that they lose interest in having sex with their partners. A leading drug company that surveyed men between the ages of 45 and 65 who were married or partnered with someone in that age range found that the majority did not feel these women were any less desirable to them than they were at a younger age.

Getting rid of wrinkles temporarily with cosmetics or a face-lift destroys the evidence of aging. Looking young again might help some deny the passing years and keep old age at a distance. But wrinkles and loose skin are merely metaphors reflecting the natural cycle of life, which eventually proceeds toward death. This is a time when we must begin screening for cancer and other diseases that occur with advancing age, so that we prevent them from interfering with the rest of our lives. We are challenged by the stress not only of a changing body, but by the challenges of our work, our children growing up and leaving home, and our aging parents, who might need more of our care.

This section of the book is focused on what happens to our bodies as our estrogen levels diminish, how many years that process takes, and what it means in short- and long-term changes in our health. Estrogen can afford us protection against heart disease and osteoporosis. In some women, that protection might be counterbalanced by side effects of hormones. We need to know how to adjust our lifestyles, our diets, and become more health conscious. We need to know about risks of heart disease, how we can prevent osteoporosis, and how our gastrointestinal system can be fixed when it is overworked.

The only way we can make sensible decisions about whether or not to use hormonal replacement therapy as our own estrogen diminishes is to become very well informed about what happens to our bodies, what the symptoms of menopause mean, what the long-term risks of this therapy are, and what options we have. And we do have many options. There is no one course of action for all women. We are all unique individuals, and who we are says a great deal about what we should do.

One thing is certain, however. If you have been putting off quitting such bad habits as smoking, overeating, and being sedentary, put them off no longer. The years of abuse are catching up fast now, and you are even more vulnerable to complications from poor lifestyle choices when your hormones are fluctuating.

We need to know how to preserve our health assets; how to continue to grow emotionally, intellectually, and socially; how to foster our creativity and reach out not only to our families but also to our communities, our workplace associates, the world at large. It is these links to others that will help our emotional and physical health and permit us to grow during these important years.

Three fifths of your life is behind you, but almost half of your life is still ahead of you. The symptoms of menopause disappear after a while, the body adjusts to less estrogen, and women experience a period of vigor, health, and sharpness of mind and drive. Margaret Mead so rightly described this time of life when she said, "There is no more creative force under the sun than that of a woman with postmenopausal zest."

··22··

The Three Phases of Menopause

With baby boomers in ascendancy, about a million and a half women enter menopause every year. Those who suffer from severe symptoms like hot flashes caused by the decline in estrogen levels consider it a national emergency. The steeper the drop in estrogen level, the more severe are the menopausal symptoms. Fortunately, not everybody experiences the full syndrome, and fewer than 10 percent truly require treatment. The most important consideration at this time is to realize that these are short-term symptoms that will eventually disappear but that there are long-term consequences that will not—the increased risk for heart disease and osteoporosis, for instance.

The Wyeth-Ayerst Laboratories, which make hormonal drugs used for therapy, conduct an annual menopause survey. Women and men between 45 and 65 years of age were surveyed in 1997 about their attitudes about menopause. The report found that baby boomers seem to be approaching menopause with the same zeal they experienced raising their families and climbing the corporate ladder. Close to nine of ten women feel that menopause can be the start of a new phase in their lives. Women who have already completed menopause are even more likely to view menopause as a positive, rather than a negative, experience. Overall, women look forward to this new phase as having to worry less about pregnancy, having their children independent, spending more time on themselves and with their spouses. And having no more menstrual periods! According to the survey:

• 92 percent feel they can now better appreciate their own sensuality because they better understand themselves and their needs.

• 84 percent of women do not believe that menopause makes a woman feel less feminine.

• 81 percent disagree with the idea that women feel less attractive and desirable once they experience menopause.

• Eight out of ten say they have become more comfortable with their bodies as they have grown older.

• 89 percent say they are more confident about themselves and their sexuality.

Menopause is not a single event but a process over a period of many years, and it can be divided roughly into three phases: perimenopause, menopause, and postmenopause. Over the years, the 2 million or so follicles in the ovaries are exhausted. Some of them have ovulated, and others have undergone atresia—a process of shrinking and disappearing. When there are no longer any viable follicles left, menstrual periods stop and estrogen and progesterone produced by the ovaries are gradually reduced until only small amounts are secreted. Actually, what usually happens first is that the capacity to ovulate declines, and many of the perimenopausal cycles are anovulatory, meaning the bleeding is due to the drop of estrogen alone. That is why in perimenopause bleeding can be irregular. Since progesterone is only produced when ovulation occurs, it is estrogen decline that is responsible for the symptoms of menopause, and usually the sharper the decline, the more severe the symptoms.

Perimenopause

Perimenopause is the two to ten years when menstrual periods become irregular but don't stop altogether. The time between periods might suddenly become longer, or shorter, and sometimes alternates between the two. Bleeding might taper off to just a day or so a month—or become so heavy as to require a curettage (D&C) to prevent anemia. Such hemorrhages can result from excessive estrogen levels, unopposed by progesterone. The Massachusetts Women's Health Study, observing more than 2,500 women between the ages of 45 and 55, indicates that on average, perimenopause begins at age 47.5 and lasts 3.8 years.

Menopause

The actual menopause is the year or so in which the menses stop. In most women menopause occurs between the ages of 50.1 and 51.5. Women who smoke reach these milestones a year or two sooner. About 30 percent of women experience menopause between the ages of 40 and 45, and perhaps less than 1 percent between the ages of 35 and 40. It is difficult sometimes to point to the exact year this happens because for several years thereafter a reprise of menstrual bleeding could occur. However, whenever postmenopausal bleeding does occur, D&C is necessary in order to rule out hyperplasia and endometrial cancer. Bleeding can also be caused by contact on intercourse, and that is most frequently due to cervicitis, an inflammation of the cervix.

Postmenopause

Any time after menopause is considered postmenopause. Some researchers consider this to extend only from five to ten years after the last menstrual period and call life after postmenopause the advanced phase. Others feel that postmenopause is forever. Indeed, the symptoms of menopause can recur twenty years later if a woman is under particular stress (acute illness or emotional turmoil). There is no end to the "change of life."

Premature Menopause

Some women, like 36-year-old Sophie, have a premature menopause. We don't know exactly why this is. It may be familial, but Sophie said her mother had died young, and she had no maternal aunts or older sisters. It could have been the stress of late childbearing—she had had a baby six months before—or the stress of family problems compounded by her company's decision to eliminate her job. Sophie had been divorced from an earlier marriage, and she and Jack married two years before. Each had a child by a previous marriage who lived with them. When they planned to have a child together, both had good salaries, and they believed they would be able to do it by both of them taking paid maternity leave. When Sophie lost her job, this changed.

Sophie came to see me because she was having hot flashes and because she had done something so out of character that it scared her. Sophie had been trying to do some freelance work at home. The two older children were arguing, the baby was crying, the television was blaring. All of a sudden, while trying to mediate the argument between the children, she got dizzy and unable to concentrate on what she was trying to say to them. Her heart pounded, her head was burning, and she began to scream. The children stopped in their tracks, and Sophie ran out of the house.

She walked quickly for several blocks, taking deep breaths, and tried to focus her mind on what had just happened. She was not prone to such outbursts. Yes, there had been lots of pressure lately, but Sophie believed she was a strong and capable woman. She could handle it. As she crossed a street and a car slammed on its brakes and blew its horn, Sophie came crashing back to reality. She saw the enraged face of the man who had almost run her down, and saw her own reflection in the car window. She apologized to the man and turned back toward her house. She was overwhelmed with guilt at having left her children, and she began to run. The older children were quietly reading, and the baby was sleeping in the portable bassinet, which her son was gently rocking with his foot as he read his book.

I saw Sophie the next day, and after I took her history, I examined her thoroughly. She told me her periods had not been regular since she had the baby. Her examination and electrocardiogram were completely normal, but her follicle stimulating hormone (FSH) was high, so it was possible that she might be undergoing menopause. When estrogen (and progesterone) levels in the blood decline, the levels of FSH rise, and testing this hormone level can determine if menopause is occurring. FSH above 40 units is considered high and is diagnostic of menopause.

On temporary estrogen therapy, Sophie felt like a new person. Not only did her hot flushes, palpitations, dizziness, and insomnia disappear, she felt more vigorous and less tired. The series of crises in her family life had taken a toll, and she had not acknowledged how tired she had been all these months.

There are times when menopause begins very early, as in Sophie's case. Her ovaries might have taken a vacation for a while, what is called a temporary ovarian failure. Her symptoms could have been a result of the childbirth, or perhaps the beginning of menopause. Sophie never got her own ovarian function back and continued on estrogen until she was 55, when the dose was tapered and stopped as a part of her decision, after a thorough discussion with me about pros and cons of continuing the hormone and an assessment of her own individual risks for heart disease, osteoporosis, and breast cancer.

THE PHYSICAL SYMPTOMS OF MENOPAUSE

We cannot predict which women will suffer the full gamut of the menopausal syndrome. Women with early menopause, either natural or as a consequence of surgical tampering with their ovaries, tend to have more severe symptoms. Stress is likely to make symptoms worse, and even in post-postmenopause, after the hot flashes have completely subsided, stress and illness might bring out a temporary return of the symptoms.

Fears about menopause, just like any other stress, can magnify the physical symptoms. At the same time, more severe symptoms might further feed the fears. Sometimes, women are not prepared for the symptoms and interpret normal menopausal events, such as the flashing, as something pathological, indicative of disease. When you do not know what to expect you imagine the worst. A sudden feeling of being disoriented, moments when your heart seems to jump out of your chest, can be truly frightening. Fortunately, very few women experience the entire spectrum of symptoms. Most have occasional flashes, sweats, or palpitations. These feelings are a normal part of the experience of menopause and eventually go away.

There is a theory that women who have vasomotor symptoms (hot flashes and profuse sweating) might be more sensitive to hormonal changes than women who are symptom-free. Another theory is that women living in societies where menopause is viewed in a positive way might have just as many hot flashes but not pay much attention to them.

From past studies and other available data, it is suggested that menopausal symptoms are similar in the North American countries, but Japanese women experience fewer symptoms. Earlier studies show that Mayan Indian women had no symptoms of menopause, but 80 percent of Dutch women reported hot flashes. In non-Western cultures such as Japan and Nigeria, joint pain and body stiffness are the most commonly reported manifestations of menopause. In Western culture, the association of these symptoms with estrogen decline remains less well-known.

Menopause affects all women differently. Some sail through and hardly notice it. Others are rendered helpless. The majority of women—about 60 to 70 percent—have only mild symptoms such as occasional hot flashes; 10 to 20 percent have no symptoms whatsoever. A small proportion suffer such intense symptoms, such as heart palpitations, frequent mood changes, unrelenting insomnia, and overwhelming sweats, that they need to be treated. The best therapy is the use of replacement hormones, but this cannot be used, and might not be needed, by all such women. The next chapter is devoted to hormone replacement therapy, and should help to guide you to your own decisions. Following here are some remedies that sometimes work without using hormonal therapy.

The Hot Flash and Hot Flush

The heat is the flash. The color is the flush. Most women have one or the other, many have both. A small proportion of women (10 to 21 percent) have neither. The hot flash is the sudden sensation of heat, which can start in the upper chest and travel up the neck to the face and head. The redness that spreads in the same pattern is called the flush. What makes the hot flash so uncomfortable is its suddenness. This is not like being in a warm climate in August where you get used to the heat. This hits you like a blast furnace, and you want to tear your clothes off or stick your head under the cold water faucet—immediately! The hot flash lasts only a couple of seconds and is usually followed by an outbreak of perspiration all over your body.

A woman with these vasomotor symptoms—the body's response to a perturbation to the heat regulatory center of the hypothalamus—can be intolerant of the cold but suddenly feel hot when everyone else is freezing. Temperature changes are acutely felt. Night sweats might soak the bedsheets. You may throw off the covers, then pull them up again. This may wake you up, keep you awake, and ruin that night's sleep.

Less than half the women in the Massachusetts Women's Health

Study reported hot flashes or night sweats. Those who did have them reported that they occurred mostly at the beginning of perimenopause, reached a peak at menopause, and then diminished.

Two important factors increase the likelihood of hot flashes during perimenopause. One is having had your ovaries removed surgically—oophorectomy. The second is smoking tobacco, which acts as an antagonist to estrogen. These findings are from studies that suggested that other factors contributing to such symptoms are psychological stress, a history of PMS, and flushing early in life.

Remedies. When you get hot flashes, take heart in the knowledge that it is a temporary condition. When hormone replacement cannot be used, physicians may prescribe Bellergal, clonidin, or progestins for the hot flashes. Various vitamins (such as vitamin E), as well as naturally occurring estrogens in plants (phytoestrogens like soy beans, yams, and ginseng), and herbs such as black cohosh, are used by alternative health providers. (There is more about this in the next chapter.)

You can also feel more comfortable by dressing like an onion, with layers of clothing. You can peel off a layer or two when you feel hot and put them back on when you are cold. Silk or cotton underwear is helpful because the fabric breathes.

Insomnia

Insomnia and restless nights translate into fatigue, irritability, and bad temper. In a bleary-eyed day, it is difficult to think clearly and function smoothly as a perfect hostess or a high-powered executive. It is difficult, but it is being done every day by most women.

Sleeplessness can remain almost unnoticed, or it can progress to become a chronic ordeal. Either you cannot fall asleep or, more commonly, you wake up early or repeatedly during the night and early-morning hours. If sleep deprivation persists, there can be emotional consequences as well as a true suppression of your immune defense system, leaving you vulnerable to viruses and bacterial infections. If antibiotics are used frequently, vaginitis and repeated bouts of yeast infections can occur. Women experiencing this sequence of events might easily feel their bodies are failing them.

Try to limit your evening meal to a small snack of non-spicy, easily digestible food; consume no caffeine-containing drinks; limit your fluid intake during the four hours before your bedtime; and take a short, relaxing walk or engage in mild exercises a few hours before bedtime. Some women say meditation or yoga helps, as do soothing herbal teas such as chamomile.

A prescription for a mild tranquilizer or a sedative before bedtime might help if your doctor has ruled out any other possible causes for the symptoms.

Heart Palpitations

If you have palpitations frequently, you should get an electrocardiogram (EKG) during the attack if possible. Ask your doctor about putting a twenty-four-hour monitor on you to try to "catch" an attack for diagnosis. A newer gadget will allow you to record events only if your attacks are infrequent. If the palpitations are part of estrogen deficiency, they will disappear with hormone medication and there will be no need for repeat EKGs.

Vaginal Dryness

Other symptoms of estrogen deprivation are more persistent. A dry vagina results when diminishing levels of estrogen produce fewer secretions. This may interfere with the enjoyment of sex. In fact, vigorous, unlubricated intercourse might result in pain, bleeding, and even lacerations. A dry vagina can also be conducive to cystitis, especially after sex.

Lubricants, such as KY jelly, Replens, and Astroglide, are available to remedy dry vagina. Before use, make sure that you are not allergic to the one you choose. If no pharmacy is available, egg white is an excellent lubricant and is nonallergenic to most people. Another useful and natural product is plain yogurt.

THE MENTAL AND EMOTIONAL SYMPTOMS OF MENOPAUSE

Hormones do affect our brains and our emotions. A small percentage of women might experience wide mood swings during menopause, and some might even have temporary lapses in memory. This can be very disconcerting, especially for high-powered women arguing a case in a courtroom or making a speech.

There is research in progress to look at this issue. We do know that the hippocampus, the part of the brain associated with new learning and memory, is estrogen-responsive. We also know that the brain is not static, that it is capable of being modulated and improved—that it is plastic, in a sense. It can be influenced by our hormones, but it is also capable of adapting to or overcoming any change our hormones might stimulate. A temporary lapse as our hormones shift is not a federal case, and most certainly we do not want to add fuel to the male argument that women cannot be trusted with power in high office because their hormones make them irrational or forgetful.

From the beginning of time, there has been controversy about the connection of mood changes and a woman's reproductive function. The word *uterus* itself comes from the Greek *husteron,* which means uterus. Hippocrates later used the term *hysteria* to describe "disordered behavior" exclusive to women. This was related to the migration of the uterus, which he believed then to be free-floating in the body. While the concept of hysteria is no longer used, episodes of psychological dysfunction are still associated with various points in a woman's reproductive life cycle, namely in the postpartum, premenstrual, and menopausal periods. It was not until 1981 that the World Health Organization removed "involutional melancholia" from its International Classification of Diseases.

Memory Loss

Some women become aware at the time of menopause of failing memory and of difficulty in decision making. This is especially painful to a woman whose livelihood depends on these qualities, such as a teacher, writer, business executive, or attorney. Although many of these problems might be related to general aging and changing life situation, I have been impressed by how a month of estrogen replacement can reverse the mental and emotional deterioration. These symptoms are not universal, and they affect only a small proportion of menopausal women and are perhaps related to the suddenness of estrogen fall, such as occurs when ovaries are surgically removed, rather than the low estrogen level itself. When estrogen levels are allowed to decrease gradually, the same woman who reacted violently to menopause will tolerate the natural low postmenopausal levels without symptoms.

Mood Swings and Depression

Emotional ups and downs sometimes occur during this period. Women might overreact to seemingly minor problems and then feel intense guilt or shame for the outburst. This sequence is common in women who have been emotionally stable in the earlier parts of their lives. Your family and friends might be clueless about what they might have done to set you off, and you might feel helpless to explain it yourself. This time can be like having severe PMS every day. You might cry more easily and feel angry more of the time. Such occasional outbursts or moods tend to be cyclical, and they pass, sometimes as quickly as they came. (If you are sad or depressed all the time, then you might be clinically depressed, and that needs to be treated. Refer to chapter 20.)

Contrary to popular belief, menopausal women do *not* suffer depression as frequently as younger women from age 25 to 44. The mood swings that occur during menopause are cyclical and do not normally lead to a lasting depression. They are prompted by a hormonal fluctuation.

Some women might go into a depression in their forties or fifties if the physical symptoms of menopause affect them intensely and if they are not prepared to cope with them. The biological changes can instill an exaggerated fear of aging, getting sick, or losing their minds. If this is combined with other stresses, such as grown children leaving home, caring for ill and aging parents, divorce, or being downsized out of a job, then menopause can be part of the dynamic of this kind of depression. An important loss or a blow to your ego, such as being replaced by a younger worker, can understandably add to the effects of chaotic hormones.

Most psychiatrists believe that many symptoms women experience at menopause are related to these other life events. However, nonpsychiatric clinicians who treat large numbers of women (internists, endocrinologists, gynecologists, and family physicians) see a marked rise in depressive symptoms in their menopausal patients and observe the symptoms stop when estrogen is given. Both groups could be correct. Any period during which hormones fluctuate—such as they do during adolescence, postpartum, premenstrual, and perimenopause—can potentially create emotional disturbances.

Depressive symptoms and the syndrome of clinical depression are not the same. Psychiatrists are likely to be more stringent in their definition of depression than general medical doctors. At menopause there might be an increase in depressive symptoms, but perhaps not in the full-blown syndrome. Thus, both groups have accurately described menopausal women through their own clinical experience. The principal physician should understand both views and accept this process as a continuum with varying symptoms as women pass through transitions into postmenopause.

There is scientific support for depression's having a chemical basis directly related to the way estrogen affects blood chemistry. It is also likely that some women enter perimenopause with borderline chronic depression and experience worsening symptoms during this time period. These women might temporarily require both antidepressants and estrogen to alleviate symptoms. No treatment should be given until the symptoms are thoroughly assessed and studied within the dynamic of a woman's life—emotional issues as well as other physical conditions that might be present.

Labeling becomes less important than understanding, supporting, and treating when necessary. It is extremely important for a woman to feel support from her intimate partner or spouse, too. Usually that nonserene period lasts a few months or a couple of years but disappears without treatment. However, if the moods are disturbing your life and family, see a doctor for help. Treatment is available, not just with estrogens but with many antidepressants.

WORKING WITH YOUR DOCTOR

Evelyn is 47, and she came to see me because of a few hot flashes she experienced before her last menstrual period. She is a university professor of biology and has a sophisticated outlook on health care. She feels she needs a principal physician to consider all her body systems, rather than a gynecologist to care solely for her reproductive tract.

Evelyn's in a minority. Most American women see a gynecologist/ obstetrician as their primary physician. The care given by most gynecologists/obstetricians is often limited to the reproductive tract, and a referral to another specialist is needed if the symptoms seem to fall outside the gynecologist's expertise. For heart palpitations you are referred to a cardiologist. For a headache and dizziness, to a neurologist. For insomnia and depression, to a psychiatrist. Evelyn, and other women like her, believe that the primary care physician of women should be a well-trained general internist with special training in endocrinology, office gynecology, and psychosocial skills to meet health needs of women.

Although the internist might very well refer you to specialists, the internist is better trained to appraise the effect of menopause on the total woman. A woman facing menopause has other health systems to consider: her heart, bones, and immune system; and her chances of developing cancer. All of these assessments, which should really be done at the time of menopause, are best done by a general internist or a general internist/endocrinologist, rather than by a gynecologist, whose area of expertise usually covers only the reproductive tract. Menopause is the time when total assessment of all organ systems is indicated.

Experts agree that the physician-patient relationship is the second most important relationship a woman should have outside her family and friends. Ask questions when you visit your doctor. (Surprisingly, many women do not.) Describe the kinds of symptoms you believe you are experiencing, how long they last, exactly where you feel them, and so on. Remember what we advised in the beginning of the book about keeping your own health records and supplying precise detail. This helps your doctor understand how best to treat you.

You want to know what is wrong and if your symptoms are due to menopause. You want to know how you can alleviate them and what to expect in the future. Your doctor should explain all the alternatives available to you from lifestyle changes to comprehensive hormonal therapy. You and your doctor should also talk about the most important health challenges you are likely to encounter in the coming decades.

A comprehensive physical examination is needed to answer Evelyn's question, "Should I take hormones?" I need to know her own and her family's health history and also run some lab tests for cholesterol and other lipid values, thyroid function, and levels of follicle stimulating hormone (FSH). She would need an electrocardiogram, mammogram, perhaps bone density measurement, and a chest X ray. If indeed her symptoms are those of menopause she has many different options if her symptoms are severe. If they are not, then with good nutrition, sleep, and exercise, there should be no reason for her to suffer greatly.

Placing every woman on estrogen is wrong. Every woman is different, faces different risks, and has different individual requirements, and the decisions about treatment must be made on an individual basis according to each woman's health, lifestyle, and risk factors.

Menopausal symptoms can be managed without hormonal therapy with the help of an exercise program, good nutrition, refreshing sleep, meaningful work, and support from your physician and from your family. These interventions help a woman function without interruption in the family and at her job, to remain balanced and even-tempered.

Many vegetables, such as soybeans, contain *phytoestrogens,* which bind to estrogen receptors in the body and might be responsible for the mildness or absence of menopausal symptoms experienced by Asian women (who, incidentally, also have a very low incidence of breast cancer). It is theorized that the phytoestrogens, by binding to some of the estrogen receptors, control the menopausal symptoms, and by occupying some of the receptors in the breast cells, block the cancer-promoting effect of estrogen. This, of course, is only a theory for which there is yet little hard evidence.

Treatment with hormones to possibly prevent long-term effects of estrogen deprivation is another matter and, according to some of the new clinical studies, need not be decided there and then at menopause. These choices are included in subsequent chapters.

There are gaps in our knowledge about menopause and a woman's health challenges within this phase of her life. Gaps that require intensified research. We still need to develop a simple, reliable, and *inexpensive* instrument for prescreening for osteoporosis. We need to develop estrogen substitutes that would have all the beneficial effects and none of the risks. Now that we can speak frankly about menopause we must demand more attention and more funds for basic and clinical research in these important areas of our health.

It is important to remember that most menopausal symptoms are not here to stay. They will disappear in time. The best thing you can do for yourself during menopause is talk with your doctor, your family, and learn as much as you can about what is happening to your body. There are also support groups that can be extremely helpful and satisfying. By talking with other women, you get information *and* support about coping with symptoms. To find such a support group, check with your doctor, your clinic, or a women's health center in your vicinity.

··23··

Replacing Hormones:
Should You or Shouldn't You?

The last twenty-five years have seen wide pendulum swings in the use of replacement hormones to treat menopausal symptoms. Estrogens have been regarded as fountains of youth and benefactors of health on one hand, and as carcinogenic killers on the other. We have seen physicians flatly refusing to administer estrogen to any of their patients and we have heard of others who would give estrogen to every woman approaching menopause. Both attitudes imply an all-or-nothing solution to the issue of hormone replacement and are inappropriate and unfair to patients.

The American College of Obstetricians and Gynecologists recommends hormone replacement therapy for every postmenopausal woman for the rest of her life unless there is compelling medical evidence against it. However, no other medical association offers such a unanimous opinion. Many women's health advocates who are against hormone replacement complain that because menopause has now been labeled "estrogen deficiency disease" the acceptance of estrogen replacement therapy as the most logical way to "cure" the disease has become standard procedure. Yet *menopause is a natural part of life, not a disease*. Ovaries might continue to produce estrogen in low levels until a woman is in her eighties, and adrenals might continue to produce estrogen precursors forever. Synthetic hormones, therefore, do not replace something that is missing, critics say, they add to what is there.

Those who are in favor of replacement therapy claim that women who take hormones have 50 percent less heart disease and are subject to greatly decreased mortality from all causes. Critics point out that the FDA has not recommended the use of estrogen for prevention of heart disease, and the risk of heart disease would be eliminated if the same women changed their lifestyles, ate properly, exercised, and quit smoking. All risk factors for replacing hormones or not replacing them need to be weighed carefully.

The 40 million women in America turning 50 at the turn of the twenty-first century need to understand the short- and long-term ramifications of hormonal therapy, as well as their own risk factors for osteoporosis, heart disease, and breast cancer. They need to learn how their lifestyle needs to be moderated so that they can live long, healthy lives and avoid heart disease, osteoporosis, and breast cancer.

Jenna came to see me when she was 55 and asked for hormones. "Why?" I asked. Jenna is a tall, big-boned woman who wore size 10 shoes, loved her work, had no history of heart disease, no family history of heart disease or osteoporosis, did not smoke, and worked out at least four times a week.

"Well, my husband is afraid I'll lose interest in sex," she said. Because she said this without any apparent irony and in all seriousness, I responded the same way and asked her many questions about possible menopausal symptoms such as loss of libido or dry vagina. Jenna had no symptoms, but she did admit that her work had been more intense and she had less time to spend with her husband lately. We decided that Jenna needed no help from hormones, but needed only to reassure her husband about her interest in him.

"See you next year," I said, explaining that the need for hormone replacement should be reevaluated continuously. "Your body and your needs can change," I reminded her.

On the other extreme was a patient I'll call Gloria, who I suspected would most definitely need a program of hormone replacement, but she continuously resisted my recommendations. Gloria was barely five-foot-two, was extremely thin, and although she was emotionally strong and a hard worker in her nonprofit agency to help the homeless, she was a prime candidate for osteoporosis. Although she assured me she usually remembered to take calcium each day, I knew she had not started out early in life by drinking lots of milk. I also knew she did not exercise because she worked fourteen-hour days. I found myself always wanting to take her to dinner or give her food. She reminded me of a bird, darting around, picking up a seed here or there. Her resistance to hormone replacement came from a fear of breast cancer and from knowing many women who had developed complications from badly managed hormone treatment. I hoped I would be able to convince Gloria to reconsider before she fell and broke a hip.

Each woman is unique. One might need short-term hormonal therapy for menopausal symptoms like hot flashes, or long-term therapy to prevent osteoporosis and heart disease. Therapy can be given in a variety of doses, forms, and combinations. It can be used cyclically or continuously. It can be started and stopped, then started again.

Not all women at menopause need hormones. While two thirds of menopausal women experience hot flashes, most of them do not suffer greatly and adjust to them. Only about 10 percent are so disabled by symptoms that interfere with work and family life that they need hormonal therapy.

And it's not as simple as just asking your doctor if you should take hormones. Your doctor cannot know the answer unless she or he has given you a comprehensive workup, taken an in-depth health history and a family history. You and your doctor together need to evaluate your menopausal symptoms as well as your risk for heart disease and osteoporosis.

Your principal doctor, if an internist, is the best one to give you this kind of comprehensive overall examination (see the previous chapter). An endocrinologist, a doctor specializing in the glandular systems, is a specialist you might seek out if you are unsure of your principal physician.

Short-term (less than five years) use of replacement hormones for menopausal symptoms has not been proven dangerous. It will relieve severe symptoms like the hot flashes, mood swings, insomnia, and vaginal dryness. Sustaining the estrogen levels in your body keeps your heart and bones in good health and increases life expectancy. There is some evidence that it can help prevent Alzheimer's disease and strokes, although the FDA does not recommend it for these purposes. However, all these advantages dissipate after the hormone is stopped. Estrogen also seems to decrease the risk of colon cancer, diseases of the retina, and dental deterioration. It also helps with the memory and delays the onset of Alzheimer's dementia.

Yet taking hormones for more than ten years *increases* the risk of breast cancer. Uterine cancer is seven times higher in women on estrogen. While adding progestins to estrogen generally protects the uterus from this cancer, many women dislike taking progestin because it can produce logginess, depression, and breast tenderness.

Estrogen replacement therapy (ERT) is the use of synthetic estrogens alone. Hormone replacement therapy (HRT) comprises estrogen and progestin (and sometimes male hormone as well).

Whether or not to take hormone therapy is a highly individual decision that a woman must make only after she has a good understanding of her own health and lifestyle, and what she can expect from taking hormones. It is critically important to discuss this with your principal physician, as well as your gynecologist if he or she is an important part of your medical team. And most important, remember that you can always stop taking hormones, change the dosage, and change the balance of estrogen and progestin in order to find the right therapy for you.

LONG-TERM ADVANTAGES: PROTECTION FOR THE HEART

Heart disease is the leading cause of death in women in this country, responsible for 355,000 fatalities every year. It kills more women than breast cancer, endometrial cancer, and osteoporosis combined. While heart disease is also the leading killer of men, it is not always diagnosed quickly enough in women. A heart attack has a worse prognosis for women than for men, frequently because of atypical symptoms that are misdiagnosed. In addition, women are older by the time they have their first coronary, and have by that time often collected other illnesses, so-called comorbidities. Because of this, they are sicker by the time they are treated. Heart disease is rare in women before menopause, but it catches up quickly after the age of 50. (Chapter 24 is devoted to heart disease in women.)

Even though the FDA has not recommended the use of estrogen as a cardiovascular preventative, there is ample evidence today that the administration of any estrogen has shown a profound improvement in the status and survival of women with coronary heart disease. All well-conducted studies conclude that estrogen therapy decreases the risk of coronary heart disease in women by about half.

It's almost as if nature decided to keep the female portion of humankind healthy long enough to ensure childbearing and survival of our species, then let us loose. About a half of the beneficial effect of estrogen is primarily channeled through its effect on blood lipids (fats). (Refer to page 359 for an explanation about blood lipids and cholesterol and their effect on the heart.) Estrogens lower the bad cholesterol, low-density lipoprotein (LDL), and raise the good cholesterol, high-density lipoprotein (HDL), which protects us. LDL acts like an oil truck distributing fat to the tissues and plugging up the arteries with fat deposits. HDL is like a sanitation truck, cleaning up the plaques and carrying them off to the liver, where they are processed for elimination. There is also an additional beneficial effect of estrogen on the ability of the blood vessels to dilate.

Although most research has shown that estrogen offers protection against heart attacks, recently reported results of Heart and Estrogen/progestin Randomized Study (HERS)—the first large randomized trial of HRT given for 4.1 years to postmenopausal women with coronary heart disease—came as a surprise. It showed no overall cardiac benefit for hormone replacement therapy. Estrogen combined with progestin given to women already ill with heart disease was associated with 50 percent *more* heart attacks and deaths than placebo for the first year of therapy. However, having survived that first year, women who took the hormones had 40 percent *fewer* heart attacks than those on placebo over the last 2 years.

Needless to say, HERS stirred up a controversy. One interpretation was that perhaps the initial effect of the HRT is to enhance clotting (3 percent incidence of clotting problems), while the favorable effects of estrogen on the bad cholesterol and on good cholesterol (see above) are slow and take time to reverse the progression of atherosclerosis (the basic cause of coronary heart disease). It is conceivable that if the trial lasted longer it would demonstrate a marked benefit in the subsequent years.

Another reason that the HERS trial gave conflicting results is that it included a progestin called medroxyprogesterone acetate (MPA) as part of the Prempro preparation (0.625 mg of conjugated estrogen plus 2.5 mg medroxyprogesterone acetate) because all women had intact uteri. MPA is known to reduce the beneficial effects of estrogen on the heart and blood vessels. It is possible that the harmful effects of that progestin affect the heart earlier than the beneficial effects of estrogen. We don't know what the effects would be if other progestins were used, such as norethindrone acetate (Aygestin) or micronized "natural" progesterone in capsules (Prometrium) or in a vaginal gel (Crinone). It is also possible that better results would be obtained if the dose of both the estrogen and progestin were reduced. No studies have so far determined the optimal and minimal cardioprotective dose of estrogen.

The research team recommended that women with coronary heart disease should not take HRT as the first choice treatment for prevention of future heart attacks but should consider other preventive means such as weight control, smoking cessation, control of blood pressure and possible diabetes, and medications such as aspirin, beta-blockers, and cholesterol-lowering agents (niacin and statins). However, since preventive benefits accrue from *prolonged* HRT women who have been taking estrogen/progestin should continue to do so. In other words, hormones might be good preventive agents but not good as treatment.

Three other trials are under way involving women with established coronary heart disease. They are Women's Angiographic Vitamin and Estrogen (WAVE) trial, the Women's Estrogen/Progestin and Lipid Lowering Hormone Atherosclerosis Regression Trial (WELL-HART), and the Estrogen Replacement and Atherosclerosis (ERA) trial. These trials should help determine if HRT prevents the *progression* of heart disease. The Women's Health Initiative a comprehensive research study of women's health, initiated by Dr. Bernadine Healy, then Director of the National Institutes of Health, when complete after 2005, will help us define the role of HRT in *prevention* of heart disease.

PREVENTION OF OSTEOPOROSIS

Everybody loses bone density as they age. We used to think that the bone density peak occurred at about 35. Now we know it occurs even earlier, in the twenties. After it peaks, bone mass remains constant for fifteen years or so, then it goes downhill. For five years after menopause, women lose bone rapidly, about 2 percent a year (the rate of loss for men is half a percent a year). Although some men do get osteoporosis, there is no dip or cycle in their hormonal level. There is a gradual loss of testosterone as they age. Osteoporosis is a disease of childhood and adolescence with manifestations at an advanced age. Those teenagers who drink plenty of carbonated sodas and avoid milk and other calcium-containing foods are at a greater risk of osteoporosis than those who consume adequate calcium.

Osteoporosis is a major public health problem, characterized by thinning of bones and propensity to fractures. About 8 million women in the United States suffer from it, with fractures of spine, wrists, hips, ribs, and pelvis. An additional 24 million have accelerated bone loss, which makes them vulnerable to fractures. (Chapter 25 is devoted to osteoporosis.) Estrogen is the most effective agent for preventing bone loss. It is the gold standard against which all other therapies are measured.

Calcium intake, while crucial during young life to prevent future osteoporosis, is not a substitute for estrogen in prevention of bone loss during menopause. Calcium, however, seems to augment the effect of estrogen so that a smaller dose of estrogen can be used. However, in women five years or more after menopause, calcium intake again helps prevent bone loss.

It was thought that once osteoporosis had progressed to the stage where bones are actually breaking, estrogens could no longer restore the bone lost. However, it has recently been found that fifteen years postmenopause, continuous estrogen therapy in women with osteoporotic fractures significantly increased vertebral bone density on an average of 5 percent per year, as compared with calcium alone. Furthermore, the older the woman, and the lower the initial bone density, the more spectacular the response. *So even fifteen years after menopause estrogen can still increase bone density.* There are other methods of treating osteoporosis, but estrogens play a central and crucial role as they are both a preventive and a treatment.

In order to know if you need hormonal therapy to prevent osteoporosis, you need a comprehensive evaluation of your own potential risk factors for getting it, and a bone density test around the time of menopause. At this date, few internists are equipped to provide such testing, but most major medical centers and teaching hospitals have such diagnostic facilities (see chapter 25). Bone density and total bone mass measurements identify vulnerability. If you are prone to osteoporosis, then preventive treatment should begin. The effect on bone is strongest when estrogen is started within the first three to five years after the last menstrual period. Even if you have established osteoporosis and fractures, you might still benefit from estrogen treatment even as late as fifteen years postmenopause. Therapy should probably continue indefinitely.

THE RISK TO THE ENDOMETRIUM

Progestin is given in order to prevent endometrial hyperplasia (cell overgrowth) and endometrial cancer. It has been found that with estrogen alone there is an increase in endometrial cancer. When progestin is added, to check the cell growth stimulated by the estrogen, the incidence of endometrial cancer drops to almost zero. There are in the literature rare cases of endometrial cancer that developed despite the added progestin; it is thought they developed because the dose of progestin was inadequate or because the patient skipped taking it.

The regimens that have been based on estrogen alone are really safe only in a woman who has no uterus. As a matter of fact, whenever a woman has had a hysterectomy, it makes no sense for her to be taking progestin at all because we have no evidence that progestin has any advantages in women as far as risk of breast cancer, and it certainly has some negative effect on the lipids and the heart. Some of these negative effects are minimized when a recently introduced natural micronized progesterone (Prometrium) is used; however, this substance is associated with side effects of its own.

If you had endometriosis and if, after surgery, some tissue was left behind, estrogen can cause the endometrial tissue to grow and might indeed also cause hyperplasia and even cancer.

If you had endometrial cancer that was only partially removed you should not receive estrogen therapy. (There are some studies following women who had past histories of endometrial cancer to see if their survival is any different from those who are not on estrogen). If the endometrial cancer has been completely removed, there is no contraindication to taking estrogen.

Vaginal Bleeding

Women who have had vaginal bleeding during perimenopause without any explanation of what the bleeding is about should not receive estrogen. Bleeding could be a sign of endometrial cancer, and therefore a careful D&C should remove that possibility before estrogen treatment could be even considered.

Fibroids

The presence of large fibroids can cause intermittent or uncontrollable bleeding when hormone replacement therapy is given. If a manipulation of the estrogen and progestin doses does not eliminate the breakthrough bleeding, then a D&C might be necessary. In the face of recurrent heavy bleeding from fibroids, hysterectomy is a common procedure of choice if a woman badly needs estrogen therapy.

THE BREAST CANCER RISK

From what we know today, it is safe to say that short-term (less than five years) treatment with estrogen, such as is given for menopausal symptoms, carries no increased risk for breast cancer. Long-term therapy with estrogen, however, such as is given for prevention and treatment of osteoporosis and coronary heart disease, carries a slightly increased risk of breast cancer, and we don't know what risk or protection is offered by the combined therapy, estrogen and progestin.

Over the last few decades, the incidence of breast cancer has reached epidemic proportions. Ten years ago in the United States one woman in thirteen developed breast cancer; in 1988 one woman in ten; and in 1991, one woman in nine was diagnosed with this disease. (For more on breast cancer, see page 247.) Some of the increase is accounted for by the aging of our population. Women live longer and are exposed to any risk over a longer period of time. The increase in the diagnosis might also be due to better and earlier detection through an increased use of mammograms. Breast cancer diagnosed in estrogen users tends to be detected in earlier stages and is therefore more easily cured. Women who have had breast cancer themselves, even though it was cured, should not take estrogens for menopausal symptoms. Other forms of therapy should be used instead.

It is clear that estrogen and progestins are not carcinogens. What has not been resolved is whether these hormones, under certain conditions, cause changes in the cells already predisposed, perhaps genetically, to develop cancer. In an ideal world we would need to have genetic screening of all women considered for HRT. Until then, we must exclude from estrogen therapy women at high risk for breast cancer, and use on other patients the smallest dose that will do the job effectively for the shortest length of time.

The Nurses Study found that among past users of ERT there was no increase in relative risk for breast cancer, but among current users there was a 36 percent increase of risk. In another study a very slight increase of 10 percent was associated with a small dose and a higher increase of risk with a larger dose. A history of benign breast disease did not increase the risk. In still another study, the relative risk of breast cancer in estrogen users was confirmed to be 30 percent, but was higher among individuals with a positive family history. The risk of breast cancer understandably frightens many women away from hormonal therapy who would otherwise benefit.

OTHER RISKS

Women who have active blood clots in the veins (*thrombophlebitis*) and clots that tear off and land in the lungs (*pulmonary emboli*) should not be taking estrogen until at least a year after all thromboembolic activity has subsided. If you require estrogen for menopausal symptoms, your doctor can prescribe it at a lower dose. Wearing elastic stockings up to but not including the knees can help prevent clot formation.

Women with liver disease, either acute or chronic, should not receive estrogen because estrogens are metabolized by the liver into other substances. With a sick liver, estrogens are likely to build up in the body and exacerbate liver disease.

If you fall into any of these categories, do not take hormones. Concentrate on the alternative treatment modes.

HOW ERT AND HRT ARE ADMINISTERED

All hormones are powerful drugs and must be administered with caution, selectivity, precise monitoring, and cooperation between you and your doctor. It is not clear when is the best time to start. We usually wait for the menses to be absent for six to twelve months. However, therapy can begin any time at or after menopause. Hormone Replacement Therapy (HRT) is labor-intensive therapy that requires you to keep track of when to take your pills or when to change the patches, and you must keep your appointments with your doctor to monitor your progress regularly. There must be continuous communication between you and your doctor and visits every three to six months at first— or more frequently if there are problems or questions. This frequent contact gives you and your doctor the opportunity to assess any other challenges to your health and design a good health care program.

Estrogen can be delivered by various routes: by mouth (orally), by injection (intramuscularly), by patch (transdermally), or through a cream to the vagina (topically). Patches containing hormones are placed anywhere on the body—thighs, arms, or backside, which is the most common place. The location should be changed from time to time so as to not irritate the skin in any one location.

For each individual woman, there is a different timing, dosage, administration, and duration of treatment. When therapy is given for menopausal syndrome, initially a large enough dose should be given to wipe out the symptoms completely. Then the dose can be tapered. With time, your body becomes more tolerant of the lower estrogen level. It is usually possible to stop estrogen without undue problems before the age of 65 or 70 if the purpose of estrogen treatment is to alleviate menopausal symptoms.

The nuisance-type side effects of taking estrogen include vaginal bleeding, water retention, and breast swelling and tenderness. Some women might be more vulnerable to migraine headaches or the development of gallstones. While in most women administration of estrogen lowers blood pressure somewhat, in rare cases it can lead to hypertension.

Diabetic women can safely use estrogen because it does not cause blood sugar to rise. It actually lowers both blood sugar and insulin levels.

Estrogen and Progestin Preparations

Our estrogens can be replaced by a number of preparations. The most commonly used is Premarin, which consists of many estrogens (conjugated estrogens) obtained from a mare's urine. There are also synthetic preparations available such as Estrace and Estradiol, available as a pill and as a patch.

Our progesterone is usually replaced by the synthetic Provera (medroxyprogesterone acetate) and Norlutate (norethindrone acetate). In some of the NIH trials, micronized progesterone was used; this medication is now available as Prometrium. Pure natural progesterone cannot be used as it is poorly absorbed when taken by mouth.

Traditionally, it has been thought that added synthetic progestins weaken the cardiac protection by estrogen by about a third. Natural micronized progesterone is less detrimental.

While progestins protect the uterus, their effect on the breast is still not clear. The effect of various progestins, various doses, and various regimens on cardiovascular factors still needs to be investigated.

Here are some of the most well-known "fixed-dose" hormone replacement combinations.

Prempro contains estrogen and progestin and is taken every day. This is known as continuous therapy. You simply take a pill every day, and within a year all bleeding will cease. One package provides pills for twenty-eight days.

Premphase contains the same things as Prempro but is used as cyclical therapy. You take one pill every day for twenty-eight days, and the pill taken on days fifteen through twenty-eight also contains progestin. On this cycle, bleeding occurs regularly after you finish the progestin-containing pills. This cyclic schedule is used mostly in younger women who are about to lose their menses and who have just lost them. Some physicians dislike "fixed-dose" combinations that lock the woman into one mold; every woman is different, and may require different dosages of each component and individual adjustment.

What Is the Best Hormone Dose?

There is controversy about what dose of estrogen is best for protection against bone loss and heart disease. While 0.625 milligrams of Premarin has been accepted as the "minimal" bone-protective dose (much less than in the past), there is new evidence that as little as half that dose is effective as long as calcium intake is sufficient. In general, the smaller the dose, the safer the treatment. We don't know what the smallest dose is that protects the heart.

How the Hormones Are Administered

Pills. When estrogens are administered by mouth, they first pass through the liver, where they produce a number of proteins that might promote clotting, water retention, vascular headaches, and gallstone formation. Oral estrogens might have more of an effect on the body's lipids because of the first pass through the liver.

Patches. If you have a predisposition to phlebitis, migraine headaches, gallstones, or gas, the patch might be a better way to go. This is a drug reservoir with a membrane that controls the rate of absorption. You peel off the protective strip and place the patch anywhere on your body other than your breasts. The lower abdomen and buttock are both popular areas. The hormone diffuses through the skin to reach blood vessels, and achieves consistent blood levels of estradiol and estrone.

Good adhesion of the patch is critical, and a new patch should be applied twice a week. The patches might cause skin irritation, which can be avoided by rotating the sites and using areas with tougher skin, such as buttocks. Estrogen patches can be combined with oral progestins.

Injections. Delestrogen is an intramuscular long-acting preparation of estrogen that can be given every two weeks. Delalutin is an intramuscular long-acting progestin. The usual cycle for a woman with an intact uterus is to receive Delestrogen alone at the beginning of the month and fourteen days later a combination of Delestrogen and Delalutin. Withdrawal bleeding occurs at the end of the month.

Topical Hormones. If you are not a candidate for hormone pills, you might still benefit from a number of estrogen-containing creams: Premarin cream, Dienesterol cream, or Estrace cream. All are absorbed through the vaginal lining and prevent atrophy of the lower reproductive and urinary tract. By building stronger vaginal support tissue, they also prevent recurrent cystitis that is so common in menopausal women.

The Ring. Recently, the FDA approved the use of Estring, a plastic ring that is smaller than a diaphragm, fits in the vagina, and that a woman can easily insert and remove. It does not interfere with intercourse and does not require progestin supplementation. In its inner core the Estring contains two milligrams of Premarin, which is slowly released over ninety days. It must be removed and a new ring inserted every three months.

CONTINUOUS AND CYCLICAL HORMONE REPLACEMENT THERAPY

There are a number of ways estrogen is used for relief of menopausal symptoms. The most traditional method of administering estrogen was designed a long time ago by Dr. Ephraim Schorr at Cornell Medical College. His regimen attempted to closely simulate the natural hormonal dynamic in the three phases of the menstrual cycle: the estrogen-only phase in the first part of the month (the first ten to fourteen days); the combined estrogen-progesterone phase to approximate the postovulatory part of the menstrual cycle (the next ten to fourteen days); and finally the last five to six days of the month, when menstrual bleeding occurs and no hormones are given.

This method of administering HRT is called *cyclic,* since it mimics the hormone levels that are present during the normal menstrual cycle (as in Premphase). This method is preferred in the case of a young perimenopausal woman who is suffering from menopausal symptoms and who might still have spontaneous menstrual bleeding off and on. Two other methods are more appropriate for an older woman in whom estrogen is given to prevent osteoporosis and/or heart disease.

Over the last decade, continuous combined estrogen-progestin has become fashionable. You can take a very small pill of estrogen daily, or a patch twice a week, and a small amount of progestin, also every day, continuously. The continuous combined therapy is popular because it is easy to do. Take one of each pill, or place a patch on your stomach twice a week. You do not need to keep a calendar of days. This method is like Prempro.

During the first eighteen months of the continuous combined treatment, there might be intermittent bleeding. After a year, however, the lining of the uterus atrophies and shrinks, and there is no longer any bleeding—and no longer any overgrowth of the endometrium, thus eliminating the risk of cancer. It's a safe treatment. The downside is that during the first eighteen months there might be a great deal of bleeding on and off. Many women get discouraged and annoyed with having the uterus lining sampled over and over again to make sure that the bleeding is not a portent of cancer.

The other problem is that not only does the lining of the uterus atrophy with this onslaught of progestin, but the vagina shrinks as well, and many women experience vaginal dryness and discomfort with intercourse. A very serious possible complication of this regimen is the long-term effect of progestin on blood lipids that can detract from the beneficial effect of estrogen on the heart.

Other ways of administering combined estrogen and progestin consist of continuous daily estrogen with progestin given for ten to fourteen days every month or every two months. This regimen is used for long-term therapy for some women in order to prevent osteoporosis and coronary heart disease. In younger women close to menopause, this regimen frequently results in intermittent bleeding, and it is very inconvenient because a woman constantly subjected to endometrial sampling or a D&C.

Traditional cyclical therapy, especially for women who have been in early menopause or shortly after menopause, restores the usual balance of hormones a woman has during her young adult life. This regimen also allows for evaluating further need of treatment. During the pause, if the symptoms return with great intensity, it is an indication that you still require the hormone. However, as you get used to lower levels of estrogen the pause becomes less and less symptomatic, and that might be a signal that you could start tapering your medication and stop.

THERAPY WITH MALE HORMONES

We are all born with both male and female hormones, but only one predominates, according to our sexual identity. Male hormones—androgens—are produced in a woman by the adrenal gland and by the ovary. The ovarian androgen is testosterone, which increases the sex drive, the appetite, muscle strength, and a sense of well-being. Studies in the 1980s showed that after oophorectomy, some women have low libido despite estrogen replacement therapy. It was suspected this was caused by lack of testosterone. And, indeed, the administration of testosterone restored sexual desire in these women.

Androgen therapy has not caught on in this country, although it is widely used in Europe, Canada, Australia, and New Zealand as part of hormone replacement therapy for women. The combination of estrogen and testosterone has been found useful in women who are incapacitated by an osteoporotic fracture and are bedridden and frustrated. As a mood elevator, testosterone acts as a stimulus to get out of bed, ambulate, exercise, eat better, and follow the physician's instructions more enthusiastically. Androgens have been used in women (usually in combination with estrogens) for the following purposes:

- To lift the mood of menopausal women suffering from depression.

- To improve libido when it is decreased in the course of menopause, especially if it is early menopause caused by an oophorectomy or chemotherapy.

- To improve the libido when it is affected by depression or antidepressive, antihypertensive, and other drugs.

- To increase the appetite, sense of well-being, and muscle strength of a woman who has a debilitating disease or is recovering from a heroic surgery.

- To strengthen bone mass in a woman with osteoporosis.

- To stop the vaginal spotting and decrease the breast tenderness that can occur with HRT.

How Androgens Are Administered

Androgens, like other hormones, can be administered by pill, patch, or injection. Of oral preparations, testosterone or methyltestosterone tablets can be swallowed with liquid or placed under the tongue. The Estratest tablet half-strength (Estratest HS) was approved by the FDA and is now available. It contains small amounts of conjugated estrogens and testosterone. In accordance with the principle of using the smallest dose that does the job, physicians begin therapy with one tablet three times a week and use estrogen alone for the remaining four days of the week. If appropriate, the Estratest dose is increased every day. If a woman has an intact uterus, progestin is added.

Creams and Lotions. Vaginal 1 percent testosterone cream or gel is applied to the clitoris and surrounding vulva daily or twice daily, primarily for the libido and sexual responsiveness. Alternatively, an alcohol-based lotion is applied to the nongenital skin. Most of these topical preparations are available through special pharmacies, such as the Wisconsin Women's Health Pharmacy, but can also be compounded by the local pharmacist.

Side Effects of Androgens

When male hormones are used in women potential side effects need to be kept in mind. Additionally, we still do not know yet how androgens affect the risk for breast cancer or heart disease. Androgens do affect the blood lipids and can change the balance of good and bad cholesterol, putting a woman at a higher risk for the formation of plaque in her arteries—and, thus, a heart attack.

It is important to keep the dose of androgens low, especially at the outset of the treatment. When used prudently in combination with estrogen, androgen therapy can enhance the total health of some women. Further studies are needed regarding the best dose of existing and new preparations. Side effects include:

• Oily skin, acne, or hirsutism might occur from excessive amounts of androgens in fewer than 1 percent of women, most often in dark-haired, dark-complected women.

• Erotic dreams of both a heterosexual and a homosexual nature might occur during sleep.

• Weight gain might result because these hormones will stimulate your appetite.

• Enlargement of the clitoris has not been observed with low doses of testosterone therapy, but it is a theoretical possibility.

• Toxicity to the liver might occur from high doses of methyltestosterone.

• Vaginal dryness might occur with high doses.

• Aggressiveness, or the so-called testosterone toxicity, has been observed in some women.

ALTERNATIVES TO HORMONE REPLACEMENT THERAPY

If you cannot or will not take estrogen, what can you do about menopausal symptoms? Fortunately, you have alternatives to treating the symptoms.

If you are suffering from hot flushes, sweats, insomnia, and palpitations (the so-called vasomotor manifestations of menopause), you have a choice of a mild sedative at night. Mild medications such as Bellergal (anticholinergic), Clonidine (an adrenergic antagonist), or progestin alone (Provera) also help relieve symptoms. Many women get relief from mild hot flashes with 400 milligrams of vitamin E once or twice a day.

Alternatives include medications like Fosamax for osteoporosis, vaginal creams for dryness, and tamoxifen and other medications for heart disease. While estrogen is the only medication that treats and helps prevent all of the complications of menopause, it is good to have choices based on your individual health. Some of these alternatives are included below and in other chapters in this book.

For all women of menopausal and postmenopausal age, it is important to keep up with exercises and proper nutrition, including a good supply of calcium and other vitamins and a diet high in vegetables and fruit, low in fat, and moderate in protein. A refreshing night's sleep and an active, fulfilling life, interspersed with relaxation and rest, are good prescriptions for any stage of life, especially this one.

Phytoestrogens: Estrogen-rich Foods

Because women in Japan report far fewer menopausal symptoms than women in this country, researchers are paying more attention to the effects of diet and nutrition on these symptoms. Although women in Eastern cultures might not report such symptoms as readily as Western women, the diet connection is given strength because women in Japan, Indonesia, India, and Taiwan also show less heart disease, breast cancer, and hip fractures than North American women. Factoring out the genetic and cultural differences, the variable seems to be the soy-based diet popular in the East.

A randomized placebo-and-estrogen controlled trial of an extract of black cohosh (a wild plant called Cimicifuga racemosa) reported in German literature recently that this preparation relieved symptoms of menopause to a similar extent as estrogen.

Australian studies have shown that soy-based flour, compared with wheat flour, reduced hot flashes more effectively in women eating both.

Several other studies focused on the soy group found similar results. Researchers also found that phytoestrogens reduced bone loss in the spine and thighbone as effectively as estrogen.

Although it is much too soon to come to any conclusions about how much of these elements should be included in a woman's diet, most of the researchers believe that a well-balanced diet with lots of fresh fruits and vegetables, and whole grains, with some tofu or soy milk added, would ease the transition through menopause.

Phytoestrogens are weak estrogens present in many plant foods. Most plants have some phytoestrogens, but the ones with the most estrogenic activity in humans are the ones, such as soy products and legumes, containing isoflavones. Phytoestrogens are present in yams and other vegetables, as well as in green tea.

Foods containing phytoestrogens include:

- Olive oil
- Soy products
- Whole-grain cereals
- Oats, oat bran, rice bran, wheat germ
- Rye, barley, corn
- Dried seaweed
- Beans and legumes
- Sweet potatoes, squash, carrots
- Fennel, asparagus, onions
- Apples, pears, cherries, pomegranates
- Sunflower seeds, hops, alfalfa
- Licorice
- Milk

Ancient Alternatives

Although the medical establishment previously ignored the study of plants and herbs, there is now a great deal of research into these alternative therapies. The Chinese have been using herbal preparations for six thousand years, and now Western science is taking a more serious look at them.

These alternative preparations have not found their way into the proverbial "doctor's bag" because there have not been any well-conducted, randomized, double-blind studies attesting to their efficacy and safety. Recently, the National Institutes of Health funded an investigation of Chinese herbs and other alternative drugs used in menopause at several medical centers. For example, Chinese herbal medicine would aim to correct the imbalance in the body caused by the hormone deficiency. It would prescribe a concoction made of several different herbs— such as ginger, white peony, hare's ear, thistle, and others—to be taken several times a day and in a variety of forms.

The herbal preparations you find in herb shops and health food stores might not be properly calibrated, however, and an overdose can occur. Unapproved herbal mixtures taken as medication have resulted in death in some instances.

There are many books on alternative medicine. In fact, in the past two or three years, bookstores have begun to carry almost as many titles about alternative medicine as traditional medicine.

Modern Alternatives

There is no *one* medication that can target all the conditions that estrogen helps with. However, there are a number of treatments that can substitute for estrogen for specific indications. Bellergal, clonidin, progestin, vitamin E, and some phytoestrogens might help hot flashes. Group discussions among perimenopausal women and supporting attitudes of the woman's family and workplace associates can do wonders for her well-being.

Dryness of the vagina and discomfort on intercourse can be relieved with various nonhormonal creams and lubricants.

For prevention of osteoporosis, adequate calcium and vitamin D intake and moderate (not excessive) protein in the diet are essential. Alternative medications for osteoporosis are now available: alendronate (Fosamax) and raloxifene (Evista), both taken by mouth; and calcitonin, taken by injection or nasal spray. It is important to avoid certain bone-loss-promoting medications, like corticosteroids and excessive thyroid. If these medications must be taken, osteoporosis can be prevented by coadministration of alendronate, and perhaps by the addition of small doses of androgens.

There is a lot you can do to prevent heart disease other than taking estrogen: adhering to a low-fat diet, exercising, abstaining from active and passive tobacco smoke, controlling your blood pressure and diabetes with the help of your doctor, and using folic acid and antioxidants like vitamin E. If you have coronary heart disease or are prone to it, but cannot use estrogen, there are cholesterol-lowering medications to be considered by your doctor, including niacin and powerful *statins*. Raloxifene was found to have a similar effect on the fat profile (cholesterol, LDL, and less so on HDL) to that of estrogen. It has been approved by the Food and Drug Administration in 1997 as an alternative to estrogen.

··24··

The Female Heart

When you ask an intelligent and otherwise well-educated woman what she considers her greatest health hazard, nine times out of ten she will say breast cancer. In truth, more women die of coronary heart disease than of breast, cervical, endometrial, and ovarian cancers *and* complications of osteoporosis combined.

Every year 350,000 women die of coronary heart disease in this country. If strokes and vascular diseases are included, the figure rises to 500,000. That's half a million deaths from cardiovascular disease. Because the incidence of coronary heart disease is low in women before menopause, it is hard for a woman at midlife to think of heart disease as a real threat. We still need a great deal of consciousness-raising—the kind we did for breast cancer awareness—to bring female heart disease out of the closet.

Hundreds of thousands of women die, leaving their families bereft and ignorant about what caused their heart attacks. One woman of 54, Peggy, got moderate chest pains while watching television with her husband one night. She began to feel a tightness of breath, she was nauseated, and she began to sweat. She told her husband she did not feel well and went into the bedroom to lie down. It must have been something she ate, she told him. When the pain got worse, she called her husband, who came into the room and asked what he could do. He brought her a glass of water and sat down on the bed and stroked her forehead for a few minutes before returning to the living room. About a half hour later, he returned to the room and found her dead. Peggy's husband always wondered if the television was turned up so loud that he did not hear her call for help.

Peggy lived in a suburban blue-collar neighborhood and was not sophisticated about health care, although she had always visited the family doctor when the children and her husband were sick. Although she did not smoke, neither did she do any exercise. She was a buxom woman who had put on weight above her waist in recent years. She also ate high-fat meats and not enough fruits, vegetables, and whole grains. She considered canned peas an adequate "vegetable" to serve with dinner.

Peggy's three grown daughters and her sisters and brothers blamed the husband for not getting help, and family disputes raged for years after Peggy's death. The husband was clueless about why his wife had a heart attack. The family doctor had never told Peggy about diet or weight, or any of the cardiovascular risks of menopause, never tested her for a predisposition for diabetes, and had never asked her if anyone in her family had heart disease.

At the same time, Peggy never asked her doctor about her health, nor did she tell him much about her symptoms or history throughout her life. If she had been suffering from menopausal symptoms, nobody knew about it. And to this day, her daughters, two of whom have the same body type, and all of whom eat the same way, are not aware of the need to educate themselves or change their lifestyle so they do not inherit their mother's condition. They do not learn about it from their friends or neighbors, or see it on the television shows they watch, or read it in their newspapers. If they are lucky, they might happen upon a physician who will educate them.

Another woman, Vida, 60, was also overweight and smoked more than a pack of cigarettes a day. Vida worked as a secretary in a high-pressure office and drank coffee continuously during the day. She had been under a doctor's care for recent symptoms of what seemed to be an asthmatic condition, which could have been caused by the smoking, or it could have been a result of her gastroesophageal reflux, or it could have been caused by the stress at work. She had a heart attack one day a few minutes after eating a cheeseburger and fries at her desk.

Peggy and Vida are not exceptions to the rule. They are, in fact, very typical, although most heart attacks occur in women in their sixties, seventies, and eighties. Most menopausal women do not understand how a lack of estrogen affects their hearts, their bones, or anything else. They do have a vague understanding that their moodiness and sudden hot flashes are caused by hormonal changes. Otherwise, the majority of women are ignorant about the long- and short-term implications of estrogen deficiency. Until recently, their doctors rarely, if ever, bothered to explain any of it to them. And if women themselves do not understand how their bodies are changing, their families know even less.

For a long time physicians have been erroneously taught that coronary heart disease is a man's disease. Women do have less coronary heart disease before menopause than men, but if they smoke or have uncontrolled diabetes, they lose their biological advantage over men and can develop coronary heart disease even before menopause. Heart disease occurs in women at an older age than men because we are protected until menopause by estrogen. It is estrogen that reduces the levels of the LDL, or bad cholesterol, that forms arterial plaque. It is estrogen that keeps the HDL, the good cholesterol, high.

Heart disease presents differently in women, too. Angina, or chest pain, appears to be the first warning of heart attack in women, where the attack itself is often the first warning a man gets. However, because chest pain could be caused by any number of things, the pain is not reported to a physician as quickly, and if it is, the diagnosis of heart disease takes longer in women. Women can have silent heart attacks, which are later detected on routine electrocardiagram. Many of the diagnostic tests that on men give reliable results, such as the exercise tolerance test and the nuclear uptake studies, are frequently unreliable in women. This results in a woman's disease being more advanced by the time she is treated. Treatment outcomes will thus be less positive for procedures such as angiography, angioplasty, and bypass surgery in older patients.

A WOMAN'S DEVELOPING CARDIOVASCULAR SYSTEM

In the early years the female heart is healthy unless affected by either of two disorders, congenital heart disease and rheumatic heart disease, both of which are more common in girls than in boys. A child might be born with a congenital heart defect, and some of the severe forms of congenital heart disease are apparent at birth or soon after.

In the early adult years, from 18 to 40, the most common heart condition in women is *mitral valve prolapse* (MVP), much more common in women than men. A prolapsed mitral valve is a valve that does not do its job. This valve is a swinging door that is supposed to go in only one direction. When the muscle that controls the door is weakened, it lets the door flop backward. Hence, the condition is also called leaky valve or floppy valve (or flail valve).

That backward bulging of the valve can be heard with a stethoscope as it produces a distinctive clicking sound. The diagnosis of mitral valve prolapse is established with an echocardiogram, an ultrasound device that visualizes the inside of the heart, the chambers, and the valves. The valvular defect can be slight, moderate, or severe. Most people with this condition have no symptoms whatsoever. In others, mitral valve prolapse might be associated with palpitations and shortness of breath.

In one study, one college girl out of ten was diagnosed as having mitral valve prolapse. Whereas many studies correlate the presence of mitral valve prolapse with symptoms of palpitations as well as many "hysterical and psychosomatic" features, mitral valve prolapse seldom causes a serious problem. An exception is if the valve becomes infected as a result of a dental or other invasive procedure. Bacteria released into the bloodstream tend to localize on a deformed valve, causing infective endocarditis, with fever, emboli, and sometimes death. Patients with MVP are thus encouraged to take prophylactic antibiotics shortly before visits to the dentist and before any invasive surgery.

Coronary heart disease is due to narrowing and occlusion of coronary arteries that feed the heart. This condition is also called ischemic heart disease, emphasizing the lack of oxygen that results from such an occlusion. Because of its high prevalence, this is what we generally mean when we say "heart disease." By middle age, Caucasian women between 45 and 54 have far fewer heart fatalities compared with white men the same age: 47.8 per 100,000 women die compared with 162.2 per 100,000 men. This difference narrows as women age. However, after the age of 65, about a third of American women develop some manifestations of coronary heart disease.

It is during the premenopausal years, in the young adult and midlife years, that you can influence the risk factors of future heart disease by changing your lifestyle to circumvent heart disease. Evaluate your risks and change the things you can change, such as your weight, what you eat, and how well you exercise. Most heart disease is highly preventable.

Racial Differences

Heart disease mortality is two-thirds higher for black women than white; even though the death rate for both is declining, it is declining only slightly for black women. It is thought that the decline of mortality from coronary heart disease—in men and women—is related to less smoking, more physical fitness, better nutrition, and better medications (lipolytic—fat-lowering—agents).

Blacks who are poor have the highest rates of heart disease. For example, for black women in Harlem, a predominantly black neighborhood in New York City, the rate was 3.38 times the national rate for white women. A study reported in the *New England Journal of Medicine* in 1997 reported that while it is a known fact that blacks have higher rates of cardiovascular diseases, there might be an environmental difference among the rates of heart disease among blacks in this country. Higher rates of heart disease were found among blacks from the South. The study, which was done with census reports and death certificates, was surprising in its finding that blacks and whites in New York had about the same rate of risk for cardiovascular disease. However, black New Yorkers born in the South had much higher risk than black New Yorkers from the Caribbean. This latter group, in fact, had lower rates than whites. (Men and women were not separated out for the study.)

The lowest mortality rate from heart disease is among Hispanic, Native American, and Asian/Pacific Islander women. However, there are

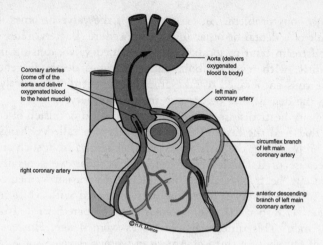

Coronary arteries
(come off of the
aorta and deliver
oxygenated blood
to the heart muscle)

Aorta (delivers
oxygenated
blood to body)

left main
coronary artery

circumflex branch
of left main
coronary artery

right coronary artery

anterior descending
branch of left main
coronary artery

©H.R. Muinos

Figure 22. The heart.

no conclusions yet about whether this is due to genetics, socioeconomic factors, or diet.

How the Heart Works

The heart is a pump composed of four chambers separated by valves that keep the blood flowing in one direction. The two atria, right and left, are the vestibules, and the two ventricles, right and left, are the main chambers, which are highly muscular. The muscular heart tissue is the myocardium. These are powerful pumps, especially the left. Valves act as doorways from one chamber to the next, and they normally open in only one direction to prevent backflow of blood.

Systemic arteries, those that feed the body, carry oxygenated, and therefore red, blood, while the systemic veins carry the blue, or deoxygenated blood. The opposite color scheme marks the pulmonary circulation, pulmonary arteries and veins. The right atrium receives the deoxygenated blood from the systemic veins, contracts, and directs the flow through the tricuspid valve into the right ventricle. The right ventricle pumps that blood into the pulmonary arteries. In the lungs this deoxygenated blood gets rid of the carbon dioxide and acquires oxygen, which it carries via the pulmonary veins to the left atrium. The left atrium conveys this oxygenated blood to the left ventricle, which is a powerful pump that distributes this red blood via the aorta to the rest of the body. This continuous recycling of blood through the network of arteries, arterioles, veins, and capillaries keeps the body nourished with blood and oxygen.

The heart beats between 60 and 100 times a minute, sixty minutes an hour, twenty-four hours a day, 365 days a year for many, many years. Because the heart must keep beating for the rest of your life, supplying

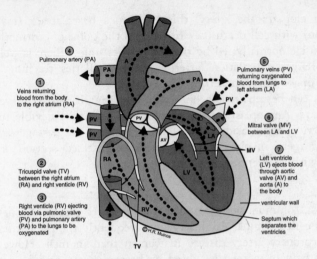

Figure 23. Blood circulation.

the muscular pump with much-needed oxygen is a priority of the first order. The faster or harder the heart beats, as it does with exercise, the more oxygen it consumes. And oxygen can get to the myocardium only through the coronary arteries. It is important, therefore, to keep your coronary arteries relaxed, wide, and free of constriction either by spasm or by plaques. A heart attack is called a *myocardial infarction,* which literally means the myocardium—heart muscle—is not getting any oxygen and therefore dies.

CONDITIONS OF THE HEART

Coronary Arteries and Heart Disease

Coronary arteries are arteries that feed the heart muscle, the myocardium. After the oxygenated blood leaves the left ventricle and reaches the aorta, the very first branches that come off the aorta are the coronary arteries. In other words, the heart must make sure that its own muscle is fed oxygenated blood before the rest of the body will get its share.

Plaques are fatty deposits that can form in any blood vessel, but when they involve the coronary arteries they have greater impact on health. Plaque narrows the diameter of the coronary artery. During exercise, when the myocardium demands more oxygen than the narrowed coronaries can deliver, the pain nerve endings are irritated by the accumulated lactic acid and you feel pain, or *angina.* The myocardium seems to cry out in anguish. Coronary heart disease is also called ischemic heart disease, meaning "no oxygen in the blood."

If the plaque ruptures from the artery wall, the debris and blood clot and clog up the artery, this leads to a heart attack (myocardial infarction) with cell death (*necrosis*) beyond the point of obstruction. The heart muscle normally fed by that vessel dies unless there is well-developed collateral circulation (arterioles and capillaries reaching it from another major blood vessel).

This can be repaired in only two ways, but it can be prevented in many ways. Angioplasty is a procedure of inserting a flexible tube into the artery, pushing aside the plug, and making the passageway wider. Bypass surgery involves grafting over the diseased section of artery, usually with segments of a vein.

Angina

The most common symptom of coronary heart disease is chest pain, which is called angina. Angina is more frequently the presenting symptom of coronary artery disease in women than in men. However, not all chest pain in women is caused by heart disease; over 55 percent of women who present with chest pain have no evidence of coronary artery obstruction, compared with 43 percent in men. The difficulty of diagnosis of cardiovascular disease in women is compounded by a high incidence of silent angina in women. In silent angina there is no pain, although an electrocardiogram can detect the signs of ischemia.

In 35 to 65 percent of women experiencing typical angina, the angiography (X ray of the blood vessels) will document a narrowing of a segment of a coronary artery, which is clear confirmation that the pain was related to that narrowing of the vessel. However, in less than 20 percent of women experiencing atypical angina will the angiogram document such narrowing. Does it mean that what these women are experiencing is not angina, not heart pain at all? There is a controversy attached to that. Some investigators believe that angina in women is due to narrowing of tiny vessels (microvasculature) of the heart that cannot be visualized on the angiogram. This is sometimes called Syndrome X, or microvascular angina. Other investigators do not believe there is such a thing and ascribe the pain to psychological factors.

Coronary heart disease should not be confused with other causes of chest pain. As most emergency room personnel know, chest pain can also be caused by extreme heartburn, as well as other conditions. Physical exertion and the use and abuse of chest muscles are the most common causes of chest pain in women, especially in younger women. Strained chest muscles—for example, from playing tennis after not having played for several months—can be erroneously interpreted as angina.

A condition called *costochondritis* might cause chest wall pain. This condition was at one time very common in European laundresses, whose job was to rub the laundry against a washboard all day. The movement exacerbated the inflammation of the costochondral junctions—cartilages in the ribs—and actual bulges would appear at those sites.

Myocardial Infarction

Myocardial infarction is the clinical term for a heart attack. It literally means that the cells of the heart muscle are dying because they are receiving no blood supply. Occurrence of silent or unrecognized myocardial infarction is more common in women than in men. While the myocardial infarction occurs later in life in women than in men, once it occurs it is associated with increased in-hospital mortality (39 percent vs. 31 percent), increased chance of reinfarction, and increased incidence of heart failure. If the clots can be dissolved with a procedure called *thrombolysis* within a few hours after a heart attack, this benefits both men and women, but it can cause more complications in women, especially bleeding, the most severe of which is brain hemorrhage.

The same conditions caused by similar lesions are manifested differently in women than in men. In the past, it was not unusual for myocardial infarction to be diagnosed after the fact on the basis of changes in the electrocardiogram on annual examinations. A woman might have no recollection of unusual pain or other symptoms in the intervening year.

RISK FACTORS FOR CORONARY HEART DISEASE

Estrogen Deficiency

Estrogen deficiency is the number-one relative risk factor for coronary heart disease in women. This means that if you have other risk factors, at menopause—when you are no longer protected by estrogen—this risk factor is combined with the others to increase your risk.

Family History

If you have relatives with coronary heart disease, you are at risk for the disease yourself. There is growing evidence that family history might determine who will or will not benefit from lowering the cholesterol in their diet. We have apolipoproteins, molecules that transport cholesterol in the blood. These are in large part determined by heredity and seem to play an important role in how our bodies respond to diet.

Age

Age is certainly a powerful risk factor for both men and women. In men, however, the cardiovascular morbidity and mortality plot against age is a linear crescendo from about age 20 on, while in women it is low until menopause. Then it increases dramatically.

Smoking

Smoking is a more serious risk for women than for men. It causes blood vessels to contract, and because women's blood vessels are smaller to begin with, they leave less room for blood to flow. Even the passive smoke of someone you live with can be a risk.

Hypertension

Hypertension is an important risk factor, especially untreated hypertension. High blood pressure exerts an increased force on the blood vessels, making them more prone to arteriosclerosis. This same stress that hypertension exerts on the coronary arteries of the heart is also borne by the blood vessels of the brain, making us susceptible to strokes, and on blood vessels of the kidneys, causing eventually kidney failure (see chapter 28).

Diabetes

Diabetes is a more potent risk factor in a woman than in a man. If the diabetes is uncontrolled, and other risk factors are present, the female biological advantage is wiped out even before menopause.

Weight Gain

Weight gain is also an independent risk for women, especially at midlife. In men, massive obesity is a risk factor. In women, being even ten pounds overweight increases the chances of coronary heart disease. This is especially so when the type of obesity is "central," above the waist rather than around the hips. A recent study confirmed that in middle-aged women there was an almost direct relation between body mass and overall mortality and three to nine times increased risk of coronary mortality (see page 136 for more information about obesity).

A High-fat Diet

Years of too much fat and cholesterol will already have put you at risk, but without estrogen, your risk will be increased. All that fat has been clogging up your arteries, and now, without estrogen to keep your arteries open, you are at greater risk for heart problems. It is during midlife, and probably even before that, that lifestyle will determine your propensity to develop or not develop coronary heart disease in the future.

A Sedentary Lifestyle

Lack of exercise deprives your heart of oxygen, makes it easier for your arteries to get clogged, and keeps bad cholesterol high and good cholesterol low. This list goes on and on. Throughout this book you can find information on how and why the sedentary lifestyle is a killer. Refer to chapters 5 and 10.

Use of Oral Contraceptives

Past history of the use of contraceptives while young does not carry increased risk of coronary heart disease, but current use in an older women does, especially if she smokes. A woman over 35 who takes oral contraceptives and smokes has a seven times higher risk for heart disease than a woman who does not smoke.

Stress

In studies of men, coronary heart disease is correlated with stresses associated with so-called Type A behavior, an overly conscientious, hard-driving attitude inherent in life in the fast lane. Women now have similar stresses in their jobs, plus the additional stress of fulfilling the multiple roles of workers, wives, and mothers. However, no long-term studies are available about women in the fast lane.

The studies we do have of women and stress indicate, however, that there are specific stresses that are conducive to coronary heart disease. The Framingham Study found that female clerical workers with little control over their work environment, repetitive job patterns, scant recognition, and underutilization of their skills have higher rates of coronary heart disease than homemakers with no outside jobs. Working women with three or more children are very vulnerable. Having a nonsupportive boss, little job mobility, feelings of suppressed hostility, and being married to a blue-collar worker are also risk factors. Single working women have the lowest incidence of heart disease, according to the study.

If you have one or more risk factors for coronary heart disease, you need a total clinical assessment by your internist, who is well trained in cardiology and can administer a comprehensive diagnostic workup. This includes a medical history, scrutiny of your family history, and a careful physical examination. You should be screened for hypertension and diabetes. Blood pressure, if elevated, must be brought down. If diabetes is diagnosed, it requires treatment and close monitoring. A referral to a cardiologist should be made if sophisticated procedures such as cardiac catheterization need to be performed.

GENDER DIFFERENCES IN CHOLESTEROL LEVELS

We all know that too much cholesterol is bad, but only some of us know the difference between the two types of cholesterol, and that women have a different response to one of them. The low-density lipoprotein (LDL) is the bad cholesterol, and high-density lipoprotein (HDL) is the protective cholesterol. (The easy way to remember is: L is for "lousy," and H is for "healthy.")

Our favorite metaphor (page 336) compares LDL cholesterol to an oil truck that delivers fat to the body and leaves fatty plaques in the walls of blood vessels, and HDL, the good cholesterol, to a sanitation truck that travels in the vascular system and cleans up the debris and the fatty components of the plaques and carries them back to the liver for processing. HDL is therefore protective of heart disease.

Triglycerides, the neutral fats in the blood, might also be more of a risk factor for women than they are for men if they are truly elevated, such as over 300.

In men the most important prognostic factor is high LDL, the bad cholesterol. In women, a low level of HDL is a more serious risk factor than elevated LDL. While many things, like high-fat diets, can elevate the LDL, the HDL can be increased only by estrogen and exercise. One could theorize that exercise, by increasing the metabolism, speeds up the uptake of lipids by the HDL and the speed of processing them out of the system, but this is only a hypothesis—mine. A small amount of alcohol, one drink a day, might also help women keep their HDL levels up. A high HDL level in a woman, which is good, raises the total cholesterol value. This is why total cholesterol in women can be safely a bit higher than in men.

High levels of the bad cholesterol (LDL) are undertreated in women, according to a study reported in the *Journal of the American Medical Association*. Fewer than one in every ten female heart patients received treatment to lower her cholesterol to a safe level. Standard treatment is taking drugs to lower the cholesterol, eating properly, exercising, and controlling hypertension and diabetes.

The author of the study, Dr. Helmut G. Schrott, an associate professor of preventive and internal medicine at the University of Iowa, reported that women are not being treated aggressively enough by their doctors, or they are not taking the medications prescribed for them. It was his feeling that most of the blame lay with the doctors. There is still a pervasive belief, even in the medical establishment, that women are not as vulnerable to heart attack as men.

Blood lipids are affected by hormones, lifestyle, and to some extent by genetics. Both men and women with genetically determined high levels of lipoprotein(a) are extremely susceptible to coronary heart disease. Lp(a) is a form of the so-called bad cholesterol that becomes plaque on arterial walls. Fortunately, this compound can be suppressed by estrogen.

A study of 600 women under 65 in Sweden showed that those with the highest levels of Lp(a) were almost three times more likely to have a heart attack or angina. The study, published in 1997 by the American Heart Association, found that high levels of Lp(a) both before and after menopause had the same consequences.

Lp(a) typically rises after menopause, when the estrogen levels decline. In the Framingham Heart Study of 3,000 women, investigators found increased Lp(a) levels in women who developed heart disease. However, women who take hormone replacement therapy generally have stable levels of the protein.

Lp(a) is a highly variable factor in the body chemistry. Levels of Lp(a) are determined by a person's genes and appear to be unchanged by diet, exercise, or "stating"—the fat-lowering drugs.

In addition to the effect of estrogen on the lipid metabolism, estrogen acts on estrogen receptors in the smooth muscles of the blood vessels and dilates these vessels. It also inhibits thrombosis, helps the natural process of dissolving clots, and might also act as an antioxidant, neutralizing the free radicals and preventing oxidation of LDL cholesterol. Oxidized LDL is what gets deposited in the vessel walls as plaque.

THE DIFFICULTIES OF DIAGNOSIS IN WOMEN

It is unfortunate that most of the diagnostic screening and testing for heart disease has been studied only in men, so we have no information from long-term studies on women. Both men and women are urged to get annual blood pressure testing and regular tests for cholesterol levels (every five years if they are normal).

The Cardiac Stress Test

The difficulty of diagnosing coronary heart disease in women is compounded by the relative unreliability of cardiac stress test in women. About 10 to 15 percent of all positive tests on women are false positive: the test appears to indicate coronary heart disease that the woman does not really have. There is also about a 10 percent rate of false negative tests.

An EKG (electrocardiogram) is first taken while the patient is resting and then at various stages of exercise. From the difference between the EKGs the cardiologist determines if there is ischemia (lack of oxygen) in the heart muscle or destruction of the muscle, and where in the heart muscle the damage resides. That exercise EKG might also uncover an abnormal conduction predisposing the patient to arrhythmias.

Angiography

The gold standard in the diagnosis of coronary heart disease is coronary angiography, an invasive test that allows visualization of the blood vessels. A catheter is threaded through the blood vessels to the various heart chambers and a radio-opaque dye is injected to follow the flow through the pertinent arteries. The aorta and the two coronary arteries can be visualized when dye is injected into the left ventricle. Cardiologists can measure the extent of narrowed or blocked arteries.

GENDER DIFFERENCES IN TREATMENT

The most important difference in heart disease in women vs. men is that it is being treated differently by physicians. It is often perceived as less important in women, and they are therefore not treated well enough or quickly enough. Additionally, doctors believe women often complain of chest pain or palpitations from a variety of unimportant or psychosomatic causes, and they tend not to always take them seriously.

Women undergo fewer invasive cardiovascular procedures, raising the question of whether the rate of use is inappropriately low in women or inappropriately high in men. Although women seem to be more functionally affected by chest pain, fewer symptomatic women than men undergo diagnostic coronary arteriography and therapeutic coronary angioplasty or coronary bypass surgery. Forty percent of men with a lesion documented on radionuclide study, but only 4 percent of women with a similar lesion, were referred for coronary angiography.

An excuse for performing fewer procedures on women has been that women are usually older than men by the time they first come to the attention of cardiologists and other internists; being older they have accumulated more illnesses called *comorbidities*, some of which might contraindicate the use of certain procedures. In a more recent paper (1998), however, an analysis of cardiac procedures was done for each decade of life, and for each decade women received less attention and fewer procedures and treatments than men.

Thrombolysis is a treatment useful in dissolving clots if administered within a few hours after a heart attack. It benefits both men and women but is associated with more complications in women, such as excessive bleeding. Women are less likely to be eligible for thrombolytic therapy because they don't get help soon enough after the onset of the symptoms.

After angioplasty, a procedure designed to open up the clogged coronary arteries, women's arteries close up again more readily than those of men. Women's arteries are smaller.

After a coronary bypass procedure, the in-hospital mortality for men is 2.6 percent; in women it is 4.6 percent. Once patients pass successfully the perioperative period, survival is similar for men and women. By the time women undergo coronary bypass surgery, they are typically sicker than men, and more often require emergency surgery. Women also appear to be referred for revascularization at a later, more symptomatic stage of illness.

Aspirin and beta-blockers are equally beneficial in prevention of reinfarction in women and men. We still do not have sufficient information to know whether taking aspirin will help in preventing heart disease in women. Low doses of aspirin in some studies show significant reduction in the risk of heart attack, but how well this works for women is not yet completely known.

Exercise and rehabilitation. Physicians refer fewer women for exercise rehabilitation, even though it is equally successful in women and men. Women who are referred tend to have poorer compliance and attendance because of their more coexisting illnesses, family responsibilities, and perhaps other psychosocial factors.

LOWERING YOUR RISK FOR HEART DISEASE

Cardiovascular disease does not have to be the leading cause of death of women in the United States. It is highly preventable. Hormone replacement therapy and lifestyle changes can lower your risk significantly (see chapter 23).

Dr. Paul Kligfield, at the New York Hospital–Cornell Medical Center Cardiac Health Center, has advice for rehabilitation of cardiac patients. He counsels them to stop smoking, manage stress, learn about proper nutrition, and gain confidence in their own strength. Dr. Kligfield has worked out a scientific method of getting patients involved in a gradually increasing exercise regimen while he monitors metabolic rate, heart rate, oxygen efficiency, and other systems. He also teaches them stress management and takes them to a local restaurant, where they learn how to eat properly.

The Importance of Diet

The more animal fats in the diet, the greater the risk of clogging the arteries and making the heart work harder. You do need some fats, however, or you will lower your good cholesterol (HDL) level too much. People who cut too much fat from their diets also tend to compensate by eating too many carbohydrates, which can also have a negative effect on the blood lipids. A good diet contains 30 percent or less of fat, but some investigators believe there should be no more than 20 percent. The important thing is that most of the fat should come from vegetable sources like olive oil, rather than from animal sources like butter and fatty meats (see chapter 10 for more information about well-balanced diets).

A recent association has been made between homocysteine, a naturally occurring compound found in the blood, and cardiovascular risk. Several studies connect folic acid and homocysteine. Scientists believe folic acid helps us convert homocysteine to a less harmful substance. Without folic acid—and other B vitamins—the levels of homocysteine can build up and damage the cells lining the heart and blood vessels. This makes it more likely that plaque will form. There has been much research into folic acid's role in preventing birth defects like spina bifida (see chapter 14), but investigators are also finding that it might play an important role in cardiovascular disease.

Estrogen-rich Food

Some studies have shown that replacing some animal proteins with soy protein can lower LDL cholesterol. The phytoestrogens in soybeans are thought to be responsible, but the amount of soy protein necessary to produce a beneficial effect is unclear. Researchers at Bowman Gray Medical School in North Carolina have recently begun a three-year investigation of the effects of phytoestrogens on cardiovascular risk factors in perimenopausal and postmenopausal women. A similar study is going on at Columbia University College of Physicians and Surgeons (refer to page 347 for more about phytoestrogens).

The Importance of Exercise

Your heart needs oxygen to be healthy. Exercise is the best way to deliver that oxygen. Walking, running, riding your exercise bike, even dancing will help. In my years of practice I have found it particularly frustrating to get women to maintain a consistent exercise program. The younger generations are more involved in sports and exercise, and they seem to be aware of the benefits of exercise and the risks associated with the sedentary life. But I think that the majority of menopausal women are still too sedentary.

Dr. Kligfield's rehabilitation program begins with stretching for ten minutes, followed by a half hour workout monitored by an EKG, then a cooldown with more stretching. This program starts in the hospital; later, patients come in three times a week. The goal is to improve their tolerance to exercise and increase what they are capable of doing. Patients in the program have less frequent chest pain, require hospitalization less often, and live longer.

$\cdot\cdot 25 \cdot\cdot$

Preventing Osteoporosis

Osteoporosis is like pornography. You know it when you see it. On an electron microscope you see the thinned-out bone plates. On the street you see the stooped walk of an elderly woman. There is a curve in her back, the so-called dowager's hump, her neck is extended, her pelvis is thrust forward, her hips and knees are flexed, and her abdomen protrudes because of the shrinking space in her bone structure. Osteoporosis can exist, however, at an early stage when you cannot see it, but could diagnose only by measuring bone density.

The old definition of osteoporosis was that it was a "condition" characterized by a decrease of bone mass and bone density such that fractures were likely to occur. The 1993 National Institutes of Health definition calls osteoporosis a "disease" and adds the criterion of bone density more than 2.5 standard deviations below that of a normal healthy young adult of the same gender. This definition applies to many millions of women who have no symptoms at all and designates them as having a disease simply because they have lost considerable bone compared with what they had as young women. This definition is irksome to some feminists who believe that one should not call something that happens normally to the elderly a disease. On the other hand, studies confirm that women with bone density of 2.5 standard deviations below the bone peak are at manifold higher risk of fracture than women with bone density above that value. Some investigators call this a *fracture threshold*.

Whatever the label, osteoporosis is a serious public health problem that can lead to disability, deformity, and death. It costs society billions of dollars and is preventable through early intervention with diet, exercise, medications, and hormones.

Osteoporosis is literally porous bones. It is a condition of decreased bone mass affecting women sometimes during and most often after menopause. This disease causes bones to become susceptible to fractures. Decreased bone density leads to crush fractures and wedge fractures of the vertebrae, and also fractures of the ribs, wrists, pelvis, and hips. With time, this breakdown of the bone leads to the postural changes we see in the stooped woman in the first paragraph.

Osteoporotic bone consists of frail supporting beams that lose their connections with other beams and end abruptly, as if suspended without reaching the opposite beam; there are big holes in between. When osteoporosis affects the spine, the vertebrae collapse, leading to pain and eventually to stooped posture, bulging abdomen, and difficulty in walking. The most severe consequences of osteoporosis, however, result from hip fractures. About 15 percent of elderly hip fracture victims die within the first six months from direct complications of the fracture. After a hip fracture over half of women are disabled and wind up in long-term nursing homes or other protected environments. Only 25 percent of women return to their prefracture lifestyle (see chapter 27).

An average, white 50-year-old woman in the United States has approximately a 16 to 17 percent lifetime risk of suffering a hip fracture. The risk is higher in a woman who starts with lower bone density. While insufficient bone density is the major risk factor for hip fractures, there are other risks, such as the propensity to fall; the direction and force of the fall; loss of balance, vision, and hearing; and deteriorating reflexes. Environmental risk factors include poor lighting, scatter rugs, and cramped quarters. Grandchildren's toys on the floor are also dangerous.

Two critical things you should know about osteoporosis. First, the steepest bone loss occurs right at menopause, after which bone loss continues more gradually. Second, prevention is better than treatment. What's the use of closing the barn gate after all the sheep have escaped? Bone density reaches a peak in a woman's young adult life, in her twenties; levels off until the late thirties, when it begins to drop; then, at menopause, makes a steep descent. Poor calcium nutrition and lack of exercise in childhood and adolescence translate into a lower bone peak and inadequate bone reserve at menopause and thereafter, when fractures are apt to appear. Osteoporosis is a pediatric disease with consequences in advanced age.

Osteoporosis is, indeed, a two-stage process. Clinical osteoporosis is when fractures begin to occur. About 8 million women in the United States suffer from osteoporotic fractures. Preclinical osteoporosis is decreasing bone density. Here, you are on the edge of disaster, waiting for the fractures to begin. Poised on this edge in this country are 24 million women.

According to the Commonwealth Fund Commission on Women's Health, from 1989 to 1991 an estimated 20 percent of women 50 and over had osteoporosis of the hip, and 50 percent of women had a moderate degree of bone loss (osteopenia) at the hip. Annually, 1.3 million fractures in women over 45 are attributed to osteoporosis. Of that total, 210,000 are hip fractures, which carry high rates of institutionalization and death. Osteoporosis can also cause vertebral and wrist fractures, which can occur even with minimal trauma and are painful and debilitating.

Osteoporosis affects one third of all postmenopausal women and three fourths of women between 65 and 75 years old. It was the twelfth leading cause of death in this country in 1989, and the projected public health cost is $10 billion a year in the year 2000 ($20 billion by 2020). Osteoporosis causes loss of employment, pain, disfigurement, disability, dependency, despondency, and death. With baby boomers approaching menopause, the coming century faces an epidemic of osteoporosis and its complications.

Osteoporosis should not be confused with osteoarthritis, the most common form of arthritis, which affects 16 million Americans—mostly women—over the age of 45. Experts have long speculated that estrogen plays a role in this form of arthritis because it is so prevalent in women who have gone through menopause. (Refer to the "Osteoarthritis" section in chapter 27 for more information about osteoarthritis.)

NONPREVENTABLE RISK FACTORS

Bone deterioration caused by loss of estrogen after menopause is the major risk factor for osteoporosis. Other risk factors you can do little or nothing about are:

Family History
Genetic research has only recently focused on the susceptibility to osteoporosis. Mechanisms for a genetic effect on bone loss and preservation have been suspected for some time. Australian researchers have identified a gene that is responsible for absorption of vitamin D and calcium; individuals with mutations of that gene are more likely to develop osteoporosis. More recently, a gene for a substance called cathepsin O has been identified in osteoporosis by Dr. Fred Drake of Smith Kline Beecham collaborating with the Human Genome Project. Cathepsin O stands for the osteoclast, the cell that resorbs bone. Cathepsin is probably involved in spurring on the osteoclast to do its bone-devouring job.

Small Bone Structure
Your stature is largely inherited, and there is not much you can do about it except make your bones strong through diet and exercise. A thin bone structure is a double whammy. First the slight frame means you have little bone reserve, so you might lose it more quickly down

to the danger level. Second, absence of body fat deprives you of the second best estrogen factory in your body. Fat is where a compound from the adrenal gets converted into estrogen. At greater risk are women with small bone structures who smoke, do not exercise, and do not ingest calcium. Women who are underweight for their height are also at increased risk. A tall and lanky body build is also a risk for osteoporosis. Ironically, women with the greatest bone mass seem to be at greater risk for breast cancer than women with small bone mass who fracture their bones more easily. This came from a study of 7,000 women at four medical centers. A previous similar study revealed that women who suffered wrist fractures had low rates of breast cancer.

Race

Race is an important risk factor. There has been a myth in existence that African American women are not susceptible to osteoporosis. This is not entirely true, but it depends on the bone structure of the woman. The heavier her bone frame the less susceptible she is. A thin black woman with a shoe size of six and a half or less is as susceptible as her white sister is to osteoporosis. White women generally have lower bone mass than black and Mexican American women, accounting for a higher risk of osteoporosis. White women also lose bone more quickly than black women. Asian women, especially the Japanese, are at even greater risk. Investigators speculate that it is not the color of the skin but the structure and strength of the skeleton that make the difference. The sturdiness of the skeleton is determined genetically and by exposure to heavy, weight-bearing exercise throughout one's life.

RISK FACTORS YOU CAN PREVENT

Surgical Menopause

Treasure your ovaries and keep them out of harm's way. Do not allow the surgeons to yank them out without a good reason, or the radiologists to expose them to radiation unnecessarily. Your ovary is the number-one source of estrogen, and no pharmacological imitation is ever as good as the real thing. While less estrogen is produced after menopause, there is still some. If you should require a hysterectomy, question the surgeon carefully about what he or she will do with the ovaries. Of course, if the ovaries are diseased you must agree to take them out. The ovary can be a site of the most fatal gynecological cancer, cancer that is difficult, almost impossible, to detect while it is still curable. Surveillance might require annual checkups and assessments using pelvic ultrasound examinations and still be ineffective; but the average woman's chance of developing an ovarian tumor is one in seventy, hardly an indication for castration of all females.

Cigarette Smoking

As if you didn't already have enough evidence to encourage you to quit, here's more: Tobacco robs you of your own estrogens and inhibits the action of estrogen on many organs, including your bones. In 1994, the *New England Journal of Medicine* published an Australian study of twins, one of whom smoked. The smoking twin (one pack a day) had an average bone mass deficit of 5 to 10 percent, which is sufficient to increase the risk of fractures.

Improper Nutrition

Lack of calcium in the growing years is directly related to loss of bone mass, and many women do not get enough calcium after childhood. In adolescence they lose interest in drinking milk, and they do not replace the milk with calcium-rich foods such as yogurt, cheese, or green vegetables, nor do they take supplements. Too much protein, caffeine, and phosphates from soft drinks are also detrimental to your bones.

A Sedentary Lifestyle

Walking, running, and riding a bike all help build strong bones. Bones need a workout to make them strong. Weight-bearing exercise builds bone. Bones that are not being used get reabsorbed by bone-eating cells called *osteoclasts*. On the other hand, when you walk you are putting stress on the bones of your legs, pelvis, and spine. That stress causes an electrochemical (sometimes called "piezoelectric") current to bring in more calcium and bone-building materials to accumulate at the areas of stress. Bone-building cells called *osteoblasts* go to work and bone deposition begins. These two processes, bone formation and bone resorption, keep occurring throughout your life. In adolescence, formation dominates over resorption. Later, at the bone peak, both are equal. At menopause and in older age, resorption predominates and we lose bone. The stress of weight bearing stimulates bone formation.

Use of Certain Medications

Steroid medications—which are used for the treatment of autoimmune conditions, connective tissue disorders, and chronic asthma—are harmful to bone and stimulate bone resorption. Such drugs can actually cause osteoporosis. Drugs like prednisone, a potent corticosteroid, can hurt bones in several ways. They can directly cause the bone to break down by stimulating the work of the osteoclasts, the cells that break down the bone, while at the same time inhibiting the work of the osteoblasts, the cells that build new bone. Corticosteroids also neutralize the effect of the sex hormones, thus reducing bone density. Medications used in thyroid and convulsive conditions, heparin, tetracyclines, and other medications have similar effects.

SCREENING FOR BONE DENSITY: NOW OR LATER?

We document osteoporosis with bone density tests. These tests are relatively expensive and, despite recent legislation, are not always covered by health insurance. We are faced with the public health dilemma of how to screen the population of a million and a half women annually at about $200 a test. To predict the need for bone density measurement, formulas of clinical and chemical risk factors have been compiled. Unfortunately, these profiles are not precise and don't match with bone density reliably. Our inability, therefore, to accurately and cheaply predict who is prone to a painful, disabling, and costly hip fracture makes our decisions about estrogen treatment difficult.

Most researchers feel that menopause is the best time to start the screening and treating in order to prevent the rapid bone loss that occurs at this time of the woman's life. A few investigators recommend that screening and treating, if necessary, start ten to fifteen years after menopause to protect women from hip fractures that are more serious, resulting in more morbidity and mortality than vertebral fractures, and are more prevalent in the seventies, eighties, and nineties rather than in the fifties and sixties.

The argument goes that we should not be wasting our big therapeutic guns on vertebral fractures in the fifties when we might need them for the true hazard later on. This argument is supported by studies that show that bone loss after menopause is a steady loss that keeps on in advanced age.

Another argument for screening later is that at 70 it might be more possible to assess other fracture risks more accurately. A 70-year-old woman who is losing her balance, her vision, and her hearing might be more prone to osteoporotic fractures than her hale and hardy sister, who exercises every day.

The proponents of screening later quote the effectiveness of estrogen at 65 as a possible proof that one does not need to hurry. For instance, one study demonstrated that giving continuous estrogen to postmenopausal women even at age 65 made an appreciable difference in their bone mass. After two years the estrogen group exhibited a significant increase in vertebral bone density—on the average, 5 percent in bone mass density per year. What's more, the older the woman, the more spectacular was the response.

Another argument is provided by analysis of a group of postmenopausal white women who were part of the Framingham study. Estrogen users were protected from bone loss if they took the medication for at least seven to ten years, but women who had taken estrogen for ten years beginning at menopause at 50 until age 60, and then stopped, showed no advantage in bone density at age 70 over women who had never taken estrogen. In other words, the bone-protective effect of estrogen wears out ten years after it is stopped. Which might mean that, once started, treatment should be continued indefinitely. And if one starts treatment at 70, the cumulative dose of hormones will not be as high and some of the long-term side effects of treatment can be prevented. This policy might also be more cost-effective. Another recent study—of 740 women in a retirement colony in Rancho Bernardo in California—also documented that estrogen started at 60 and continued indefinitely was almost as good for the bones as the continuous estrogen treatment started at menopause.

Perhaps both sides are right. Whenever a woman appears in the doctor's office, at menopause or twenty years later, we should screen her and consider treatment if she is susceptible. Perhaps the screening should be done at both points of her life, at menopause and then again at 75. Still, by postponing the screening until later years, one does not prevent the early major and steep bone loss that occurs at menopause. Prevention is always better than treatment.

How Bone Density Testing Is Done

Bone density checkups are critical once you enter menopause. There are two ways to do this. Bone densitometry, which has been with us for over a decade, tells us how much bone we are left with, a static measurement of current bone mass. This is like knowing how much gas there is remaining in the tank. It does not tell us how fast we are consuming it. Bone density measurement is the most valuable baseline assessment of the state of bone of the individual. We need biochemical markers—the cross-links—to assess the rate of bone turnover and to measure effects of treatment.

Bone densitometry techniques are not designed to pinpoint the cause of bone loss but to allow the clinician to quantitate the degree of bone loss. The combination of bone density measurement and levels of cross-links in urine enable us to know if there is sufficient ongoing bone loss to cause a nontraumatic fracture, to assess the risk of future fractures, to provide a baseline, and to monitor and follow up treatment.

In the past, bone density was measured using simple single photon absorptiometry (SPA), a method that measured the density of your forearm bone, the radius. SPA, however, cannot distinguish bone from soft tissue and is used for those sites, such as the radius, at which skeleton is surrounded by uniform soft tissue. Since most serious fractures involved the spine and the hip, a more accurate method was developed, namely the dual photon absorptiometry, which was later perfected as dual energy X-ray absorptiometry, called DEXA or DPX (depending on the manufacturer of the equipment).

Dual photon absorptiometry is able to distinguish bone from soft tissue and can measure bone density of the spine and thighbone. DEXA or DPX is now the method of choice for bone density measurements.

Its accuracy and precision are superior to any other technique. Radiation exposure is also the lowest.

Photons that penetrate your spine or hip register on a sensitive record that gives you a picture of your spine as you lie on a table. The computer calculates the density of each bone as grams of the mineral (calcium) per square centimeter. From that record the doctor can see if your bones are above or below the fracture threshold.

Your bone density is compared with the expected density for a young normal adult, and also a woman of your own age, weight, and race. For example, a 42-year-old woman had 91 percent of the expected peak bone density for a young woman and is not at an increased risk of fracture. Another woman, 58 years of age, measured well below the bone density of a young woman and is very susceptible to fractures.

Another method of measuring bone density and integrity is quantitative ultrasonography of the heel, approved by the FDA in 1998. The advantages of this system include lower cost, portability of the small instrument adaptable to almost any clinic or doctor's office, and assessment of the integrity of the bone architecture that the more expensive DEXA and DPX do not do.

Cross-link Testing

Urine tests for so-called cross-links can tell us how fast we are using up bone. Cross-links, also called N-telopeptides (NTX), are breakdown products of bone. As bone turnover occurs, some of the digested bone components appear in urine. Cross-links are more specific for bone than other chemicals that used to be measured in the past. The test can be repeated accurately every three months, so we can evaluate more quickly if a treatment is working. Every woman is different in the way she responds to different treatments.

PREVENTION WITH HORMONE REPLACEMENT

If a woman is not at increased risk for osteoporosis there is no reason to treat her, but there is every reason to observe and follow her. If she is identified as susceptible to osteoporosis, we have a choice between estrogen replacement therapy and alendronate, a medication that improves bone strength.

The smallest estrogen dose possible together with sufficient calcium supplements and lifestyle changes including exercise comprise the best regimen we have now that protects you from osteoporosis and other estrogen-deficiency conditions, such as heart disease. We don't know how long we should continue estrogen for preventive protection of women from bone loss and fractures. But present practice is to treat for ten to fifteen years, then taper off and stop. Others will continue on a small dose indefinitely, especially if they are extremely susceptible. The invigorating and antidepressant effect of estrogen helps women ignore the bone pain and exercise more enthusiastically with an indirect beneficial effect on the bone.

Although estrogen is the most effective prevention of osteoporosis, many women cannot take it because of a strong family history of breast cancer or because they themselves had breast cancer.

ALTERNATIVES TO HORMONE REPLACEMENT

Until very recently, estrogen was the only FDA-approved viable option for the majority of women susceptible to osteoporosis. Now, a most important treatment agent is FDA approved for the use in osteoporosis. This is *alendronate*, a bisphosphonate marketed under the name Fosamax.

Bisphosphonates

Bisphosphonates interfere with the function of mature osteoclasts, which break down bone. Alendronate is 1,000 times more potent than an earlier bisphosphonate, *etidronate*. It increases bone density and mass while also slowing the rate of bone loss. After six days the drug gets buried inside the bone tissue and no longer affects the osteoclasts, so it must be taken continuously.

An international clinical trial of alendronate in various dosages was carried out in almost 1,000 osteoporotic women. At the end of two years, lumbar bone density increased by about 7 percent, while women taking placebos lost 0.5 percent of spine density. At three years, the increase in spinal bone mass still held. So did the hipbone mass response. In the final three-year analysis, alendronate increased bone density in the spine, neck, and hips. It was effective regardless of age, race, and baseline bone density. Alendronate reduced incidence of vertebral fractures by 48 percent and slowed progression of vertebral deformity and loss of height.

The presence of food, however, impairs alendronate absorption, so you cannot take the pill less than one hour before breakfast. You must take alendronate with a full glass of water, and after you take the alendronate you must not go back to sleep or even recline as it can cause esophageal irritation and heartburn. Remain sitting or standing until it is time to have your breakfast. Calcium and magnesium impair absorption, so calcium-rich food and supplements must be taken at a different time—with the evening meal or before going to sleep.

On the horizon there are other bisphosphonates being tried and used.

Sodium Fluoride

Fluoride had been used in the past to stimulate bone growth, but it had side effects after being used for a long period of time. These included nausea, brittle bones, leg pain, and gastric bleeding.

Cyclical, intermittent use of a new slow-release sodium fluoride, called Slow-Fluoride, was studied in ninety-nine postmenopausal, osteoporotic women. After four years, 85 percent of the women on Slow-Fluoride were still fracture-free, compared with only 57 percent of those who did not take the medication. Most important, there were no significant side effects, no gastric ulcers, no microfractures, no pains in the extremities.

This study indicates that slow-release sodium fluoride and calcium citrate administered for four years stimulate the proliferation of osteoblasts, the bone-building cells, inhibit new vertebral fractures (but not recurrent fractures), augment spinal and femoral neck bone mass, and are safe to use in combination. There are not enough long-term data, however, to let us know if it is potentially toxic. Also, the new bone, reported as being normal, still might have some hidden defects. Besides, the compound's main effect is on the spine; the effect on the hips is only secondary. Fluoride-treated bone is more resistant to resorption. That is why it increases bone density; but this diminishes bone plasticity and might make it less biomechanically competent than normal bone. It is likely that the slow-release fluoride will be approved by the FDA in the near future.

Calcitonin

Calcitonin is a hormone produced by special (parafollicular) cells of the thyroid gland. It "tones up" the calcium level in the blood and pulls it into the bone-forming area. Salmon calcitonin is much more potent than human calcitonin, and therefore it is salmon calcitonin that has been used for prevention and treatment of osteoporosis. It is broken up, however, by gastric acid and cannot be used orally; it must be either given by injection or inhaled through the nose.

After almost a decade of experience with injectable calcitonin, the intranasal calcitonin was approved by the FDA in 1997 for use in osteoporosis. It is a weaker antiresorbant than alendronate; its effect on bone mass density is an increase of about 1 percent. Its advantage is that a woman using multiple medications, or who has a kidney or liver abnormality, can tolerate it. It can be used any time of the day, and it does not irritate the esophagus.

When it is given by injection, calcitonin is administered every day or three times a week. It has been used in the treatment of osteoporotic fractures because it also has analgesic, pain-relieving properties. The nasal preparation is now available in the United States. While weak, it offers a viable alternative to alendronate.

Tamoxifen and Raloxifene

Tamoxifen, an anti-estrogen that is given to breast cancer patients to inhibit the regrowth of the cancer, has an effect on the bone that is like that of estrogen, though weaker. It is an alternative to estrogen for osteoporosis. Tamoxifen has the disadvantage, however, of stimulating overgrowth of the endometrium and, occasionally, encouraging endometrial cancer.

Raloxifene, manufactured by Eli Lilly as Evista, was approved by the FDA in the fall of 1997. It is an excellent alternative. Like tamoxifen, raloxifene inhibits breast cancer, but, unlike tamoxifen, does not encourage the endometrial overgrowth. It does have the beneficial estrogenlike effects on the bones and the cardiovascular system.

Combination Therapies

In the future, using smaller doses of two or several antiosteoporosis medications in combination might help women achieve the greatest benefit at the least risk of side effects. It has been shown that a combination of estrogen with a bisphosphonate (etidronate or alendronate) doubles the bone benefit.

Alendronate and raloxifene combined promise to work better than either one of these separately.

Because taking estrogens for longer than ten years increases one's risk of breast cancer, several investigators recommend that after ten years of estrogen therapy, it be stopped and substituted for by alendronate for osteoporosis or alendronate plus raloxifene for osteoporosis and cardiovascular effects.

PREVENTION AND TREATMENT WITH EXERCISE AND DIET

Behavior modification is one of the most difficult therapies to enforce. It should start early, well before menopause. As I said earlier, osteoporosis is a disease of adolescence with manifestations in late adulthood. The major behavioral changes that must be introduced early are calcium intake and physical activity. *No matter how much calcium and vitamin D you consume, it will do you no good unless you exercise.* In paralyzed patients on respirators, whatever calcium they get is excreted in the urine.

Physical Activity vs. Real Exercise?

When I suggested a 63-year-old patient get some exercise, she told me she got plenty of exercise picking up after her grandchildren, for whom she was the nanny. She described how she was constantly following the children around, carting their toys back to the toy box, cleaning up after them, and so on. When she got home after her day's work, she collapsed in front of the television. Many women tell me how "active" they are and describe their hectic jobs, traveling, schlepping heavy brief-cases, and carrying tote bags. Yes, these women are active, and they are busy. But they are not getting the kind of exercise that is a requisite of good health.

Physical activity is any body movement produced by muscles that results in increased energy expenditure. Exercise is physical activity that is planned, structured, repetitive, and purposeful.

From the time of childhood through their teens and adolescence, girls and women must engage in weight-bearing activities, like walking. African women in Africa seldom suffer from osteoporosis. The ingrained habits and necessities of heavy labor and walking, sometimes encumbered by carrying loads on their heads, not only confer graceful gait and posture but also strong bones. The bone is a living tissue, constantly resorbing and reforming depending on the current mechanical stress. Our sedentary lifestyle allows the bones to resorb without the stimulus to reform.

Both the level of daily physical activity and a lack of organized exercise are potent risk factors. A computer operator and a psychiatrist are both at risk. The grandmother nanny needs to spend a solid half hour on a bike or perhaps walking at a pace that will stimulate her aerobically and strengthen her bones. Any physical activity is better than sitting in a chair all day, but there needs to be activity that counts as exercise and makes a difference in your health. It needs to be a "program" of exercise to which you make a commitment.

Minimize the bone breakdown of menopause by continuing to exercise and by ingesting calcium. Vigorous aerobic weight-bearing exercise, for at least thirty minutes a day, is the minimum recommended by the American College of Sports Medicine. Walking one to two miles daily, in about half an hour, preserves some bones. Walk briskly, as if you were running, swinging your arms, turning the torso, bouncing on your feet. When you run or walk keep your arms loose, unencumbered by bags and packages. Brisk walking does not mean slowing down for window displays. Walking during daylight helps you manufacture vita-min D in your skin that is essential for absorption of calcium from the gut.

The National Council on Women's Health, an organization devoted to education in women's health, is in the process of revising its booklet on additional exercises to prevent osteoporosis. Its phone number is 212-746-6967.

See chapters 5 and 10 for more about exercise programs.

The Critical Lifetime Role of Calcium

The best thing you can do for your daughters and granddaughters is insist that they get enough calcium in their diet or in supplements.

The more bone they build, the higher will be their peak and the more reserve they will possess when their bone mass starts to go down in later years. Peak bone mass is attained in the twenties, and you should enter menopause with the highest peak bone mass to which you are genetically programmed. High calcium intake, especially in adolescence, helps achieve this. Reduced calcium intake aggravates weakness associated with a low peak.

For postmenopausal women and women on estrogen therapy, calcium is not a substitute for estrogen, but taking it can decrease the dose of estrogen necessary to preserve the bone. And five years after menopause, calcium supplement can prevent further bone loss, especially in the hip and radius.

Too much protein can cause calcium to leach from your bones and be excreted in the urine, so decrease the amount of meat in your diet; anything more than the equivalent of one hamburger and one 4 ounce piece of fish a day is too much. Protein means not only red meat but also fowl, fish, eggs and dairy, and vegetable protein. High phosphate such as is contained in soft drinks also prevents calcium absorption.

If you have a predisposition to calcium-containing stones in the urinary tract, supplements can compound this problem. Calcium can also interfere with the absorption of other drugs and minerals, including iron, zinc, fluoride, beta-blockers, and bisphosphonates such as Fosamax. There are some side effects to calcium supplements, especially if more than 1,500 milligrams a day are taken this way. For example, intestinal bloating, gas, and constipation can occur with calcium carbonate. Drinking more fluids might offset this side effect. Some people can tolerate calcium citrate better than calcium carbonate. A new preparation called CCM (calcium citrate malate) is absorbed best.

Vitamin D intake should be about 400–800 international units a day unless you enjoy sunlight frequently. This supplementation is especially necessary in the winter and in the higher latitudes. Vitamin D is needed to absorb calcium in the intestine. Without vitamin D, calcium would be totally excreted in the stool.

Refer to chapter 4 for more complete information about the amounts of calcium needed at various times of life, the best food sources, and how supplements are compounded.

··26··

Protecting Your Digestive System

The digestive system is at our mercy. Some people are born with stronger "constitutions" than others. However, just as the heart is hurt by bad habits such as smoking, a sedentary lifestyle, and poor nutrition, so is the digestive system harmed. And the harm is cumulative as we age. If our diets are high in fat and low in fiber, our gallbladders and colons will eventually rebel and cause us grief.

Everything we eat, drink, or even inhale affects the dynamics of the digestive system. Not only do we get heartburn, bloating, or indigestion, we can get ulcers, gallstones, constipation, colon polyps—or cancer. Most (but not all) of these conditions are caused by eating or drinking the wrong foods and liquids, by not exercising enough, and by not understanding how to prevent problems.

Women and men are afflicted in similar ways, but women are more prone to certain gastrointestinal conditions such as irritable bowel syndrome and gallstones—and for some women, gastroesophageal reflux, a condition in which the stomach acids back up into the esophagus, is often confused with indesgtion or asthma.

Fat will raise the cholesterol in your blood, thus increasing the risk for heart attack and several cancers; but before it even gets to your blood the fat might cause problems. The gallbladder has to process all the fats you eat, and if you overwork that organ, you can develop gallstones.

Fiber in the form of cereals, whole grains, and fresh fruits and vegetables helps flush the fats and waste products from the body with more efficiency. When there is no fiber to transport the waste matter though the colon and out of the body, it stays in the colon, where it contributes to the growth of polyps. These polyps, if undiscovered, can become cancerous. A tendency to constipation might be hereditary, but constipation, more common in women, is frequently caused by lack of fiber as well as by a sedentary lifestyle.

Exercise is critical to bringing oxygen to your digestive system and keeps the process going, especially through the lower intestinal tract.

Smoking increases your risk of stomach cancer and ulcers. These two conditions are especially high in smokers, as are cancers of the entire upper digestive tract. You might think the smoke is going only to your lungs, but it is contaminating the upper part of your digestive tract as well—including your mouth.

Drinking too much alcohol is especially harmful to women because we lack certain stomach enzymes that are required in the conversion of alcohol to less toxic substances. As a result, we get drunk faster. Alcohol is toxic to the stomach lining and other organs, including the liver, where cirrhosis ultimately begins. Excess alcohol is directly responsible for cancer of the esophagus, bleeding of the stomach lining, ulcers, and destruction of the pancreas and liver.

By the time cancer of a digestive organ causes symptoms, it is frequently too late for effective treatment. Tumors in the system are usually slow-growing, solid tumors, and might not be discovered until they have spread outside the digestive tract and caused problems elsewhere.

HOW THE DIGESTIVE SYSTEM WORKS

The digestive tract begins with the mouth and teeth and continues as throat; esophagus; stomach; small intestine, which includes the duodenum, jejunum, and ileum; and ends with the large intestine, known as the colon. The liver, gallbladder, and pancreas are also involved in the process.

Everything we eat consists of water and three main components: carbohydrates, fats, and proteins. Throughout the digestive system, the lining of the digestive tract secretes juices that help break down food into smaller molecules. For the three major components of food to be absorbed through the intestinal tract, the carbohydrate needs to be broken down to simple sugars, mostly glucose. Fats (triglycerides) are molecules composed of three fatty acids anchored to a core of glycerin. When ingested, fats are broken down into their component parts before they can be absorbed. The liver metabolizes these fatty acids and glycerin, then sends them as lipid particles to organs that can burn these high-energy molecules for energy or store them for future needs. Proteins must be broken down into amino acids.

In the mouth, the teeth help break up the food into smaller pieces and the saliva coats the pieces for easier swallowing. Saliva contains a major enzyme called *amylase,* which starts the digestion of starches into

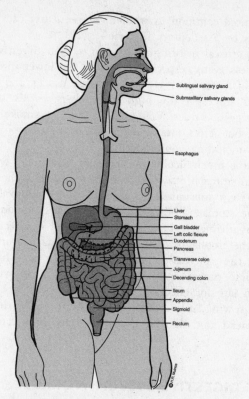

Sublingual salivary gland
Submaxillary salivary glands

Esophagus

Liver
Stomach
Gall bladder
Left colic flexure
Duodenum
Pancreas
Transverse colon
Jujenum
Decending colon
Ileum
Appendix
Sigmoid
Rectum

Figure 24. How the digestive system works.

glucose. The muscles of the throat and esophagus facilitate the swallowing process to propel the food down into the stomach. In the stomach, a very muscular sac, major grinding and milling action takes place, exposing the food contents to another important enzyme, *pepsin,* which breaks up proteins into amino acids. Pepsin does its job best in an acid environment, and the stomach obliges by producing a very powerful acid in its juice.

In the small intestine the basic constituents are absorbed. They pass through the intestinal wall into the surrounding small blood vessels, the capillaries. When they are absorbed into the bloodstream, they are carried to the liver for major restructuring (metabolism) to be apportioned according to the need for fuel and structural repair work. The liver is like a kitchen in this respect. It gathers ingredients, sorts them out, mixes them with homegrown compounds, and sends them out to the body.

By the time the intestinal contents reach the end of the ileum, what remains is water along with nondigestible residues. The most important job now for the colon, or large intestine, is to absorb the excess water and reduce the residue to a small volume to be excreted as stool. The body has developed many mechanisms of conserving water, and the absorptive qualities of the colon are just one.

The colon is the last part of the gastrointestinal or digestive tract. It looks like a large question mark pinned up in place within the abdomen by a ligamentous double sheet called the *mesentery*. The beginning of that question mark, lying in the right lower quadrant of the abdomen, is called the *cecum*. It is into the cecum that the end of the ileum empties. Attached to the lower end of the cecum is a thin, wormlike structure called the *appendix*. The appendix sometimes gets inflamed, causing *appendicitis*, a condition that, before antibiotics became available, was very serious and meant that the appendix needed to be immediately removed surgically. Whereas there is no difference in the incidence of appendicitis in women and men, the diagnosis of appendicitis in women is more complicated because of the proximity of ovaries and Fallopian tubes. It is not unusual to confuse the signs of appendicitis with those of a ruptured ovarian cyst, especially if the appendix happens to be located behind the cecum. This misdiagnosis can be life-threatening if an inflamed appendix ruptures and causes a generalized infection in the abdominal cavity.

The cecum continues up on the right side of the abdomen as the ascending colon. The ascending colon goes up until it reaches the liver and then turns, forming the hepatic flexure, the bend around the liver. After the hepatic flexure, the colon becomes horizontal, going across the abdomen (transverse colon) to the left, turns around the spleen (splenic flexure), descends straight down to the left lower quadrant of the abdomen (the descending colon), makes a few loose loops (sigmoid colon), goes straight down (the rectum), and ends at the anus.

Both the small and large intestines are tubes with at least three layers of muscle that have the ability to contract as necessary. These contractions and relaxations travel like a wave along the intestine, propelling the contents along. This movement through the entire digestive system is called *peristalsis*, and this is what keeps everything moving in the right direction.

While the job of the small intestine is to absorb nutrients from digesting food, the job of the colon is to absorb the water. If the peristalsis is slowed, more water gets absorbed and the stool becomes hard and infrequent, resulting in constipation. If peristalsis is too swift, water is not entirely absorbed and the stool turns to liquid and is more frequent.

Who Takes Care of the Digestive System?

Your principal doctor can diagnose most digestive problems, but you will need to visit a specialist for endoscopic testing and treatment with surgery.

- **A gastroenterologist** is an internist who specializes in diagnosis and treatment of diseases of the digestive system.

- **A colorectal surgeon** is a surgeon with special training in treatment of diseases of the colon, including the rectum and anus.

- **A hepatologist** is an internist who specializes in diseases of the liver—and often has advanced training in gastroenterology as well.

UPPER GI PROBLEMS

We are inundated with commercials on television for remedies for acid indigestion. Think of all those images of people looking pained as they describe the "hard-to-digest" meal they just ate and then running for the remedy. Even worse are the ones that tell you to take the antacid before you overindulge on a high-fat, spicy meal. Many of us use these self-medications indiscriminately, in the wrong amounts, and at the wrong times. Many people also use them instead of improving their diets or visiting their doctors to find out what is really wrong—always a bad idea.

Diagnostic tests for the gastrointestinal system have improved enormously with the widespread use of endoscopic testing. Using flexible fiberoptic tubes, doctors can now literally see inside the digestive tract and take samples of tissue, bacteria, or digestive fluids for pathological study.

With proper diagnostic testing, what is often thought of as routine heartburn might actually be esophageal reflux, or any number of ailments that need to be treated professionally.

Gastroesophageal Reflux Disease (GERD)

The esophagus is a thick ten-inch-long tube connecting the throat with the stomach. It is generally shorter in women than in men regardless of height or weight. It is also the site of the fastest-growing cancer. Until recently, few physicians could diagnose precisely the problems related to this part of the digestive tract. It has been discovered that reflux can be the cause of some symptoms of asthma, laryngitis, and chest pain. It causes special problems to pregnant women and women with scleroderma, a condition that causes skin and fibrous tissue to harden.

Gastroesophageal reflux disease (GERD), or simply "reflux," became one of the hot topics of the medical community in 1997. It is one of the most underdiagnosed and misdiagnosed conditions in existence. Heartburn, a burning sensation in the chest after or during a meal, is a common symptom experienced by people who overindulge in spicy, hot food. But heartburn can also be a symptom of reflux.

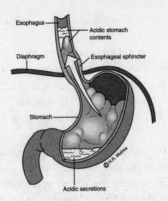

Figure 25. Gastroesophageal reflux.

Reflux is caused by a weakening in the sphincter muscle that separates the stomach from the esophagus. This sphincter's job is to keep everything flowing in one direction. But if it becomes weak, or fails to function, the acid in the stomach refluxes, or washes back up. (It is something like the mitral valve of the heart that allows blood to backflow when it isn't working.) This causes the esophagus to become irritated and inflamed by the stomach acids. Over the long term, this can cause the esophagus to ulcerate, then scar and form a stricture, or become narrow so that swallowing becomes difficult. In rare cases, the cells lining the end of the esophagus can become malignant.

Stomach acid is like battery acid, and it can eat away or actually corrode the inside of your digestive tract. If you put a piece of paper into a container of stomach acid (which is hydrochloric acid), the paper would dissolve. Some of us have more potent stomach acid, and some of us have less durable stomach linings. The digestive system, too, is unique to each of us.

Reflux can be prompted by certain conditions, such as pregnancy, weight gain, straining during a bowel movement, or even wearing clothes that are too tight. As many as 25 percent of pregnant women—but probably closer to 80 percent—are estimated to be bothered by reflux, especially during the late stages of pregnancy. This is not only due to the pressure on the digestive tract because of the enlarging uterus. The excessive estrogen levels can weaken the sphincter muscle between the esophagus and stomach. Caffeine and nicotine can also do this.

Women with scleroderma are also more prone to reflux. In nearly 80 percent of women with scleroderma, the esophageal sphincter becomes weak.

Pain can also occur after you have gone to bed, frequently in your back or neck. When you are lying in bed, the condition can be complicated if the stomach contents back up into the trachea and enter your lungs. This would cause nocturnal asthma or even aspiration pneumonia (see page 457).

Sometimes the reflux is accompanied by a hiatal hernia. Such a hernia is formed when the uppermost portion of the stomach pushes through the diaphragm. The sphincter for the diaphragm and the esophagus are at the same level, so there is added pressure. Hiatal hernia is common in women, especially overweight women and during and after pregnancy.

To determine if the esophagus is strictured or if there is a hiatal hernia, an X ray can be taken of the upper digestive tract. This is known as an upper GI series, for upper gastrointestinal. However, an exam with a fiberoptic endoscope, a flexible tube with a camera on the end, would be needed to see inside the esophagus and stomach to locate inflammation or ulceration of the lining of the esophagus. This way, a biopsy can be done to reveal the extent of the damage and rule out malignant transformation, such as development of cancer.

Sometimes endoscopic procedures can be used to dilate the esophagus if it has narrowed because of stricture. If reflux is not relieved by such adjustments, and if it is causing stricture, bleeding, or respiratory complications, then surgery is called for.

Treatment of Reflux. Reflux can be treated with medications, changes in lifestyle, and sometimes with surgery. Neutralizing the acid is usually the first step, and liquid antacid remedies are better than pills. These can be taken up to an hour after eating. In addition, there are H2 blockers (Tagamet and Zantac, for example) that inhibit acid production and can alleviate some symptoms. There are stronger drugs for more severe cases such as pump inhibitors (Prilosec).

Prevention of Reflux. Eat only three meals a day at fairly consistent times so that you do not overwork your digestive system. The stomach acids are secreted over the three or four hours following a meal. Also, don't eat right before you go to bed. Let at least three or four hours go by between eating and lying down to sleep. Cut way back on fats, since they slow down the digestive process. A high-fat meal stays in the stomach longer and causes more acid to accumulate. That half pint of coffee ice cream is not the wisest bedtime snack! A good diet with low fats, only moderate proteins, and high complex carbohydrates such as fruits and vegetables and cereals, is more easily digested and also relieves constipation (constipation makes reflux worse). Smoking and caffeine should be avoided, too.

Don't wear tight clothing that increases pressure around the abdomen.

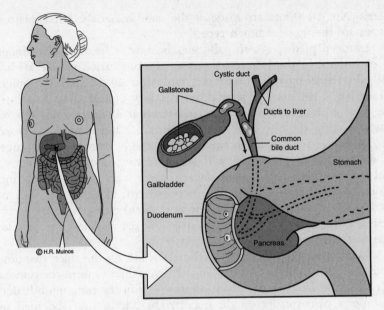

Figure 26. Gallbladder with stones.

The Stone-prone Female Gallbladder

Gallstones are three times more common in women than in men. These stones can be as small as a grain of sand or as big as a golf ball. They are actually little balls of hardened cholesterol that become painful as they attempt to pass through strictured bile ducts. The gallbladder must sometimes be removed surgically. *Cholecystitis* is inflammation of the gallbladder. This is what occurs when the stone or stones get stuck and cause the wall of the gallbladder to become irritated and swollen.

The gallbladder is a small organ shaped like a pear that lies under the liver with just its bottom (fundus) peeking up from underneath the liver on the right side of your abdomen. It is a pantry for the storage of bile, a complex substance produced by the liver. Bile is made of bile acids, cholesterol, and chemicals (including lecithin) that assist with the metabolism of fat. The bile also contains bilirubin and whatever metabolized toxins and drugs are being shed by the body. The gallbladder, much like the sigmoid colon, the part nearest the rectum, removes water from this material. The more water is absorbed, the denser and more concentrated the bile becomes. The slower is the flow of bile, the more water gets absorbed.

When we eat foods containing fat, the gallbladder sends the bile through the cystic duct and the common bile duct into the small intestine in order to digest the fat. Sometimes the bile is so concentrated that the cholesterol or calcium bilirubinate becomes crystallized into stones. Not all stones are made of the same materials, but cholesterol stones are the most common type.

Estrogen predisposes to gallstones because it increases the amount of cholesterol in the bile and decreases the proportion of bile acids in the bile, rendering bile "lithogenic" (stone-prone). In addition, progesterone has a tendency to slow down the flow of bile. Any slowing of the flow is associated with more reabsorption of water from the bile ducts, making the bile even more concentrated and more stone-prone.

Whenever there is an increase in the level of estrogen (and progesterone), such as in pregnancy, with administration of oral contraceptives, and with hormone replacement therapy, there is an increase in the incidence and risk of gallstones. An increased risk of gallstones does not accompany transdermal (through-the-skin patch) estrogen because transdermal estrogen does not reach the liver first the way oral estrogen does (the first liver pass of oral medications).

When a stone gets stuck in the cystic duct—the duct that leads from the gallbladder to join the hepatic (liver) duct to form the common bile duct that lands in the small intestine—or in the common bile duct, it causes a pain you feel in the upper right side of your abdomen and sometimes under the ribs on that side. Frequently the pain radiates through to the back of your torso just under your right shoulder bone. The pain comes from the spasms of the gallbladder trying to rid itself of the stone. This can bring on nausea and vomiting. The severe pain is known as biliary colic, and is sometimes as severe as labor pains.

This condition usually follows a fatty meal, which causes the gallbladder to work overtime. It contracts vigorously to send the stone on its way so it can get on with its current business. If the stone moves through the duct to the intestines, the pain subsides. However, when a stone lodges at the end of a bile duct, the bile cannot pass through from the liver and backs up into the blood. This can cause jaundice, and you will know something is wrong by your yellowish complexion. In addition to the inflamed gallbladder and biliary jaundice, an infection (*cholangitis*) of the entire bile duct system (within the liver, too) can occur, and the pancreas can become inflamed as well.

When the cholecystitis becomes chronic, as it does when women experience many episodes of pain and inflammation, the wall of the gallbladder thickens and it is no longer able to concentrate the bile.

Because the symptoms resemble those of other digestive conditions such as spastic colon, it is necessary to make a careful and thorough evaluation and exclude all other possibilities. The most helpful test is an ultrasound of the abdomen, which will show stones in the gallbladder.

Treatment with Surgery (Cholecystectomy). Some gallstones simply pass through the system and are eliminated, and some can be dissolved with medications, but when this does not work, surgery is the best alternative. Removing the gallbladder, of course, offers a complete cure for gallbladder disease. Such surgery is called *cholecystectomy*. Without a gallbladder, the liver keeps working and producing bile but bile is not concentrated. This means it is absolutely essential to stay on a low-fat diet, because the capacity of the liver to produce an adequate amount of bile on sudden demand is limited. The surgery is far from simple. There are many possible complications, including bile peritonitis, scarring of the common bile duct, and the dreaded cholangitis, an infection and inflammation of the biliary tree, which is the system of connecting ducts involving the liver, gallbladder, and small intestine.

The standard, open abdominal procedure, is major surgery requiring a couple of months of recovery. The advantage of traditional surgery is that the surgeon can explore the area to be sure that all stones are removed from the bile duct area.

A newer technique is laparoscopic surgery, which introduces surgical instruments into the abdomen through several small incisions. Recovery is much quicker. This surgery is best if the case is uncomplicated by scarring of the gallbladder, and should be done only by a surgeon with a great deal of experience in the procedure. Laparoscopic surgery might also turn into standard surgery at any time during the procedure if the surgeon observes that the condition is more complicated than first determined.

Since 1990, when the first laparoscopic surgery was done for gallstones, it has become the most common way—90 percent—to remove the gallbladder. While it seems to be the current gold standard for cholecystectomies, critics believe it has also become responsible for many unnecessary surgeries. Since that time the number of cholecystectomies in the United States has risen by more than 40 percent in some areas of the country. While it is a fairly safe surgery, the potential for fatal complications is three times higher than with the conventional surgery.

Treatment with Medication. The medical treatment of gallstones consists of dissolving the crystallized cholesterol stone with a medication that changes the chemical balance of the bile. If the stones can be dissolved this way, medication might be continued to prevent formation of new stones. Normally, this type of treatment works only when the disease is not extensive.

The Smaller Female Liver

As I mentioned before, the liver is like a kitchen. It has hundreds of separate functions that revolve around assimilating all the foods and nutrients, separating them, storing them, detoxifying harmful substances, and producing important chemicals to add to some of the foods it receives before dispersing them to other parts of the body. The chemicals it produces include bile, proteins for the blood, clotting components, and urea.

The liver can also regenerate itself, so that if part of it is injured, more new tissue will replace it. It can, however, be harmed by toxins and viruses. Long-term use of certain medications for high cholesterol, seizures, or blood pressure can become toxic to the liver, so periodic tests are needed to measure levels of these drugs in the blood. Toxins found in the workplace can also be harmful to the liver. These include cleaning fluids such as carbon tetrachloride when inhaled in sufficient amounts. Also PVCs (polyvinyl chloride), which is used to manufacture plastics. If you work where these chemicals are used, check the safety regulations at the workplace to be sure proper safeguards are in place to protect your health.

Liver disease is essentially the same in both men and women, but women are more prone to lupoid hepatitis, a chronic autoimmune condition.

Postmenopausal women are susceptible to hemochromatosis, an inherited disease that causes iron to accumulate in the liver, pancreas, skin, heart, and other organs. It is caused by the intestine's inability to regulate the amount of iron absorbed from foods. Menstrual blood flow protects younger women because the excess iron leaves the body with the blood. Hemochromatosis is controlled by periodically removing the blood (*phlebotomy*) in order to maintain less toxic levels of iron.

Hepatitis, or inflammation of the liver, happens when the cells of the liver break down. This most common liver disease is caused by viruses, but alcohol and drugs can also cause it. It can be chronic at a low level for long periods, or it can appear as a severe attack. Untreated, some forms of hepatitis will eventually lead to cirrhosis. There are several types of hepatitis—labeled A, B, C, D, and E. Hepatitis A is caused by contaminated food or water and does not lead to chronic disease. Hepatitis B is transmitted sexually, by sharing contaminated needles in drug use, and vertically to the fetus in pregnancy (see chapter 11). Hepatitis C has recently been recognized as the most common cause of liver failure. Hepatitis D, or Delta, is more rare, caused by a virus that strikes only in the presence of hepatitis B. The hepatitis E virus infection is rare in this country, but is more common in Asia, particularly India. It has extremely devastating effects on pregnant women.

Because a female's liver is smaller than a male's, it is less capable than a man's of metabolizing alcohol. In addition, women have diminished quantities of a stomach enzyme called *aldehyde dehydrogenase,* which breaks down alcohol. The alcohol is dissipated in women more slowly, therefore, and the same quantity persists in the blood for a longer period of time. More than one drink a day in a woman can be conducive to cirrhosis. In men, the minimal dose for cirrhosis is two drinks.

Primary Biliary Cirrhosis. This is primarily a woman's disease—90 percent of sufferers are women—and begins between the ages of 40 and 60. Most common in women of middle age. This condition destroys the small bile ducts and is thought to be an autoimmune disorder. The symptoms are severe itching on skin all over the body because the excretion of bile acids is faulty. It is complicated by the blockage of bile flow. Scars form in the liver, and eventually cirrhosis with liver failure sets in.

Cancer of the Liver. There are two kinds of liver cancer: primary and metastatic. Primary liver cancer means the cancer starts in the liver cells. This cancer is the leading cause of death in Africa and Asia. In the United States, it is much less common, but where it does exist, it is two thirds more common in men as in women. Primary liver cancer is usually found in people with chronic viral hepatitis (especially types B, C, and E), or alcoholics. In Asia, primary liver cancer is caused by a chronic hepatitis virus that is transmitted "vertically" from the mother to the baby through the placenta or through contamination with maternal blood during delivery.

Metastatic liver cancer is the most common form in this country. This is a cancer that originated elsewhere, such as in the breast, and then spread to other organs, including the liver.

Treatment for Liver Disease. Any damage to the liver is serious. The degree of damage can be determined by a liver biopsy. This is an office surgery by a physician who can insert a needle into your liver and bring out a piece of tissue to be examined by a pathologist. The biopsy is quite painless and safe.

Depending upon what the pathologist finds, the condition can be diagnosed and treatment planned. The toxic or benign conditions can sometimes be treated by avoiding the offending toxins, such as alcohol, but most serious conditions can only be fixed by removing the liver. Since we cannot live without our liver, this means transplant is the only hope. Cancer of the liver has been treated with chemotherapy, which can slow the disease, but rarely cures it.

LOWER GI PROBLEMS

Anytime a woman has pain or bloating in the lower abdomen, or below the waist, we must consider symptoms not only of the digestive system but also of the nearby reproductive system. Pain and bloating, for example, could be symptoms of problems in the ovaries as well as irritable bowel syndrome. A physical examination for such symptoms should always include a pelvic exam.

The lower gastrointestinal system problems include constipation and diarrhea, gas, and bloating. Chronic problems can lead to colitis, diverticulosis, polyps, and cancer.

Constipation

Women are twice as likely to use over-the-counter laxatives, have less bulky stools than men, and in general suffer more from constipation. The hormone progesterone might be partially responsible. It has been shown to delay the emptying of the gallbladder, but studies are not definitive on this. In a clinical study of chronic constipation, women's stools were softer just before and during menstruation, when more prostaglandins are present. A woman's colon responds to dietary fiber differently than a man's colon, but so far no definitive studies have added to this insight.

Diet and exercise, and drinking plenty of water, are key elements in preventing constipation. Once it is present, your doctor might prescribe stool softeners. However, over the long term, such use will not promote health. Good nutrition, with lots of fresh fruits and vegetables, is important to aid the transit of digested material from the body. As are plenty of fluids.

Irritable Bowel Syndrome (IBS)

This condition is called spastic colon, mucous colitis, irritable colon, functional bowel disease, or even, incorrectly, nervous stomach. There is an abnormality in the contractions of the muscle layers of the colon. The peristaltic wave might be too slow or too fast. Or a disorderly function might result in simultaneous contraction of one layer of muscles on top of the other within the same segment, resulting in abdominal pain. The spastic colon is twice as prevalent in women of all ages than in men. This might be because women are more likely than men to seek medical treatment.

Women with IBS rarely enjoy going out to dinner, rarely go anywhere they cannot be sure of access to a suitable rest room. The manifestations of spastic colon are intermittent or persistent diarrhea, intermittent or persistent constipation, and alternating constipation and diarrhea, with or without abdominal cramping, pain, gas, and bloating.

For the most part, IBS is a benign condition that comes and goes. A person might associate episodes of spastic colon with unusual food; spicy, hot, or very cold food; and with times of emotional stress and depression. Typically, the symptoms occur after a meal and are relieved by a bowel movement.

Estelle's face betrayed anxiety and pain when she came to see me. Estelle is a former model, rail-thin, who now works in the catering business. Her two children are in college, and Estelle and her husband entertain a great deal. At 50, Estelle believes she is paying the price for all those gourmet meals she prepared and, alas, eats!

"What hurts?" I asked.

"The cramps in my stomach," she said, grimacing in pain. "They come and go, but boy, when they come, I could scream in pain." Estelle told me she woke up in the middle of the night with cramps and nausea. When she tried to move her bowels, she only passed gas, which gave her some relief, but not much.

The previous evening's meal did not appear to be the problem— chicken breast braised in wine, an arugula salad with vinaigrette, and some grilled zucchini and potatoes. Her husband had eaten the same food, and he had not gotten sick. Estelle's history revealed that she had had similar episodes in the past, usually at times of great stress or anxiety, but never this bad.

While she was on the examining table, she moaned and brought her knees up to her chest as a spasm overwhelmed her. I pushed on her belly, and it was soft. There was no "guarding," an involuntary tightening of the muscles. There was some tenderness on the left side. Listening for bowel sounds with the stethoscope, I heard a normal pitch. A pelvic exam confirmed that her ovaries and uterus were normal.

I suspected irritable bowel syndrome, but this diagnosis can be made only by eliminating all possible causes of the pain: appendicitis, ruptured ovarian cyst, gallbladder inflammation, gallstone, or kidney stone. Intermittent episodes of abdominal pain and diarrhea would make me suspect this, but her abdomen is completely flat and nontender between spasms. Besides, Crohn's disease usually starts causing symptoms at a young age. Everything pointed to a problem with the colon. It is unlikely she had ulcerative colitis because there was no rectal bleeding. Cancer of the colon was unlikely at her age, but we could not rule that out. We ordered a colonoscopy to see inside the sigmoid colon, and a Hemoccult to check for hidden blood in the stool. The colonoscopy showed no polyps or other problems, and it was likely she had an irritable colon. Lactose intolerance is often mistaken for the irritable bowel syndrome, but I knew Estelle did not have this condition.

Normally, the lining of the large intestine secretes mucus that facilitates smooth passage of the fecal matter. In IBS, there is an excess of mucus, resulting in some mucus appearing on top of the stool, or even alone. This is why the condition is sometimes called mucous colitis.

A full clinical evaluation includes a complete blood count and chemistry profile. Urine and stool analyses to check for infection. Flexible colonoscopy to rule out mucosal disease of the bowel.

Treatment of IBS is primarily prevention, and treating the symptoms. Constipation is prevented by an increase of fiber foods such as fruits, vegetables, and whole-grain breads and cereals in the diet. Bulk-type fiber-substitute laxatives and stool softeners are sometimes helpful.

Diarrhea is prevented by avoiding hot, spicy foods or ice-cold foods, excessive amounts of alcohol, and other irritants.

Abdominal discomfort is relieved by rest, applying a hot water bottle to the abdomen, or by moving the bowels. Some medications will release the spasm of the bowel muscles and bring relief. Muscle relaxants and antidepressants can also help symptoms. Hypnotherapy has been used successfully in the psychiatric approach to treatment.

Estelle's acute episode passed with a heating pad to the abdomen and a diet that gradually progressed from nothing by mouth for several hours to juices, gelatin, and applesauce, to a full diet eventually with plenty of fiber but less spicy and salty foods. For the future, Estelle learned how to control her symptoms. With a better diet and a daily workout, she has avoided the gastronomic indiscretion so common in her occupation.

Recently a correlation has been established between the irritable colon syndrome and a history of sexual abuse in children.

Diverticulitis

In some women, IBS is complicated by the presence of diverticula. These pockets or pouches develop in the wall of the colon and protrude outward into the abdominal cavity. The diverticula form when there is high pressure within the segment of colon, and the high pressure pushes the lining through a weak spot (where blood vessels penetrate the muscular coat) to form a pocket. Diverticulosis is the presence of diverticula, and diverticulitis is the inflammation of these diverticula. Most of these pockets appear in the sigmoid colon. A diminishing number appear in the descending, transverse, and ascending colon. Diverticulosis is associated with the high-fat, low-fiber diets found in Western industrialized nations.

Diverticula are more common in women, and especially in older women, who are at greatest risk after 65. Women more often have diverticula on the left side (sigmoid colon area), have more of them, and have more severe pain.

Most people who have diverticula have no symptoms whatsoever. Others might have pain, usually on the lower left side of the abdomen. If diverticula are inflamed, they can cause fever, nausea, vomiting, and occasional rectal bleeding. Diagnosis is made with endoscopic testing.

Treatment consists of a high-fiber diet to restore a normal muscular function of the colon. Treatment of an acute attack of diverticulitis is usually conservative. Rest the colon by not eating and forcing it to work. Intravenous feeding and antibiotics are usually prescribed. A neglected diverticulitis may result in the formation of an abscess or perforation of the colon. In such cases, surgery might be needed to cut out the involved section of colon and sew the healthy sections together. Once healed, the shortened colon adapts and the digestive process goes back to normal.

Inflammatory Bowel Disease (IBD)

The first time inflammatory bowel disease occurs it can seem like a stomach virus that brings on diarrhea, fever, or abdominal pain. The two major forms of this disease are ulcerative colitis and Crohn's disease. Inflammatory bowel disease (IBD) is characterized by periodic inflammation of both the small and large intestine, or only the large intestine. About half a million people in the United States suffer from this, and a large portion of them are women. There is no cure, and no way to prevent it has been discovered. It is interesting, however, that the disease is more common in countries that are economically developed. The first attack usually comes between the ages of 15 and 40.

Diagnosis of Crohn's disease is difficult because the symptoms mimic other conditions—such as irritable bowel syndrome, a more common but less serious ailment. Bacterial infections are also suspected, such as salmonella, which comes from food such as spoiled eggs that are contaminated with the bacteria. Stool culture can identify these.

With endoscopic testing, the inside of the colon can be observed. Ulcerative colitis is inflamed tissue in the rectum and sigmoid colon, but does not usually involve the small intestine. The disease usually affects only the innermost layer or mucosa of the colon.

Crohn's disease looks a bit different, with patches of diseased tissue adjacent to normal tissue. With this disease, damage extends into the walls of both the large and small intestine.

Inflammatory bowel disease seems to run in families, because from 10 to 25 percent of the patients have a relative with Crohn's or ulcerative colitis. British researchers found that families with two or more siblings with IBD were more likely to have certain common genes that play a key role in the immune system. Other researchers believe a trigger is a reaction to an environmental assault by bacteria or a virus.

The immune response system has been studied. When the lining of the intestine is hurt by bacteria or bits of food, this can provoke an immune response. But for some reason the wrong rescue team comes to the call for help. Suppressor T cells, which inhibit inflammation, are supposed to come, but instead the T-helper cells arrive and promote the inflammation and weaken bowel walls.

The symptoms can be treated, however, and recent advances have improved the lives of many people with IBD. Therapy can reduce inflammation and, in many people, bring on remission. Steroid suppositories treat inflammation directly if only the colon is affected. When disease is farther away from the anal opening, oral medications are necessary. Steroids, such as prednisone, can be used for a month or two to induce remission, but longer use can cause dependency, osteoporosis, hypertension, diabetes, and cataracts, all more common in women in the first place.

Inflammatory bowel disease can also be treated with drugs to modulate the immune system.

There is no particular diet that has been proven effective in preventing or treating IBD, but mild symptoms can be controlled by avoiding foods that cause diarrhea, such as spicy foods, ice-cold foods, and excessive alcohol.

When all else fails, surgery is the treatment of last resort, and is the only way the disease can actually be cured. About 25 percent of people with ulcerative colitis have their entire large intestine removed. A colostomy is generally required. This is rerouting the intestines so that waste is excreted outside of the body into a pouch. There are more sophisticated surgical techniques now so that it is possible to rebuild the intestinal tract in such a way that fecal matter can be rerouted but still excreted through the anus.

Colon Cancer

Colon cancer is another preventable disease that kills men and women equally, but is more often overlooked in women. At age 50 everyone should begin screening for this disease with annual digital rectal exams, Hemoccult tests for hidden blood, and a colonoscopy to examine the inside of the colon endoscopically. While there is a strong genetic component in this disease, it is primarily a disease of age. The longer your colon is used and abused, the more likely polyps will form. The polyps can be benign, but if they stay in the colon long enough they will eventually become cancer.

Although the cause of colon cancer is unknown, epidemiological studies point to high-fat, low-fiber diet as a possible inciting agent. It has also been discovered that the use of aspirin, NSAIDs (non-steroidal anti-inflammatory drugs), folic acid, and estrogen are each associated with a decrease in incidence of colon cancer, especially the large-size tumors. It is not known if that benefit is independent or due to better health care and monitoring of the persons who take these substances.

The symptoms of colon cancer depend on its location: cancer on the left side (descending colon, the sigmoid, and the rectum) might cause blockage of the stool, obstruction, and abdominal pain; cancer of the right-sided colon (cecum, ascending colon, and transverse colon) does not usually cause symptoms until it is well advanced or has spread to other organs. The only way the right-sided colon cancer can be detected early enough for cure is through periodic Hemoccult—testing of stool for hidden blood—and periodic colonoscopy.

At all ages, women have a higher incidence of colon polyps and cancer in the right side, usually in the cecum rather than the left side where the sigmoid colon leads into the rectum. Sigmoidoscopy (examination of the rectum and sigmoid through a long tube with a light at the end that is inserted through the rectum), recommended for screening of men, is of no value to women, who should be examined through colonoscopy that visualizes the entire colon all the way to the cecum.

Charlotte, 60, was a neighbor in the rural town where we have our family farm. I often saw her when I went into the village to buy fresh vegetables from the farmer's market where she worked. She had not been feeling well, she told me, when I asked after her health. She did indeed look haggard, but her local family doctor told her she was fine, just getting older. This was the doctor who delivered her daughter forty years earlier.

I asked Charlotte a few questions to find out how thorough her doctor's examination had been. I urged her to get some diagnostic testing done, and she said her doctor had found anemia but said it was okay at her age. My look of shock must have frightened her, because she then nervously asked me if she could make an appointment with me for the following week. She was coming to the city to visit her granddaughter. I urged her to call my office. I suspected Charlotte might have felt ill at ease talking about her personal health with her male doctor, especially since he seemed to have some old-fashioned ideas about aging. (Many such doctors consider any woman past middle age as having mostly psychosomatic problems.)

When she came in for her visit, Charlotte said she had lost about five pounds recently, but she had been worried about her teenage granddaughter, who wanted to drop out of college.

"Of course, I don't do as much as I did when I was younger, but as my doctor said, old age is not a time of glory."

"When did he say that?" I asked, beginning to suspect this doctor of being a little lazy at best and incompetent at worst. "How much of a workup did he give you?" She told me he examined her and drew some blood. "I have always been slightly anemic," she said, "so the blood results just confirmed that." Slight anemia in a menstruating woman might be okay during menses, but in a 60-year-old woman it warrants further investigation.

Taking Charlotte's history was difficult because she trivialized everything that might be a clue.

"Headaches?" I asked.

"Oh, sure, once in a while," Charlotte said. "I take an aspirin and they go away."

"Stomachaches?"

"Yes, doesn't everybody? Especially after a big meal," Charlotte replied. "The doctor said I had a nervous stomach, so I have to watch what I eat."

"Did he give you a gastrointestinal workup? A colonoscopy? A sigmoidoscopy? A barium enema?" I persisted.

Charlotte told me, "The barium showed nothing two years ago, and I really do not want to go through that uncomfortable test again. I refused to take it this time. Besides, I have normal bowel movements, no bleeding, so what could that prove?"

Obviously, her doctor did not explain very much to Charlotte. He did give her a digital rectal exam and Hemoccult to test for hidden blood. He found a trace of blood, which he said was due to hemorrhoids. The more I listened, the angrier I got. Even though it is common to make such a mistake, one must not assume that the blood is coming from hemorrhoids rather than from a smaller, possibly malignant abnormality farther up the colon. "That trace of blood," I explained to Charlotte, "could indicate a lesion in your intestine. Possibly a polyp that is bleeding. It could be benign or malignant, but we can't know that unless we see it and have it biopsied."

"Not another barium enema," she said nervously.

"No, I would recommend a colonoscopy. This endoscopic tool can bend around all the curves and examine the entire length of colon." I explained that the procedure was painless, that she would get a sedative so she would relax, and that it would be over before she knew it.

"You mean they stick a tube all the way up there?" She had a look or horror and embarrassment on her face that made me smile. "What if I refuse?" she asked. I assured her that she would probably continue to feel weak and tired, lose weight, bleed from the rectum, and would not know the true cause of her discomfort. "If it is a malignant polyp, it could grow into a cancer and kill you." I hoped my bluntness would compel her to let go of her old-fashioned doctor and his techniques. "I should think you would want to be around to watch your granddaughter graduate from college," I said. She did not respond, so I continued to explain.

"The preparations are more uncomfortable than the procedure itself. You have to drink a great deal of a liquid preparation that will cause your bowels to empty entirely, and this means for a few hours you will be in or near the bathroom. An intravenous medication will relax you during the procedure, which takes about thirty to forty minutes, but leaves you fairly alert if you want to watch. You remain in the recovery room until the medication wears off, then you can go home with your daughter. If they find a polyp it can be removed then and there. If it is a large one, then you would need colorectal surgery to remove it."

As it turned out, Charlotte had a medium-size polyp in the transverse colon, halfway between the liver and the spleen. Her preop workup, including cardiac tests, showed she was in good condition to survive surgery. X rays and CT scan indicated no spread of cancer. Her tumor was removed using laparoscopy. The tumor was cancerous but it had not spread to the surrounding tissues, to regional lymph nodes, or to the liver. Biopsies of all questionable tissues revealed no invasion. Laparoscopic surgery uses a tube to visualize the inside of the abdomen. Operative instruments can be inserted through the tube to enable the surgeon to cut, sew, and perform any number of procedures. It can be used for uncomplicated removal of an appendix or an inflamed gallbladder. However, if Charlotte's cancer had spread to the lymph nodes or liver, a laparoscopic technique would not have been sufficient. Open abdominal surgery would have been needed, to be followed with a course of chemotherapy. Had she not had the surgery done, the tumor would gradually grow and encircle the colon, eventually causing intestinal obstruction.

SCREENING AND DIAGNOSING DIGESTIVE DISORDERS

Beginning at the age of 50, everybody should have periodic endoscopic screening for cancers in lower digestive tract. This way, a telescopic tool with a tiny camera can search out and identify any tumors or other abnormalities. Regular blood tests can identify possible cancers of the liver and pancreas, although malignancies of these organs are usually advanced by the time they are detected. A fecal occult blood test should be a routine part of annual physical checkups. This is a simple way to determine if there is any hidden blood in the stool. Blood that could be caused by a bleeding ulcer or a bleeding colon polyp. These conditions can be cured if diagnosed early.

Because symptoms are similar for a variety of gastroenterological conditions, most diagnosis must be made through a process of excluding all possibilities. A physical examination including an abdominal and rectal check—and a pelvic exam for women—is needed, as well as a detailed history of symptoms and lifestyle.

If no cause is found, then diagnostic colonoscopy should be done. Since the 1970s, it has become much easier to look inside the digestive system and find out what exactly is wrong. Endoscopic procedures are usually more expensive than regular X rays, but they are the most effective. In the past (and still today) barium enemas were given before an X-ray examination to look inside the abdomen. Endoscopy is much more efficient. Such tests should be done only by a gastroenterologist-endoscopist, and they should be done where there is access to the most up-to-date equipment.

Esophagogastroduodenoscopy (EGD)
This is an upper GI endoscopy that provides a thorough examination of the esophagus, stomach, and duodenum.

Before the procedure it is necessary to fast so there is no food in your esophagus or stomach. The back of your throat is numbed by a local anesthetic, and a sedative will relax you.

Endoscopic Retrograde Cholangiopancreatography (ERCP)

This is a combination of endoscopy and radiography that allows visualization of the ductal pattern from the liver and pancreas, and changes caused by inflammation or tumors. The ERCP is a good way to locate stones, which can be removed in the same process. Tubes can be inserted to bypass any blockages of ducts caused by tumors or stones.

Sigmoidoscopy

This is an examination of the sigmoid colon, the largest part of the large intestine, which is where the majority of polyps and colorectal cancers originate in men. The flexible endoscopic tube has a light and a camera that enable the physician (and you can watch on a video monitor) to see the inside of the sigmoid colon.

Since cancer of the colon usually affects the right side of the colon in women, screening with sigmoidoscopy is ineffectual for them. Sigmoidoscopy is useful only for the left-sided surveillance, and might *not* be the most effective test for women (see below).

Colonoscopy

The colonoscopy allows us to examine the entire length of the colon, and it takes more time. (This is how we examined Charlotte.) If a polyp or other condition is found through a sigmoidoscopy (described above), then a colonoscopy would usually be called for to examine the rest of the colon. People at high risk for cancer would get a colonoscopy rather than a sigmoidoscopy. Once an endoscopic exam has been decided on for a woman, a full colonoscopy should be done. If a polyp is discovered during a colonoscopy, it can be removed right then and sent to a pathologist for examination. Some polyps become malignant if allowed to remain in the colon.

A colonoscopy can be done with a flexible tube without benefit of a video monitor. Some practitioners still use the older method, which allows them to look through the tube and "eyeball" what's inside the colon. However, when the procedure is monitored on a video, more than one doctor can look at the pictures—and so can you. Without this, you will not have photocopies to take around for another opinion.

Prior to this procedure, the colon is cleansed with special laxatives prescribed by the gastroenterologist, and a mild sedative is given before the procedure. The procedure takes a half hour or more if a biopsy is being performed, or a polyp removed, or blood vessels cauterized.

Abdominal X ray

This is helpful in ruling out free air within the abdominal cavity, which shows up just under the diaphragm and, if present, could indicate a ruptured bowel or appendix. The air pattern within the intestinal tract is useful in diagnosis. Usually air is seen in the loops of the large intestine. When air is prominent in the small intestine or the stomach, intestinal obstruction is likely. Occasionally a kidney stone or a gallstone can be visualized on X ray.

PHASE IV

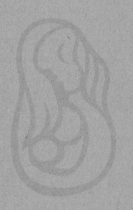

THE POSTMENOPAUSAL YEARS

AGES 65 AND UP

····

INTRODUCTION:
POSTMENOPAUSAL ZEST

This is the time of your life when you are free to just be. No more
kids at home, no more menstruation, and for some, no more of the
nine-to-five grind. This is also the time when your past catches up
with you. If you ignored your health, you might have more chronic
conditions to manage in these postmenopausal years.

In the twenty-first century, the number of people over 65 will
far surpass the number under 65. We are living longer because we
have been able to cure and treat many diseases that killed us in the
past. Contributing factors in the passing century were changes in
public health and hygiene such as sterilization of food, washing hands,
keeping flies away from food, cleaner drinking water, and keeping
sick patients isolated.

We live longer than men. And because we live longer, we are
the "pioneers" when it comes to chronic conditions of old age. Many
of these conditions are not fatal, but unless controlled, they can
detract from the quality of life. A 1993 survey by the Commonwealth
Fund Commission on Women's Health found that 31 percent of
women between the ages of 65 and 85 had one chronic condition,
27 percent had two, and 24 percent had three or more. Only 18
percent had none. Many of the debilitating conditions that afflict
mature women get little research attention because of the double
whammy of ageism and sexism.

The Center for Demographic Studies at Duke University periodically samples 20,000 older Americans. They have noted a 15 percent
drop from 1982 to 1994 in chronic disability rates in people over
65. This is measured against the ability to take care of oneself, such
as eating and getting dressed. The center attributes this to smarter
living by more Americans, rather than to better medical care. There
has been more awareness about nutrition, the dangers of smoking

and alcohol use, and the importance of exercise. A headline in the *New York Times* grabbed my attention in the spring of 1997. It read ACTING THEIR ATTITUDE, NOT THEIR AGE. This was a report about how older Americans are continuing to enjoy the physical pursuits of their younger years. The Duke University Center recently began tracking more rigorous activities like tennis, marathon running, and cycling in mature Americans.

Ironically, more people today believe they are in better shape at an older age than they ever were in their younger years. The Harvard Nurses Health Study, completed in the 1990s, showed that low-fat diets, regular exercise, and low body weight in relation to height favor longevity. But such women are not yet the norm in this country. The National Health and Nutrition Examination Survey indicated the average woman eats more fat, gets less exercise, and has a higher body mass index than those who live the longest. Obese women, in fact, rarely live to be old. As a result, when we compare a normal 60-year-old to a 40-year-old or 20-year-old, we are observing not only the effects of aging but also the effects of twenty to forty years of excess dietary fat, extra poundage, and inactivity.

We don't know all the reasons why women live longer than men. Is it because we take better care of our health? Or is it because men have only one X chromosome while we have two? The Y chromosome, found only in men, is smaller and contains less DNA information than the X. Does the Y chromosome trigger early death? Men also have no estrogen to protect them from early death from heart disease and other conditions. Still, more male embryos and fetuses die in utero, and more boys die in early childhood—well before estrogen is supposed to exert its lifesaving effect.

An oxygen-burning machine, the human body is in a long-term war against oxidation. As we age, we gradually start losing battles, but the rate at which we lose them is determined by genetic and environmental factors. While even good health care, diet, and exercise will not prevent death, they will certainly make the life we have left worth living. As the infirmities of age creep in, we adjust and adapt and keep the machine going. Any kind of machinery will rust and break down if it is not used.

All of our systems suffer some deterioration, some more than others.

• The skin becomes thinner and less firmly attached, so we lose elasticity. In other words, our body suit begins to loosen and is more easily damaged. Loss of pigment-producing cells makes us more vulnerable to ultraviolet radiation, skin infections, and burns.

• Blood vessels, too, become less elastic, and more like metal tubes than rubber tubes. They cannot accommodate to changes in blood volume, so when it increases, blood pressure rises. The heart has to work harder if arteries are clogged or there is hypertension. There is a limit to the adaptability of the heart muscle. If it dilates it uses oxygen inefficiently, fails to propel blood to the body, and eventually fails.

• By the age of 75, we have about 70 percent of our maximum lung capacity and function. We lose some of the elastic fibers that keep bronchioles open, oxygen does not diffuse as well, so less oxygen gets circulated. (This effect is worse if you smoke or have smoked.) We are more susceptible to respiratory infections. Aerobic exercise helps keep lungs in good condition.

• The thymus, a small gland in the neck that is responsible for the T cells that coordinate the immune system, degenerates with age and the immune capability loses its edge. So do the B cells, derived from the bone marrow, and thus the defensive army weakens and invaders can get in more easily. Flu shots are more important after 65 because the immune system is not as strong as it once was. We need flu shots, pneumococcus vaccine, and a tetanus-diphtheria booster. The good news is that we are not bothered as much by allergies because our hyperactive T cells have calmed down.

• Although we lose bone density, muscle fibers, and nerves, exercise keeps the musculoskeletal system performing. However, arthritis and other mobility disabilities are a common condition of advanced age.

• Reduction in bladder capacity means we urinate more frequently, and we need to get up more often at night because of this.

• While most of our hormone levels are diminishing with age, endorphin levels rise with age, and so we are less sensitive to pain.

• Sexual response might taper off slightly. It might take five minutes rather than five seconds to lubricate, but clitoral response is the same. The duration of orgasm might decline from eight to twelve contractions to four to five after age 50. There is no decline in arousability and often there is an increase. Women can have multiple orgasms well into their eighties, which few men can do at any age.

• The gastrointestinal tract is least affected by aging if we eat well and exercise. While intestines and organs lose some tone with age, they still perform as well as in youth. Production of some of the enzymes declines, constipation is more common, and calcium might not be absorbed as well. The gallbladder releases less bile to the intestine, allowing more time for gallstones to develop. The liver shrinks a bit, so it takes more time to process drugs and alcohol, but most elderly people consume less alcohol anyway.

• The sensory organs are the hardest hit by aging. Nerve cells in the ear that conduct sound signals to the brain atrophy, resulting in hearing loss, especially for high-pitched sounds. Our ability to switch our vision from far to near diminishes. We have fewer taste buds, and subtle scents are not distinguished as well. Getting regular vision and hearing checkups, and the use of eyeglasses and possibly a hearing aid, can keep you as sharp as ever. Loss of nerve cells from the cerebellum, the organ of balance situated in the back of the rest of the brain, is responsible for more frequent falls among the elderly; and so is the general slowing of reflexes.

• Brain cell loss is actually not as severe as was once thought. Evidence shows that if the brain is stimulated, the cells remain healthy. Think of all the creative minds that kept right on going into their eighties and nineties. Verdi continued to compose, Picasso continued to paint, and Agnes deMille choreographed after a stroke and worked until her death at 90. Dr. Connie Guion, the famous physician at the New York Hospital–Cornell Medical Center, attended to her patients into her eighties, even making house calls. Dr. Estelle Ramey, a Georgetown professor emeritus of physiology, is still breaking up audiences with her wit, perfect memory, and scientific insight as she nears the age of 90.

The cause of infirmity in old age is often not the body—that frequently can be fixed—but the mind that lacks information and has been conditioned by ageism and sexism in our society to believe that it must deteriorate at a certain age. Two obvious reasons are the fact that medical insurance does not cover much of the care needed for disability, and the fact that many women are often overmedicated.

See your doctor regularly during this time—at least annually, and more often if necessary—and do your best to be a good partner in your health care. Especially important is to keep tabs on your blood pressure and cholesterol. Blood pressure should be checked at every visit, and cholesterol every three to five years. Get annual mammograms, pelvic exams, and Pap smears. Surprisingly, many women over 65 fail to do this. Pap smears perhaps can be done every three years if they have always been normal, but talk with your doctors in case you have any particular health screening needs. Continue to monitor for sexually transmitted infection, since with a weakened immune system you might be more vulnerable. The number of older women being diagnosed with AIDS has increased in recent years. This could be partly because doctors who assumed these women were not sexually active didn't bother to screen for STIs.

The following chapters examine the conditions that most often occur during this phase of our lives and talk about how to prevent or cope with them. They are disorders of mobility, risks of hypertension and stroke, respiratory infections, urinary disorders, and diminished vision and hearing.

So while we all depend on our doctor and pharmacist to treat our medical conditions and to try to replace the hormones that keep us young, we frequently forget that a good lifestyle will protect us as well. And it is never too late to start. Use sunscreen and sunglasses. Eat well-balanced and nutritious meals that contain plenty of natural nutrients and vitamins such as E, C, and B complex. Don't forget the calcium. And exercise, exercise, exercise. This increases lung capacity, builds muscle and bone, conditions the heart and blood vessels, and brightens your outlook on life.

Most important of all, try to remain fully engaged in the passion of life, developing that "postmenopausal zest" we hear so much about, using old skills or developing new ones. Many women find these years the time to give something back to society. They become mentors to young women or provide financial or social support for children, the arts, and education. Women who love to read can teach literacy or read to hospital patients. I had a patient who was a teacher, and when she retired, she taught children in the hospital who stayed there for a long time. The children loved her—she taught them to use their minds and imaginations. There are organizations of retired executives who lend their expertise to businesses and workers in all fields. Shed your fear of computers. Learn something new every day.

Empowerment of the old is important. Women should wear their years as a badge of honor.

··27··

Mobility: Keeping the Body in Motion

I recently saw a cartoon in the *New Yorker* magazine that made me laugh. Three elderly ladies are sitting in a room. One of the women has a look of exhaustion on her face. Another woman remarks to her companion: "She's waiting for menopausal zest to set in."

Many of the women I have seen in my long practice do develop this zest in their lives as they age. They are out and about, fully engaged in life, and physically active. Women who do not have this zest are the ones with multiple chronic conditions resulting from failure in earlier years to nurture their own good health. These women, physically and mentally "retired" from life, are simply waiting to die.

Rebecca, 75, is one of these. She is always in pain and has such difficulty getting around that she rarely leaves the house. She relies on her family—and feels guilty about it—to bring her what she needs from the outside world. Unaccustomed to physical exercise, clumsy with osteoarthritis, Rebecca got up one day to pick up a jar of marmalade, slipped on a scatter rug, and fell. The Meals on Wheels delivery woman found her cramped up and lying on her side in the kitchen. An ambulance took her to the hospital with a hip fracture.

Another one of my older patients, Dana, was a devotee of folk dancing. She knew dances of all nations and led a group of older women and men giving community dance performances. Dana had been a fashion editor in her professional life, and in her travels in various parts of the world, she became interested in folk dancing. When retired, folk dancing became her avocation. On examination, she was remarkably young-looking, with flexible muscles and not a trace of arthritis—although she owned up to some aches some of the time.

The decline of physical condition in many otherwise healthy women is centered on the lack of exercise in their lifestyle. While exercise will not reverse aging, it will keep you healthy and fit, and feeling good regardless of age. Across the board, exercise reduced disability in all people over 70, according to a report in the *Journal of the American Medical Association*. Older people who exercised also fell asleep faster.

A seven-year study of 40,000 women reported in 1997 found that postmenopausal women who exercise outlive their sedentary sisters. Those who were active were 33 percent less likely to die during the length of the study than women who were not active. The researchers, led by the University of Minnesota School of Public Health, studied women in Iowa. Moderate activity included walking, bowling, and gardening four or more times a week. Vigorous activity included swimming or aerobics, jogging, and racket sports. However, so few women did this on a regular basis that results were not significant.

Loss of mobility is a major problem for the aging woman stemming from weakening of the bones, degeneration of the joints, loss of muscle strength, and loss of balance. Failing hearing and vision might prevent a woman from perceiving the danger ahead, and slowing of reflexes robs her of a defensive posture. The number-six killer of women is injuries and accidents, many of them related to falling or failing agility when they need to get out of harm's way. Loss of balance also leads to increased isolation because of fear of falling. The aging musculoskeletal system means the bones and muscles are not as strong or flexible as they once were, and the joints are getting creaky. However, maintaining a healthy lifestyle and keeping your body working—that is, limber and strong and flexible—can prevent most of this. Even learning how to fall—if you must—can help prevent bone fractures such as the common hip fracture.

Rebecca was an accident waiting to happen. She led a sedentary life and never took calcium until recently. But the lack of fresh air and sunlight robbed her of vitamin D, which she needed for the calcium to be absorbed. Her home was not accident-proof, and she slipped on a loose scatter rug. She has osteoarthritis as well as osteoporosis, both of which might have been prevented by a healthier lifestyle early in her life. However, Rebecca grew up in a time when women were not encouraged to be physically active and when there was not the kind of awareness we have today about the dangers of poor diet and lack of exercise.

OSTEOARTHRITIS

Osteoarthritis is the everyday, garden-variety arthritis that is most common after menopause. The joints are usually not inflamed as they are with rheumatoid arthritis, but they wear down with age. (There is a variant of osteoarthritis that does cause inflammation in some women.) Osteoarthritis generally develops slowly and gradually. Very often symptoms are not apparent to the patient, although an X ray might show signs of it. On the other hand, during the stage of "inflammatory" osteoarthritis, the patient might have a lot of pain but X rays will not show any abnormality. You are at greater risk for osteoarthritis if you are overweight, have poor posture, or have had injuries.

The term *arthritis* is commonly used to include any condition affecting the joints—pain, swelling, or stiffness. It is important to make sure you know what kind of arthritis you have—and if, indeed, it is arthritis. There are several diseases in the arthritis family, and they all require different types of treatment. Sometimes an aspirin is enough to relieve stiffness or mild pain. Exercise and physical therapy might also be required, and in more severe cases, surgery might be needed to correct disabling deformities and restore function.

Rheumatoid arthritis is an autoimmune disease that causes a severe inflammation of the joints. It affects three times as many women as men, and often begins at an early age (refer to chapter 18). Less common forms of arthritis are polymyalgia rheumatica and temporal arteritis, explained below.

Osteoarthritis is not the same as osteoporosis (see chapter 25, page 365), which is bone weakness and loss of bone density. Osteoarthritis is a breakdown of the cartilage, the structure that comes between the bone and the lining of the joint (*synovia*). Normally, cartilage acts as a buffer, dampening the effect of the force of gravity, the grinding and sliding that are part of the action around the joint. With repeated wear and tear, the cartilage wears out, and the stress is transferred to the adjoining bone. The bone thickens, and this sclerosis can be observed on X ray as excess bone, as narrowing of the joint space, and as bony spurs. However, the two diseases, osteoporosis and osteoarthritis, can coexist in one individual, as in Rebecca's case.

There were bumps on Rebecca's gnarled fingers, the so-called Heberden nodes. Her back and knees hurt whenever she attempted to stand up from her chair. Pain struck her shoulder when she reached for her favorite cup in the cupboard. Getting out of bed and getting dressed were tasks she had to steel herself to perform. Dressing in pullover sweaters was out of the question; just pulling them over her shoulders was agony. She would grit her teeth and was bathed in sweat after the effort. Some days she just gave up and sat in her bathrobe and watched TV. Being immobile most of the time, Rebecca was always cold.

The loss of natural estrogen after menopause has long been suspected of playing a role in osteoarthritis because so many women develop the disease after menopause. We still don't know how the estrogen protects the joints, but some investigators think it prevents abnormal changes in the bone such as thickening and the formation of cysts. While not everyone agrees with me, I have always believed the problem is not the bone but the cartilage. Once lost, cartilage cannot be regenerated. The bone, on the other hand, in an attempt to heal itself, thickens. The bone's thickening might be the secondary, not the primary, event. We still do not know how estrogen affects osteoarthritis. It might be a nonspecific effect. Perhaps estrogen makes a menopausal woman feel better so she can get around easier and be less aware of discomfort. This basic primary breakdown in osteoarthritis is the wearing out of cartilage.

There is currently no way to prevent osteoarthritis, which affects 16 million Americans, most of them women over 45. Studies have shown that estrogen replacement might lower the risk of osteoarthritis as well as osteoporosis.

Treatment for Osteoarthritis

Most often treatment for osteoarthritis begins with painkillers, because the pain comes and goes—and you do not need to be on these medications every day. Naturally, no treatment can begin until a comprehensive medical evaluation and examination and history have been taken. Blood and urine profiles should be taken to establish a baseline from which to monitor the effect of medications. If the analgesics, like aspirin, fail, then nonsteroidal anti-inflammatory drugs, like ibuprofen, are prescribed. Recently Celebrex, a more selective NSAID belonging to a group of substances called COX-2 inhibitors, was found to be helpful in osteoarthritis and rheumatoid arthritis with fewer gastric side effects. Another substance—glurosamine—has been found to be beneficial in osteoarthritis in some trials; with chondroitin sulfate there was less clear-cut benefit.

A study at Brigham and Women's Hospital and the Harvard School of Public Health showed that women were less inclined to want drastic surgery, such as hip replacement, than men. The women were more fearful of the invasion and preferred to suffer arthritis pain rather than risk surgery. The surgery, which would need a long rehabilitation, would interrupt their roles as caregivers to dependent spouses, they claimed. Men chose surgery earlier in the course of the disease and had higher expectations for success. The study was conducted with eighteen women and twelve men with moderately severe osteoarthritis of the knee or hip.

Physical and occupational therapy are needed to remain mobile. Range of motion and fitness walking are part of the program (see the section on page 270 on rheumatoid arthritis for more about these therapies). Other treatment can include ice packs and splints or braces to rest affected joints.

Your primary care physician can treat osteoarthritis and advise you on when a rheumatologist or orthopedic surgeon should be called in.

Diet and Vitamin D

While there are no studies yet to prove that any particular diet helps osteoarthritis, it is known that good nutrition and high calcium intake, along with a program to keep weight and cholesterol down, are musts.

There is also new evidence linking low levels of vitamin D to the progression of osteoarthritis. One study showed that people who did not get enough vitamin D in their diets were more likely to develop the disease and three times more likely to have existing disease become worse. Researchers now suspect that a repair mechanism in the bone might not work without sufficient vitamin D.

Vitamin D is stored in body fat. We can often rely on stores of vitamin D that we build up during the summer months, but in winter some older people, particularly if they are housebound, might need a daily multivitamin supplement. (Keep in mind that taking large amounts of pure vitamin D in a supplement can be toxic.) If you do not have enough vitamin D in your diet, you need to get more exposure to sunlight, which the body needs to make vitamin D. Milk is the best source of vitamin D, with fish, egg yolks, and fish liver oils following.

The Need for Exercise

A study reported in 1997 tried to determine the effects of structured exercise on osteoarthritis of the knee in older adults. Over 400 men and women over 60 were enrolled in an aerobic and resistance exercise program coupled with overall instruction in health education. According to the researchers, disabled elderly patients improved enough to get around better with less pain. The results of the study convinced researchers that exercise should be part of the treatment program for osteoarthritis. The American College of Rheumatology also published guidelines that suggest exercise should be an important part of the treatment of this very common condition.

People over 60 with osteoarthritis of the knee are stabilized if they walk briskly or work out with weights for an hour three times a week. This helped so much, according to one study, that people who exercised were able to climb stairs, get in and out of cars easily, and had less pain than sedentary people in the study. In a study at the Bowman Gray School of Medicine at Wake Forest University, people over 60 who exercised despite osteoarthritis of the knee had less pain than those who did not exercise.

POLYMYALGIA RHEUMATICA AND TEMPORAL ARTERITIS

Less common conditions that cause soreness, stiffness, and pain in the neck and shoulder are *polymyalgia rheumatica* (PMR) and *temporal arteritis* (TA). While PMR is less common than rheumatoid arthritis, occurring in 50 of every 100,000 people over the age of 50, it is three times more common than TA. The peak incidences for both conditions are between the ages of 60 and 80, and both are more common in women than in men. These conditions are rare, however, in black women, and there is a higher incidence in people of Scandinavian descent. We do not yet know why.

Both these conditions are inflammatory disorders that cause pain in the muscles and joints. TA also causes vascular lesions in the blood vessels branching off the carotid arteries. Symptoms include abnormalities in the vision, headache, jaw pain when eating, and sometimes even a stroke. We do not know what causes it, but it is thought to be a genetically defined autoimmune process that damages the elastin, the internal elastic membrane, of the blood vessels that are involved. Women with symptoms of PMR often complain of fatigue, fever, weight loss, and some joint pain. Some PMR patients also develop TA over time, so it is crucial to tell your doctor about any problems with vision or headache.

Loss of sight and total blindness can occur with TA. This most common serious consequence occurs when blood vessels and nerves to the eyes are deprived of oxygen. In 20 percent of cases, there is permanent loss of vision. Blood flow to the jaw might be cut off, so you cannot move your jaw, or you feel pain when you do. This "claudication" could occur in the arm or leg, too. Half of patients with TA have such musculoskeletal symptoms. Aortic aneurysms have been reported. A test called sedimentation rate is very high in PMR and TA.

Because the distribution of affected joints varies and changes, TA is difficult to diagnose. Temporal artery biopsy should be done in all suspected cases of TA. However, even in classical cases, 30 to 40 percent of biopsies might be negative because of the way the inflammation moves around. At this point, a negative biopsy does not rule out temporal arteritis or what is now called cranial arteritis. A new, non-invasive test for diagnosis of TA has been developed by two German ultrasonograpters. The accuracy of the test "color Duplex ultrasonography" has not been confirmed yet by other researchers.

Steroids are used to reduce inflammation and prevent blindness. Because most people who get this disease are elderly and have other conditions, treatment must be carefully planned and monitored. As many as half the patients treated with steroids could develop life-threatening side effects, such as osteoporosis. Steroids must be tapered as soon as the initial symptoms are relieved. This tapering must be guided not only by blood tests but by how well the patient is doing.

THE VULNERABLE HIP

In anthropological terms, humans pay a penalty for having evolved an upright posture. In addition to supporting the whole weight of the body when we stand on one leg, the hip is capable of many movements:

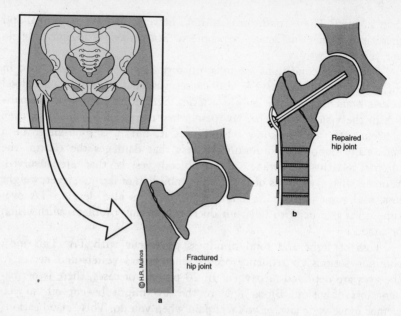

© H.R. Muinos

Fractured
hip joint

Repaired
hip joint

a

b

Figure 27. Hip fractured and repaired.

flexion, extension, adduction (bringing the thigh toward the body), abduction (moving the thigh out), and external and internal rotation (moving clockwise and counterclockwise). There is a penalty for this versatility as well. A diseased hip interferes with our freedom to move from place to place. Elderly women feel the brunt of the loss of this mobility more frequently than men. The two most common diseases affecting the hip are more common in women: hip fracture, usually associated with osteoporosis, and degenerative hip disease due to osteoarthritis.

Physicians believe that osteoporosis is the direct cause of most hip fractures in the elderly. But, of course, that is not the only reason. Body weight, the characteristics of the fall, the force exerted on the bone, and the location and direction of the fall all play a role in the chance of a fracture. Not to be left out of the picture is the overmedication of many women, making them less alert and agile.

Cartilage wears away with age, so most people eventually get a mild form of osteoarthritis after 60. But the cartilage is more likely to erode in the weight-bearing or frequently used joints, like the hip. The hip, a ball-and-socket joint, is particularly vulnerable to the changes of osteoarthritis. The disease can erode the hip socket and almost completely flatten the normally convex curve of the head of the thigh. Unlike rheumatoid arthritis, which usually affects the body's joints symmetrically, osteoarthritis can be asymmetrical and concentrate on one joint.

The disease can be hastened if there are other risk factors, such as obesity, a congenital defect, injury, infection, or a familial tendency.

Repairing the Broken Hip

Surgery performed for hip fracture is different from the procedure employed for hip replacement. In an acute situation, when the patient is brought in after having sustained hip fracture, the goal of the immediate surgery is to place a pin through the broken bone fragments so they knit together as soon as possible and the patient can move again. It is early ambulation, walking, that helps prevent blood clots in veins and lungs. Thromboembolism (clots and emboli) is the greatest enemy of patients immobilized by hip fractures.

After surgery to pin together the broken parts of her femur, Rebecca entered a long period of rehabilitation, physical therapy, and a sojourn in a nursing home. She developed phlebitis of her leg and threw a number of pulmonary emboli (clots that broke off the clot in her vein and landed in her lungs). Now on anticoagulants in addition to all the other medications she was taking, Rebecca was lucky she did not die from the complications of her hip fracture.

Hip-replacement Surgery

Most hip- and-knee replacement procedures in this country (70 percent) are prompted by osteoarthritis, according to a study reported in a 1997 issue of the *Archives of Internal Medicine.* If a painful osteoarthritis of a hip cannot be treated with medication, or if a fracture renders the hip useless, a prosthesis can replace the hip joint. This form of surgery is being used more and more as techniques improve. Patients are usually given anticoagulants before surgery to avoid clots and emboli.

The artificial hip is made of metal and plastic for the femoral shaft and the cuplike pelvic socket. Newer versions of these prostheses stimulate bone growth, eliminating the need for cement to hold them in place.

The ligaments and muscles are pushed aside or cut through so the surgeon can see the entire hip joint. The head of the femur is usually removed entirely. The cavity of the pelvic bone that normally holds the femur head is shaved and shaped so that a new plastic socket can be fitted and cemented into place.

The long femoral shaft is fitted, and the rounded head of the shaft fits into the pelvic socket. Once these are secured, the incision is closed up. X rays are used after surgery to be sure the hip replacement is precisely fitted.

Physical Therapy and Rehabilitation

Exercises are needed after surgery to strengthen the muscles around the hip. Rehabilitation of the weakened muscles might be a lengthy process until a woman is back to normal. Failure to do this after hip replacement deprives a woman of the full advantage of such surgery and increases the risk of falling—which was why she would get a hip replacement in the first place. There are examples of age-appropriate exercises later in this chapter.

FALLING AND THE FEAR OF FALLING

As all of the effects of aging accumulate, elderly women are more prone to accidents, either because they did not see or hear something, they lost their balance, or they were unable to move fast enough. Medications that cause drowsiness also contribute. While a minor fall might not be a big deal to a young person, an older person might not snap back from the injury as easily. A fall on a brittle bone could result in a fracture.

Even with good health, the sense of balance changes with age. Loss of balance is frequently the cause of falling, and having fallen once, a woman's fear of falling is reinforced. Balance can be maintained by taking a wider step; that is, planting the feet farther apart when walking. This might seem ungainly, but it is practical and will eliminate some of the fear of falling. A cane or walking stick might come in handy, too, especially when walking on uneven ground. And never walk in darkness.

Broken bones do not have to be the inevitable consequence of aging. There are things you can do to prevent it, steps to take. Muscle-strengthening exercises are in order. Weakness of legs predisposes one to falling. There are three things to keep in mind to prevent fractures.

Learn How to Fall
Hip fracture is more likely to occur if you fall to the side. Try to fall straight down or forward or backward, but with your body straight, not to the side. This might seem difficult to do, especially if you panic when you start to fall. But if you think it through ahead of time, you might remember to do it when you feel yourself falling—and prevent a fracture.

Cushion the Fall
Danish researchers found that wearing hip pads reduced fracture in more than half the older people studied. Pads available commercially look like bicycle shorts. These mostly reduce the impact of the fall by cushioning. A newer system under development transfers energy away from the hip and into the surrounding tissue in the thigh. A gellike substance in the garment shunts the energy away from the hip. The gel conforms comfortably to your body, but when you fall, it stiffens rapidly on impact and deflects the force. This approach reduced the amount of force absorbed by the hip by 65 percent and provided almost twice the

cushioning of conventional protective clothing. Hip pads are now used by some nursing homes to prevent what is one of the major causes of morbidity in these institutions.

Keep Bones Strong

Maintaining or increasing bone density is still the best prevention of hip fracture. If you do weight-bearing exercise (walking) regularly, you increase bone mass. Good nutrition, including sufficient amounts of calcium and vitamin D, is also essential. Estrogen replacement therapy is effective, and if you cannot use hormonal therapy, other medications are now available (refer to chapter 23 for more on estrogen replacement).

Restore Balance with Tai Chi

A good way to prevent falls is to improve your balance, muscle strength, flexibility, and reaction time. In a May 1996 issue of the *Journal of the American Geriatrics Society*, Tai Chi, an ancient Chinese martial art, was reported to help with all of these factors. One translation of the term Tai Chi is "shadow boxing." It is a form of meditation, a balance of yin and yang that improves balance and helps abort falls by teaching you how to cope with missteps or precarious positions.

I often see groups of people—of all ages, but mainly older women—out on the grass near the East River Drive in Manhattan doing their early morning Tai Chi. Slow, precise movements improve balance and strength. Studies show that older people who did Tai Chi for fifteen weeks cut their risk of falling nearly in half compared with those who did not take the classes. One major benefit was that patients felt less afraid of falling after practicing. Also, Tai Chi improves cardiovascular fitness and lowers blood pressure.

For information, check your yellow pages for the local branch of T'ai Chi Ch'uan, or ask at a health club, local senior citizen centers, YMCA, or YWCA.

Prevent Falls

Even though most elderly women have lowered bone density, not everyone falls, and not every faller breaks her hip. We must pay parallel attention to prevention of falling, and then prevent the kind of falls that result in a hip fracture. It makes sense to think about this and to plan your living environment to reduce the risk of falling. Most accidents happen in the home—most often the kitchen, bathroom, and stairways—and the most common cause of accidental death in those over 65 is falls.

- Avoid hypnotic drugs, sleeping pills, tranquilizers, and medications that cause sudden drops in blood pressure, confusion, and impaired balance.

• Keep your eyeglass prescriptions current, and use eyedrops if you have glaucoma.

• Exercise to gain strength and coordination of your legs and torso.

• Make sure there is good lighting in your home, especially near stairs. Consider remote-controlled light switches so that lights will go out automatically after you are already in bed. Outdoor walkways and stairs should be lighted well. Have light switches at the top and bottom of stairways.

• Keep the floors free of objects you could trip on. Use nonskid rugs.

• Use handrails on all stairs and install a grab bar in the tub or shower.

• Get up slowly when you have been lying down to avoid dizziness.

CREAKY JOINTS: THE KNEES

Our knees have been bearing our weight for a long time, and surprisingly, the knee is among the most unstable joints in our bodies. This is why there are so many knee injuries among athletes. The very shape of the knee bones means they cannot provide stability. The knee is the body's largest joint. Like the elbow, the knee joint is a modified hinge joint. It can bend up and down but has limited rotation.

For stability, the knee relies on ligaments and cartilage. Ligaments are tough bands of tissue that connect bones. Cartilage is the smooth, flexible tissue that covers the joints. We also have tendons connecting the muscle to the bone. Fluid-filled sacs called bursae cushion the friction between tendons. If the ligaments or cartilage are damaged, the knee cannot always repair itself. Ligaments take a long time to heal, and cartilage cannot regenerate.

Athletes hurt their knees with sudden twisting motions, but older people end up with bad knees because of a fall, osteoarthritis, or simply the normal weakening of muscles. A torn ligament is extremely painful. Swelling is also an indicator that something is wrong, and you might not be able to move your knee through its normal ranges of motion without pain.

Creaking sounds, pain, stiffness, and swelling are the common symptoms that cartilage is wearing away. Nonsteroidal anti-inflammatory drugs are usually needed to treat this. Cortisone injections or surgery might be needed for more advanced conditions.

The most common knee injury to women is damage to the ligament in the center of the knee. This ligament is called the anterior cruciate

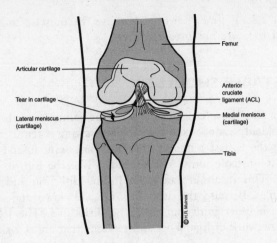

Articular cartilage

Tear in cartilage

Lateral meniscus
(cartilage)

Femur

Anterior
cruciate
ligament (ACL)

Medial meniscus
(cartilage)

Tibia

© H.R. Muñoz

Figure 28. The knee.

ligament (ACL), and it runs along the inner knee. Tears of the ACL do not usually heal on their own with rest or a brace, and they can cause chronic knee instability that often needs surgical repair. The ACL is usually reconstructed by taking a tendon from another site of the knee and creating a new ACL. This can be done with arthroscopic surgery. Sometimes draining the fluid with a needle can relieve the pressure and also provide important information. For example, if blood is present in the fluid, that might indicate a torn ligament. If fat also shows up, then a fracture might have occurred, and the marrow fat has escaped into the knee cavity. Injection of hyaluronic acid into the arthritic knee has recently been approved by the FDA. This treatment reportedly restores lubrication and viscosity of the knee fluid, and benefits the cartilage.

Exercises to Strengthen the Knee
To strengthen the muscles that support your knee, there are simple exercises you can do while lying flat on your bed or on the floor.

• Tighten your thigh muscles while pressing your knees down. Hold this tension for five or ten seconds. Then relax and repeat.

• Keep your leg straight and lift it a foot in the air. Hold this for five seconds and relax.

• Bend your knee and slide your heel up closer to your body. Then straighten your leg and relax.

If your knee ligaments have been strained, rest them temporarily by using a broad elastic support that fits your knee. Never immobilize the knee for a long time, however, because the muscles might atrophy and freeze if they are not used.

THE UNSTABLE SHOULDER

Few of us realize how crucial the shoulder joint is until it hurts or when we suddenly cannot comb our hair or swing a tennis racket. The shoulder has the widest range of motion of any joint in the body. It is also the most unstable joint. The shoulder, like the hip, is a ball-and-socket joint. This means it can move in any direction and rotate in a complete circle. Because the arm goes up and down and around and around, the shoulder joint can easily be dislocated. The joint is supported by a network of ligaments and tendons that are at risk of tearing and strain.

The shoulder is second only to the knee as the most-at-risk body part for injury on the playing fields. The anchor for the shoulder is the rotator cuff, four muscles and connecting tendons that attach the upper arm bone to the shoulder blade and clavicle. Most problems are located here. After age 40, this cuff begins to break down from normal wear and tear. Bone spurs are overgrowths at the edges of the joint, the results of wear and tear of the adjoining bones, and might pinch the nerves and cause *tendinitis*, an inflammation of the tendons of the muscles around the joint. With progressive inflammation a space might develop within the rotator cuff, which can also be inflamed. This is variously described as *bursitis, inflammation of the bursa*, or *peritendinitis*—inflammation around the tendons. As we age, arthritis might also set in and cause additional shoulder discomfort. Bone and cartilage surfaces become rough and thin, and sometimes ligaments loosen with this disease. Thus, the joints become more unstable.

Most people will develop problems with the rotator cuff as they age. As long ago as 1931, autopsy studies revealed that 39 percent of people had an injury to the cuff at some time in their lives. In a 1980s study of people who had died, progressive deterioration of the rotator cuff was found in those from 50 to 70 years of age. Most important for older women is to avoid immobilizing the shoulder so it does not get frozen. This could make the shoulder rigid and painful.

Despite the vulnerability of the rotator cuff, the shoulder generally holds up pretty well unless it is overstressed. If you stay in good physical shape and keep your muscles flexible and strong enough to support your shoulder, it is less likely to be injured. This means warming up before doing anything strenuous, and stretching afterward. If your shoulder hurts because you've been playing too much tennis, or painting the ceiling, rest and apply ice for two minutes a couple of times the first day or two. The general rule is that cold helps the acute injury, the first twenty-four to forty-eight hours, and heat helps heal an injury that is older. Nonsteroidal anti-inflammatory drugs (NSAIDs) such as ibuprofen might also help.

According to the American Academy of Orthopedic Surgeons, 90 percent of those who suffer from shoulder pain can be treated successfully with rest, physical therapy, and medication. Some might need an injection of cortisone to the rotator cuff to quickly relieve the inflammation and pain.

Diagnosing Knee and Shoulder Problems

An accurate diagnosis is needed to treat any shoulder. This includes a range of motion test and resistance tests that enable your doctor to assess mobility impairment, pain, tenderness, and any popping sounds. X rays might also be needed to determine if there is arthritis or a fracture in the bone. Some internists can diagnose joint problems—in fact, I have been teaching such a class recently to internists—but an orthopedic physician is the specialist to see for diagnosis and treatment of bone and joint diseases and injuries.

An arthrogram of a shoulder is an X-ray study in which an injected dye outlines the rotator cuff. Magnetic resonance imaging (MRI), a non-invasive test, helps distinguish cuff tear from tendonitis or bursitis. An arthrogram of the knee might outline a torn ligament.

Sometimes shoulder pain can come from somewhere else. For example, if your shoulder hurts when you are looking over your shoulder to back up the car, your spine could be the source of the pain. An orthopedist would be able to determine if this were the case.

Arthroscopic Surgery for Knees and Shoulders

Arthroscopic surgery is the most common procedure for repairing joints. Using a pencil-thin arthroscope equipped with a camera, a surgeon can scrutinize the joint while making the repairs through a small incision. Fiberoptics illuminate the interior of the joint. The lenses magnify the site and send the images to a video monitor. For larger problems, like joint replacement, traditional open surgery is needed (see the section on hip replacement surgery on page 415).

An orthopedic surgeon can shave away cartilage that has been roughened by osteoarthritis. Then the free-floating bits of cartilage that are cut away are retrieved with tweezerlike devices. Sometimes the painful inflamed joint lining of rheumatoid arthritis can be trimmed or cleaned up this way.

Arthroscopy is done as an outpatient procedure preceded by a series of preoperative tests. Depending upon your age and general health, you will need general, regional, or local anesthesia.

Complications of this surgery are very rare, less than 1 percent. The most common complications are damage to nerves or blood vessels in

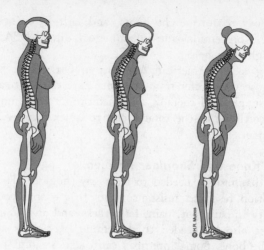

Figure 29. Osteoporosis.

the area, excessive bleeding, and postoperative infections. Such surgery can also put you at risk of complications common to any leg surgery, such as phlebitis. To prevent this, surgeons often give you anticoagulants before surgery. The most important consideration is to be sure the surgeon has wide experience in arthroscopic surgery.

You probably will not be able to stand on your leg without pain at first, and will need crutches to get around. Your knee must be elevated at home while you apply ice for the first few days to reduce pain and swelling. There is generally some collection of fluid in the repaired joint, but the body usually absorbs this in a few weeks. If not, your doctor might have to drain it through a needle.

It is important to make a commitment to postoperative exercise to speed your recovery. It takes about six weeks before your surgeon will be able to gauge the success of your surgery.

If the tear in the rotator cuff is too big for this procedure, then a larger incision needs to be made, and this might take longer to heal and rehabilitate.

THE ACHING BACK AND NECK

The spine inevitably undergoes some degeneration with age. As bone, ligaments, tendons, and intervertebral disks age, they do not always remain in perfect alignment. The upper and lower part of the spine are at greatest risk.

Vertebrae can collapse from osteoporosis-thinned bones. Bony over-growth of arthritis can narrow the spinal canal and cause pain in the legs, often the first symptom that something is wrong. When disks degenerate, they can herniate into the spinal canal and injure the nerves and collections of nerve cells (*ganglia*).

Sciatica

The most common consequence of a herniated or degenerated spinal disk is the so-called sciatica. Sciatica is pain traveling from the lower back down the thigh, the back of the knee, and even to the ankle. The pain follows the path of the sciatic nerve, the root of which is injured by the diseased disk, and can involve one side or both. In addition to pain there is frequently loss of or change in the sensation over the involved area. In the extreme, the involvement of the sciatic root results in weakness of the ankle with loss of normal ankle reflexes. Disk disease and arthritis frequently coexist.

While sciatica can happen at any age—I got it long ago from pulling my young son out of a swimming pool—it is much more common in the older years.

Arthritis of the Neck

Abnormalities in the neck (cervical spine) can also lead to pain and disability. Most commonly, this is arthritis with bony spur formation. The spurs might press on cervical nerves that travel to the arms. Typically, a woman might complain of pain and tingling in her hand when she wakes up in the morning. On questioning, the doctor learns that she sleeps with her arm elevated above the level of her head, a position she assumes involuntarily because it is most comfortable for her. With a simple maneuver of tying the hand loosely to her waist so she does not raise her hand to this position while asleep, the pain and tingling disappear—although the arthritis obviously does not.

Whiplash

Another cause of pain radiating from the cervical spine down the arm to the hand is a vehicular whiplash injury. In a car accident, the driver is more likely to anticipate the sudden movement of the car. Whiplash is more common for persons riding in the passenger seat. Most typically, the passenger is a woman, because when most couples go out in a car the husband usually drives. I was noticing how frequently this is the case one afternoon when I took the train to our farm in the country. The cars waiting at the train station had all been driven there by women. Once the husband got off the train, however, he went straight to the driver's seat and his wife slid over to the passenger seat.

Women are frequent victims of whiplash leading to a spasm of the muscles around the neck. The spasm causes the spine to assume an abnormal position that, in itself, leads to more pain and more spasm. Treatment consists of physical therapy, medication, and the use of a surgical" collar. Surgery is seldom employed even if there is an associated herniation of one of the cervical disks.

Treatment for Back and Neck Problems

When spinal cord problems cannot be treated with special exercises or by wearing braces, surgery might be needed. *Laminectomy* is the most commonly performed surgical procedure involving the spine. This procedure decompresses the pressure generated by the herniated disk on the nerves. Laminectomy is usually accompanied by excision of the disk and cleaning out of the debris created by the degenerated disk. If laminectomy and disk excision do not work, the orthopedic surgeon might perform spine fusion, which immobilizes the spine in the least uncomfortable position. The patient thus trades immobility of the spine for relief of pain.

CARE OF THE FEET

Women are nine times more likely than men to develop corns, calluses, hammertoes, bunions, and neuromas (inflamed nerves) in the feet. There is also evidence that the incidence of foot problems increases with age in women, but not necessarily in men.

Badly fitting shoes cause most of the foot problems for women. No man in his right mind (at least, not since the eighteenth century) would walk around in spiked heels or pointy toes, as women commonly do. Vanity also prompts many women to buy shoes that are too small for them. Large feet were seen as so unfeminine to the Chinese that for centuries they bound the feet of girl children. We effectively do the same thing when we jam our toes into narrow, pointed shoes and walk on four-inch heels that send our bodies into an unnatural tilt.

Since women have taken on roles other than sex goddess and baby maker, they have improved their footwear. In the 1980s we began to see women walking around in running shoes with business suits, keeping their "heels" in the bottom drawers of their desks or using them only for parties and nighttime activities. Today women tend to wear flatter heels and more rounded toes, with other changes in costume, such as pants, that allow us to shed the restrictive panty hose.

The makers of Dr. Scholl's foot products, together with the American Podiatrists Medical Association, found in a 1996 study that 46 percent of American women do not wear high heels every day. Ten years earlier, only 39 percent did not wear high heels. The majority of women agreed, however, that if high heels were more comfortable, they would wear them more.

Keep in mind also that your feet might grow larger as you age. After all, you have been standing on them for sixty years or more; they might want to spread out a bit. They might also grow if you gain weight or have children.

If you have diabetes, circulatory problems can exacerbate any foot problems you already have. Serious infections might result from the neglect of your feet. See your podiatrist frequently.

Some things to remember:

• Don't subject your feet to extreme temperatures. This means not soaking your feet in very hot water before a pedicure.

• Inspect your feet daily for signs of abnormalities such as redness, rash, or ingrown toenails.

• Exercise. Your feet are meant for walking. Walk!

• Wear comfortable and well-fitting shoes made of flexible material. There are wonderfully comfortable—and attractive—shoes available to women that never existed before.

MAINTAINING STRENGTH AND FLEXIBILITY

I knew a woman in her nineties who opened up her bedroom window every day, breathed deeply of the fresh morning air, and then did her workout. She raised her arms to her shoulders and rotated them in circles, did some side bends, then some brisk walking in place. After her breakfast and shower, she went out when the weather was good, walking to the local stores and to see her friends. She did not know much about health care or fitness then, but she instinctively knew that she needed to get her blood flowing and her muscles to flex.

Walking and swimming are the best forms of exercise for mature women. Both offer a cardiovascular workout and are easy on the knees and joints. You need exercise to assure that your heart, lungs, and blood vessels are getting adequate oxygen to aid muscle function, relieve tension, help digestion, and promote a sense of well-being. Women who exercise feel in control of themselves and their lives.

It is not difficult to incorporate thirty minutes of daily moderate exercise into doing errands on foot and taking stairs instead of an elevator. For the ambitious elderly women who strive for cardiorespiratory fitness, a supervised exercise program in a rehabilitation or sports medicine center is much safer than a solitary effort.

If you have been athletic for most of your life, it is likely you will remain so even as you age. Although we are not sure about all the genetic and environmental factors involved, we do know that remaining athletic for life will prevent much of the debility generally expected to be part of aging. Katharine Hepburn, the actress, aged beautifully and actively with swimming and tennis.

We know that all of our bodily systems do decline with age, but the systems of athletes do not decline as quickly. This applies even to amateur athletes. While more and more people are getting active, or remaining active, there is still a big lag in the number of older Americans who are athletic. Only 10 percent of those over 65 play tennis, jog, ski, or engage in any vigorous activity. About 65 percent of older Americans do little or nothing to stay in shape. This kind of lifestyle invites health problems like high blood pressure, heart disease, obesity, and worst of all, loss of the mobility that enables us to remain independent.

Walking Is Weight-bearing Exercise

The best exercise is walking, yet few people, especially suburbanites, who are used to getting around in cars, consider it a particularly interesting pastime. Ironically, sedentary people have the most to gain by simply taking a daily walk. You can burn up about 100 calories a mile with a brisk walk—while you are also strengthening your bones and reducing your risk of heart attack and stroke.

Weight-bearing exercise increases bone density, especially in the legs and back. This is essential in slowing or preventing osteoporosis. Such moderate activity is also involved in lowering blood pressure and the harmful cholesterol.

Plan your daily walk around your chores but do not encumber your hands with packages and purses. Use a backpack so you can keep your hands free and walk purposefully and energetically, swinging your arms and limbering up the muscles of your body. Enjoy your exercise.

Stretching for Fun and Flexibility

We do not hear as much about flexibility training as we do about cardiovascular exercise, or weight-bearing exercise to build strong bones. But flexible muscles are essential to long-term health and continued mobility. Joints are controlled by muscles that need to remain flexible so the joints can move freely. By increasing your range of motion, you keep moving more efficiently and greatly reduce the chance of injury. This also results in better posture, better balance, fewer muscle cramps, and less back pain. This can help you stay upright if you are about to fall.

Flexibility exercises include a variety of stretches and bends that make you feel good, too. Look for a book of stretching exercises, or talk with your doctor, or a sports trainer, about the best ones for you. Here are a few.

Calf Stretch. Runners do this before they begin. They lean on a wall, first with one leg behind them, stretched out, then the other. This stretches the muscle of the calf. Hold the stretch for ten seconds and then switch legs.

Quadriceps. While you are at the wall, stand straight and place one hand on the wall to support yourself. Bend your opposite leg behind you and hold your foot in your same-side hand while you try to raise your heel to your buttocks. Hold and relax, and then do the other leg.

Ankle and Lower Leg Stretch. You can do this sitting on a chair. First cross one leg over your opposite knee. Hold your foot in your hand and slowly turn your ankle upward. Hold it and release it.

Triceps Stretch. Hold a short towel or cloth behind your back. One arm is raised and bent behind you to grasp the top of the cloth. The other arm is bent behind you at the lower end of the cloth. Now pull the cloth in opposite directions with both hands. Flex your elbow and hold for ten seconds, and then relax. Reverse arms and repeat.

Lower Back Stretch. Lie on your back and pull your knees toward you, elevating your hips slightly. Hold this position for thirty seconds, lower your legs, and then extend your legs again, one at a time.

Lower Back Stretch. Sit in a chair with your legs slightly separated. Bend down and let your upper torso rest on your thighs, with your head hanging down between your knees. Hold this for thirty seconds, then relax.

Flexing Your Hip. While on the floor with legs outstretched, raise one knee toward your chest. With your hands behind your knee, hold your raised knee against your chest for ten seconds, then relax.

Buttocks and Hips Stretch. Sitting upright on the floor, lean on your hands behind your hips and extend your legs. Pull your leg up to your buttocks, then cross your foot over the opposite leg. With your opposite arm, hold that leg in that position for thirty seconds. Then reverse legs.

Pumping Iron for Strength

The inactive, sedentary majority of Americans lose about 30 percent of their strength and 40 percent of muscle mass by the time they reach 70. Muscle fibers shrink in size and number as we grow older. They are less responsive to signals from the nervous system. This impaired coordination and response time means our muscles tire more easily. Muscle becomes less efficient at using oxygen from the blood, and less efficient at storing nutrients.

This is downward mobility! However, the closest thing we have to a fountain of youth is strength training. A study at the University of Alabama found that nonathletic women between 60 and 77 improved their muscle power dramatically with a resistance training program. Using stationary weight machines on lower and upper body exercises for four months improved their *isotonic* strength (to lift a force) on an average of 52 percent. The *isometric* strength (to push against a force) rose by 31 percent.

In 1994, the *New England Journal of Medicine* reported on a ten-week study of sixty-three women and thirty-seven men in a nursing home. The average age was 87. The study showed that exercise training and nutritional supplementation helped frail elderly people get stronger. Muscle strength increased by more than 100 percent in the residents who took the training. This meant they improved their walking ability (gait velocity) and could climb stairs better. The study showed that high-intensity resistance training is an effective way to counteract muscle weakness and physical frailty in the elderly.

Because loss of muscle function is also associated with malnutrition, supplements were used in the study. However, this supplement seemed to have no effect unless it was accompanied by the exercise training. Muscle function might improve with vitamins alone in younger people, but apparently not in the elderly.

The training included progressive resistance training of the hip and knee muscles three days a week for ten weeks. The load of resistance was increased at each session. Sessions lasted forty-five minutes, every other day. The participants in the study who did not do the resistance training were allowed to pick an activity of their choice that was available at the home, such as aerobics, calisthenics, walking, and board games. And they increased their walking speed by 18 percent, even though that was not part of the program.

Weight lifting is also good for athletes who want to maintain their muscle strength—to keep up their golf swing, for example. You can use hand weights to strengthen your upper body. Standard advice is to do this three times a week, but if you exercise different muscle groups, you can do it every day. Each muscle group needs a full day to rest. So if you exercise the lower body one day, you can exercise the upper body the next.

WHERE TO GET INFORMATION

• The American Association of Retired Persons (AARP), the Travelers Companies, and the President's Council on Physical Fitness and Sports have published a book, *Pep Up Your Life: A Fitness Book for Seniors.* This offers three categories of exercise: strength, flexibility, and endurance. Even people in a wheelchair can accomplish the first two categories.

- Recent guidelines of the Centers for Disease Control and the American College of Sports Medicine might also come in handy. Contact the CDC at 1600 Clifton Road, Atlanta, Georgia 30333 or on-line at www.cdc.gov. The American College of Sports Medicine in Indianapolis can be reached at 317-637-9200 or on-line at www.acsm.org/sportsmed.

- The Arthritis Foundation sponsors a variety of fitness programs, including swimming, and also offers videotapes. Call 800-283-7800.

- Local community center, senior center, fitness club, YMCA, and YWCA.

POSTSCRIPT: HOW REBECCA GOT BETTER

While Rebecca was in the hospital, her son asked me to manage his mother's medical care. We assembled a team of health professionals to attend to Rebecca's various problems. A social worker was called in to help us utilize all the available resources for a senior citizen with multiple medical conditions. Rebecca was discharged from the nursing home, and a visiting nurse was hired to come to the house and supervise her medications. Rebecca had not been taking all of her medications properly, such as timing before or after meals (which she sometimes skipped). An occupational therapist helped her streamline the activities of daily living, such as getting her to use a spoon with a large handle, which is easier for Rebecca to maneuver with her gnarled hands. Loose scatter rugs were removed and new lighting was installed in her kitchen and hallways. A handrail and bar were added in the bathtub, and a rubberized mat was put in the shower booth. The therapist scrutinized Rebecca's movements around the house and equipped certain hallways and other areas with "hold-on" stations. She is to limber her joints after taking a hot shower and must walk outside several times a day. She is instructed on how to walk properly. A physical therapist taught Rebecca how to use first the walker, then crutches, and finally a cane. (Her son bought her a fancy polished mahogany cane he found in an antiques shop that she has learned to use with a certain élan.)

Now that Rebecca goes out and sees people her spirits are better. While resting on a bench she struck up a conversation with another elderly woman who has no family at all. They made a date to go to lunch together. It is good to see the sun shining, to hear the voices of children in the park, to still have her family not too far away.

··28··

Hypertension and Stroke

About 70 percent of women between 65 and 75 have high blood pressure, or hypertension. For black women, it is 80 percent by the age of 65. There is no known cause of the ordinary kind of hypertension, but its prevalence increases with age because the arteries begin to lose elasticity. However, it is no longer considered a natural result of aging. More awareness about our health in the latter part of the twentieth century means more people are doing something about regulating their blood pressure. Still, most doctor visits and drug sales in this country can be attributed to hypertension, with most of those doctor visits made by women.

A 74-year-old former newspaper reporter, Valerie, is well versed in matters of health and understands that *hypertension* does not mean "super-tension." Hypertension simply means high blood pressure. Valerie knows that hypertension is a silent killer that creeps up silently and without symptoms for years, and sometimes even decades, but is a major risk factor for heart disease, and an even more serious risk factor for stroke. She has had hypertension for at least twenty years, but has never had any symptoms.

Twenty years ago, when I first saw her, Valerie was a pack-a-day cigarette smoker. She was disappointed when, after having stopped smoking, her blood pressure came down only partially, but she accepted the fact that hypertension is a multifactorial condition stemming from many genetic and sometimes unknown environmental causes. Scrupulously, she took her various blood pressure medications, quit smoking, and cut her two predinner drinks to one. She "felt great," she said. I attributed this to her having stopped smoking, and to the pleasure she took in her retirement, visiting her grandchildren, and traveling to new and exciting places.

An enthusiastic traveler, Valerie has always equipped herself with enough medications to last her through a trip. Unfortunately, she was delayed in India, making connections and drastically changing her itinerary, and ran out of medications for ten days. Upon reaching the first available pharmacy she immediately resumed her pills. That night, however, she had a stroke. The right side of her body and face were paralyzed and she could not speak. Fortunately, her companions got her into a good hospital where diagnosis of ischemic stroke was made and anticoagulants were started. With vigorous physical and speech therapy, Valerie recovered most of her strength and also her speech.

Another patient, Ursula, was not that lucky. She could never keep her appointments with the doctor and frequently ran out of medication, which she would renew only when a cold or other minor illness would bring her back to the physician. After years of poorly controlled hypertension, Ursula had a massive hemorrhagic stroke that affected not only her brain hemisphere but also the brain stem. She remained in a vegetative state, in deep coma, not recognizing her relatives, not reacting to voices, unable to turn over in bed, unable to cough adequately to clear her lungs, and only equipped with some basic reflexes and just breathing on her own, for weeks and months. She finally died, after having exhausted the resources of her family.

HYPERTENSION: THE SILENT DISEASE

Hypertension is known as the silent disease because there are usually no symptoms until it has caused a stroke or a heart attack. However, there are some symptoms that might become apparent in some people over time. Neurological symptoms include headache, insomnia, depression, changes in libido, or changes in vision. Cardiovascular symptoms include palpitations, shortness of breath, fatigue, and angina.

The force of our blood pulsing through our arteries is blood pressure. A certain level of pressure must be maintained so that blood carrying vital elements to other organs is able to do the job. The pressure is measured by the pumping action of the heart and the resistance supplied by the arteries. There are two phases in the cardiac cycle. When our heart beats, the cardiac muscle contracts and pumps blood into the arteries. That phase of the cycle is called *systole,* and the pressure in the arteries generated by the beat is called *systolic pressure*. When the heart relaxes and the blood returns to the heart through the veins, that phase of the cycle is called *diastole*, and the pressure of blood is called the *diastolic pressure*.

A high blood pressure reading usually means the blood vessels do not fully relax. If they always remain somewhat constricted, the heart must work harder to pump the blood through them. This extra effort, over a period of time, can cause the heart muscle to become enlarged and weakened. When blood is pumped at high pressure for long periods, the force of the blood can make small tears in the lining of the arteries, and eventually plaques, which raise the resistance of the vessels. This self-perpetuating process causes further damage to the blood vessels. The damage is most pronounced in the blood vessels in the brain, kidneys, and eyes.

Hypertension means there is sustained abnormal elevation of pressure in the arteries. The sustained high blood pressure reflects defects in one or more of the regulatory mechanisms that determine the blood pressure: the nervous system, the cardiovascular system, and the hormones. Aldosterone, a hormone produced by the adrenal glands maintains a sodium balance in the body, prevents fluid loss, and protects us from dehydration. It acts on the kidney, stimulating more fluid reabsorption back into the body and thus maintaining blood pressure.

Most of the hypertension in this country is essential hypertension, also called primary hypertension, meaning we don't know its cause. About 5 percent of cases of hypertension are secondary, being caused by something else, such as kidney disease, long-standing diabetes, or a tumor of the adrenal. Renal disease is the most common cause of secondary hypertension in women. Ironically, renal disease might itself be the result of long-term, uncontrolled hypertension. This is especially true for black women. Also vulnerable to hypertension are women with lupus and diabetes. Once the underlying condition is treated, the hypertension is usually alleviated.

The Gender Difference

There are differences in blood pressure levels in men and women, and this is initially apparent in adolescence. Blacks—both men and women—are more vulnerable to high blood pressure at an earlier age. Some believe the cause is genetic as well as related to diet and stress. While young, men of all races tend to have more hypertension than women. This equalizes around the age of 55, when both sexes develop hypertension at the same rate. However, after 65 more women are likely to be hypertensive. Arteries become less elastic with age.

An increase in diastolic pressure is more common in men, but as we age, the difference narrows. The increase in systolic pressure is especially common in women. The good news about this is that women are more inclined to have their hypertension treated and their blood pressure kept under control. A study of the differences between hypertension in men and women, called the National Health and Nutrition Examination, was conducted from 1988 to 1991 with nearly 5,000 men and women over eighteen years of age. About a quarter of that population had blood pressure greater than 140 over 90, which defines hypertension. Up to age 59, fewer women had hypertension. But when they got older, they had more than men. This reversal occurs at 60 for blacks and Mexican Americans, and at 70 for Caucasians.

The Framingham Heart Study showed us that women with hypertension, either controlled or uncontrolled, had a two-to-four-times-greater risk of coronary heart disease, stroke, and death from all causes.

The Link Between Estrogen and Hypertension

Our hormones play a major role in hypertension. Because blood pressure increases with age, it is suspected that menopause and the decline of estrogen contribute to this. Nevertheless, blood pressure increases with age because of many other things: other diseases such as diabetes, long-term overweight, and smoking. Thus, we cannot blame menopause for causing hypertension. Most studies have shown that when women take hormone replacement therapy their blood pressure goes down somewhat. We do not yet have complete information about the effect of such therapy on women who already have hypertension.

During pregnancy, the levels of the hormones estradiol and progesterone increase dramatically, and in general the blood pressure is lower. This leads to the suspicion that when these hormones are diminished in later years, the blood pressure could increase. Studies have shown that 4 to 5 percent of younger women taking oral contraceptives might develop hypertension, and in 9 to 16 percent who already have hypertension it gets worse. (Most women taking oral contraceptives exhibit a slight increase in both systolic and diastolic pressure.)

It is not well understood why the pill has this hypertensive effect. Some investigators blame the progestin in the pill, others the estrogen. Others still believe that the selected few women who develop this form of hypertension are genetically predisposed.

If you are taking hormone replacement therapy, it is essential that you and your doctor monitor your blood pressure. It might be helpful to stop therapy for a few months to see what effect it has on the blood pressure.

Measuring Blood Pressure

If your blood pressure is 110 over 70, it means your systolic pressure is 110 and the diastolic is 70. The blood pressure cuff of the manometer, when inflated, cuts off the blood flow to your arm for a few moments. While slowly deflating the cuff, the doctor listens carefully to the first sound as your blood starts flowing into the blood vessels (systolic) and makes a note of the pressure reading at that moment. As the cuff is further deflated, the doctor still listens to the sound of the pulse until the noise stops when the pressures are equalized. The readings are found on the column of mercury attached to the balloon that inflates the cuff. The pressure is measured in millimeters of mercury (mm Hg).

Systolic and diastolic pressure both increase with age. By middle age, the diastolic pressure reaches a plateau, but the systolic pressure keeps going up.

- 130 over 85 = normal

- 130 to 139 over 85 to 89 = mild hypertension. Most of the people with high blood pressure fall into this category.

- 180 over 110 = severe hypertension

- Over 200 systolic and 120 diastolic is extremely dangerous

There is still considerable debate about the ranges of normal and high blood pressure, but keep in mind that sometimes a person can have isolated systolic or isolated diastolic hypertension. Systolic hypertension is most common in later years because the heart works harder to get the blood through the narrowing blood vessels.

If your first blood pressure reading is high, do not assume that you have hypertension. Blood pressure readings can vary for any number of reasons, and if you are at risk—that is, if your pressure is higher than normal—you need to check it more than once to establish whether or not you have high blood pressure. Blood pressure might be higher than normal, for example, if you have just eaten, felt anxious, or been out in the cold—or if your bladder is full. Certain medications such as decongestants, nose drops, and steroids can also elevate blood pressure. Doctors refer to the high blood pressure reading from a patient who is anxious about visiting the doctor as "white coat hypertension."

One reading should be taken while you are lying down and another while you are standing up, this latter especially if you are elderly or diabetic. In older people the arteries are like rigid tubes, and on standing or sitting most of the blood pools in the legs. This may give rise to an incorrect reading because there is lower pressure in the arms. If lower blood pressure upon standing also evokes a fainting sensation, this is called *postural hypotension*. The pressure should be measured in both arms, and if there is a difference, the arm with the higher measurement should determine the blood pressure. The size of the cuff makes a difference, too. For example, if the cuff is too small to encircle the arm properly, and therefore too tight, you might get a higher reading.

If you already have hypertension, your doctor might want you to monitor your own blood pressure, and you should always rest for at least five minutes before you do this. You will need to take two readings in succession, a few minutes apart.

Diagnosing Hypertension

Blood pressure readings alone are not the only way a doctor will look for hypertension. The doctor will look into your eyes for any signs of retinal changes. When listening to your heart, he or she will pay particular attention to the left ventricle, listening for any abnormal murmurs, as well as rhythm patterns. A neurological exam should include testing for strength, function of cranial nerves, motor and sensory intactness, balance, reflexes, and mental function.

A complete blood profile assessment is needed to check lipids, blood sugar, and other blood chemistry. A low level of potassium, for example, could be a clue because certain adrenal abnormalities that lead to hypertension are characterized by low potassium.

Your doctor needs to thoroughly go over your history to be sure nothing else is contributing to the disease such as other medical conditions or medications, or lifestyle risk factors such as smoking.

The physical exam will include palpating your abdomen to look for any mass that could suggest kidney disease, abdominal aortic aneurysm (abnormal dilatation of the aorta as a result of weakening of the vessel wall from hypertension), or an adrenal tumor. A physician will listen for sounds in the arterial walls in the abdomen and neck, and check pulses in the neck, arms, and legs. A urine analysis will indicate the condition of your kidneys and look for the presence of sugar, indicating diabetes. A chest X ray will help determine if the heart is enlarged. An electrocardiogram might detect the stress that hypertension is exerting on the heart muscle.

The results of these tests will determine the need for further tests, such as echocardiogram, which is a sonogram of the heart. X rays can evaluate the size and condition of the kidneys. Hormone levels might also be measured. Even more complex arteriograms and CT scans are done if you have renovascular disease or endocrine tumors that are causing the hypertension.

TREATMENT OF HYPERTENSION WITH LIFESTYLE CHANGES

Changing your lifestyle to get rid of the contributing risk factors is usually the first line of defense against hypertension. This would include losing weight and getting regular exercise. It also means quitting smoking, which constricts the blood vessels, and cutting down on salt, which increases the blood volume.

Each case of hypertension is unique, and you and your doctor need to evaluate the kind of treatment you need. In cases of moderate hypertension, lifestyle changes alone might suffice. A more severe case might need medications as well to bring the pressure down faster. The goal of using medications is to reduce the blood pressure with the smallest amount of drugs possible.

Don't Smoke or Drink

As soon as you inhale the smoke of a cigarette, your blood pressure goes up. Nicotine speeds up your pulse, makes your heart work harder, and does damage to the walls of your arteries. Over time it can cause hardening of the arteries. If you have high blood pressure, you should not drink more than an ounce of liquor a day, or a glass of beer or wine. More than one drink a day can increase your blood pressure.

Do Aerobic Exercise

Performed at least three times a week for twenty minutes a session, aerobic exercise has been shown to lower blood pressure. Fast walking, running, or cycling is good for your heart and might also lower your blood pressure. Exercises that constrict your muscles, the so-called isometric exercises, however, might increase blood pressure. Some weight lifting can also do this, so always check with your doctor before you begin any new exercise.

Lose Weight

Weight loss is well documented as a factor in lowering blood pressure. Women 20 percent overweight are more at risk for hypertension, as are women who have most of their weight above the waist (apple shape) rather than in the hips (pear shape). While there are plenty of thin people with hypertension, it is more common in those who are overweight. Obesity causes the body to resist the action of insulin, and thus stimulates the production of more insulin, which can contribute to hypertension. About 75 percent of the people who lost twenty pounds or more in one study brought their blood pressure back to normal with weight loss alone. Not everyone responds to this, however, especially if they have not stopped smoking or reduced their salt intake, stress, or other risk factors. Cut down on saturated fats and cholesterol, too. Anything that increases lipids works together with hypertension to damage your arteries.

Cut Down on Salt

Reducing salt in the diet brings the blood pressure down in 30 to 40 percent of people with hypertension. Not everyone with high blood pressure is sensitive to sodium, but one way to find out if you are is to cut down and see if it makes a difference. We know that societies that consume salty food have more hypertension. The ancient Chinese believed that large amounts of salt made the pulse race. A teaspoonful of salt a day (including the naturally occurring salt in foods) is enough. Processed foods are very high in salt, so avoid those, and don't salt your food at the table.

Despite the continuing debate about how much salt is too much, it is the long-term consumption of a high-sodium diet that is harmful.

Too much salt can harm women even more because it leeches calcium from the body, increasing vulnerability to osteoporosis.

The Antihypertension Diet
The National Heart, Lung, and Blood Institute has made diet recommendations based on a study of approximately 500 men and women with mild or moderate hypertension. While the participants did not lower salt levels or undertake any weight loss program, they all lowered their blood pressure. The diet is very similar to diets prescribed by the American Heart Association, the American Cancer Society, and the National Cancer Institute

Keep in mind that "servings" can be interpreted in many ways and are not necessarily the same as the "portions" that most Americans are used to. While one slice of bread might equal a serving of grains, a New York bagel would be the equivalent of about four servings.

- Grains: seven to eight servings a day
- Vegetables: four to five servings a day
- Fruits: four to five servings a day
- Nuts, seeds, and legumes: four to five servings a day
- Low or nonfat dairy: two to three servings a day
- Meat, poultry, and fish: two or less servings a day

Learn How to Handle Stress
Unless we are in a coma, we cannot avoid all the sources of stress in our lives. However, we can learn how to handle stress so that it does not take such a toll on our bodies. When we are stressed, the nervous system makes the heart beat faster and constricts the small arteries. This stress factor is especially important to women, who routinely have a higher stress load on a daily basis as they balance their roles as workers, wives, mothers, and homemakers. Role multiplicity is a horrific stressor. In later years, women are often the caretakers of spouses who are chronically ill. At a time in their lives when they think they are free to do what they want, they are tied down with nursing care and their lifestyle is greatly inhibited.

A study that measured blood pressure of 120 working women around the clock found that whenever a woman was stressed, the blood pressure went up. Most vulnerable were working mothers, whose blood pressure often remained elevated for a good deal of time.

There are many ways to help yourself reduce your body's response to stress. Meditation, yoga, relaxation therapy, and biofeedback all help. With biofeedback, for example, you can learn to lower your own blood pressure significantly. Under the guidance of a biofeedback therapist, monitors are attached to your body. These monitors record your blood pressure on a video monitor, and while you watch this monitor, you can learn, with the therapist's help, how to consciously lower your blood pressure. Many hospitals, especially cardiac centers, use biofeedback therapy. Relaxation techniques are ways of calming your body by reducing and eliminating outside interference, forcing your mind and body into a peaceful place, and allowing the tension from stress to dissipate (refer to chapter 20).

Life is less stressful if you organize your priorities, plan ahead, and solve one problem at a time. Here are some tips for heading off stress before it hits:

• Plan your day the evening before and prepare materials for it—papers, clothes—ahead of time. Do not plan an unreasonable load and do not blame yourself if you cannot accomplish all you had planned for. Sort priorities with an A, B, and C list. Just do your best and postpone the omitted items to the next day.

• Use transcendental meditation or another stress-relieving relaxation technique such as biofeedback.

• Learn to say NO if too many people expect you to do too much for them.

• Enjoy your stresses: If you are in much demand, console yourself that you must be doing something useful. Try to do something for yourself.

• Don't forget your exercises.

When changes in lifestyle do not lower the pressure sufficiently, then antihypertensive medications might be prescribed.

TREATMENT OF HYPERTENSION WITH MEDICATIONS

Drug treatment of hypertension has not been thoroughly studied in women. Most of the research has focused on men, or on both sexes without studying the differences in women. It has been found that pharmacological treatment of hypertension in men can reduce heart disease, but in women, the evidence is less conclusive. Because the side effects of some drugs cause men to become impotent, the accompanying "blurbs" carry a warning about it. It is quite possible that the drugs cause sexual dysfunction in women, too, but this has not been examined.

Not everybody responds to only one drug. Most treatment is based on using the least amount of drug necessary to bring down the blood pressure. And if one drug does not do it, then we try another. The Joint National Committee for the Detection and Treatment of Hypertension suggests that beta-blockers and diuretics be used first. Both are proven to reduce death from hypertension. Different drugs might be tried before you find the right one. There can also be side effects to consider, so it is important to talk with your doctor and understand whether the risk of hypertension should override the possible side effects of medication.

A major problem with drug therapy is that people think because there are few or no symptoms they are better, and they stop taking their medications. This is especially true if there are unpleasant side effects. The cost can be prohibitive, too, as much as $100 a month.

The major drug types used to treat high blood pressure are as follows:

Diuretics

Diuretics are commonly called water pills because they reduce the amount of water your body has been holding onto because of the hypertension. Thus, the volume of blood is lower, and there is less pressure through the vessels. These drugs increase the output of urine—and therefore, salt. These are effective, but they have side effects such as loss of potassium, which can cause cramps and fatigue. Loss of potassium can be corrected by eating foods high in potassium such as bananas, kiwifruit, or orange juice. Diuretics can also elevate blood sugar and cholesterol, as well as uric acid. They can cause weakness or loss of libido. Most of the diuretics used are of the thiazide variety.

Thiazides are diuretics that flush the important nutrient potassium from your body. On the other hand, Aldactone is a potassium-conserving diuretic. However, physicians do not like to use it because Aldactone cuts down on production of testosterone and can cause breast swelling and impotence in men. This is why Aldactone is seldom considered by physicians as a diuretic supplement. In women, Aldactone is an excellent choice, either as the only diuretic or in conjunction with Hydrodiuril. In addition to treating hypertension in women, Aldactone is a preferred diuretic to prescribe in premenstrual syndrome (PMS). Pregnant women who are carrying a male fetus cannot use this drug because it can cause feminization of the baby.

Angiotensin Converting Enzyme (ACE) Inhibitors

ACE inhibitors are relatively new and are now used widely. They inhibit the production of the hormone aldosterone, which increases blood pressure. ACE inhibitors are expensive, but they rarely cause side effects. When they do occur, they include rash, coughing, or loss of taste. Some of the new ACE inhibitors block the angiotensin receptors and have less tendency to cause coughing.

Calcium-Channel Blockers

These drugs relax the walls of the blood vessels by interfering with the way cells absorb calcium. The ability of the blood vessel to contract is reduced. The older calcium-channel blockers were short acting and needed to be taken often, but long-acting calcium-channel blockers of every variety are now available. Occasionally they cause fluid retention, which causes swelling of the ankles, dizziness, palpitations, or constipation.

Adrenergic Blockers

This class of drug includes beta-blockers, alpha-blockers, and drugs that act directly on the central nervous system such as alphamethyldopa and clonidine. Beta-blockers lower your heart rate and the amount of blood pumped. By blocking other signals from the nervous system that would normally make the vessels contract, they also relax the blood vessels. Possible side effects in women include nightmares, depression, and fatigue. In men, it can cause impotence. These are not recommended for athletic women or for those with asthma. Also, they might not work as well for black women as for whites.

Vasodilators

These are usually given in combination with beta-blockers or diuretics. Direct vasodilators cause the blood vessels to relax, but by themselves they can cause palpitations, fluid retention, rashes, or headaches. These drugs, used in more severe cases of hypertension, include minoxidil and hydralazine. Minoxidil is not used to treat women because it can cause increased hair growth. (Minoxidil is Rogaine, a drug initially used for hypertension until it was discovered to cause growth of hair in some people. Now the manufacturer has converted that disadvantage into an advantage in marketing.)

HOW A STROKE OCCURS

Hypertension is a major risk factor for stroke as well as for heart attack. When blood to the brain is interrupted the result is loss of consciousness. Depending on how long it lasts and the severity, it can result in partial or permanent paralysis of movement or speech. This is a stroke. A stroke is also known as a *cerebrovascular accident* and can be fatal. It can also put you at high risk for a heart attack. Conversely, a stroke can occur in the setting of a heart attack when the blood pressure is suddenly lowered because of heart failure or because of a medication and not enough blood is propelled into the brain.

Strokes affect twice as many women as men and are the third leading cause of death for women in this country. However, strokes, espe-

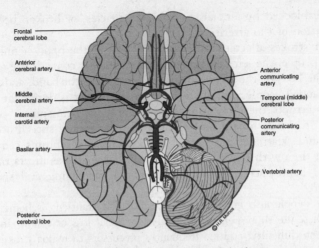

Figure 30. Arterial circulation of the brain.

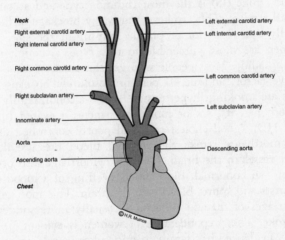

Figure 31. Aorta and its major branches.

cially in the elderly, have become less common in recent years. This could be the result of better health care in general, and most especially better management of hypertension, which strongly predisposes to stroke.

There are half a million incidents of stroke in the United States every year. It is the number-one cause of disability. In survivors over 75, women predominate—probably because we live longer than men. A little over half of the 3 million stroke victims are women, with black women overrepresented. Black women also have strokes at an earlier age.

A stroke can occur suddenly or over a period of hours. It is the result of a clot blocking the blood supply to the brain or of a hemorrhage in the brain. This can be because the blood vessels supplying blood to the brain are blocked by air, fat, or foreign particles, or broken because of degeneration of the arteries.

Most strokes affect the circulation of one of the brain hemispheres. In most people, the left hemisphere is dominant. It controls the opposite side of the body— the right side of the face, the right hand, and speech. In left-handed people it is the right hemisphere that is dominant. When a clot interrupts the circulation to the dominant hemisphere, paralysis develops in the dominant part of the body and loss of speech occurs. If therapy and treatment are started quickly, these symptoms can be reversed in time with rehabilitative therapy. If the stroke affects the non-dominant hemisphere, the effects are not as damaging and speech is not affected.

Some people also get "little strokes," called transient ischemic attack (TIA). These are short periods of paralysis, partial loss of vision, and transient speech difficulty, and are frequently precursors to major strokes. Anyone with such symptoms should get immediate medical attention.

Ischemic stroke (IS) is the most common type and accounts for 64 percent of all strokes. This stroke is caused by blockage of blood to the brain, usually due to a clot or plaque forming at the site. Postmenopausal women are most vulnerable to this type, although it can also affect a young adult. Most people who get this stroke harbor more than one causative factor, and in 40 percent absolutely no cause is found. Risk factors are smoking, hypertension, excess alcohol, family history in either or both parents, six or more pregnancies, elevated lipoproteins, not enough HDL (good cholesterol), and poorly controlled diabetes.

In a hemorrhagic stroke the elevated blood pressure flows out a major blood vessel in the brian. Cerebral hemorrhage also occurs when an aneurysm—an abnormal, blood-filled swelling of a blood vessel—in the brain bursts and spurts blood into the brain. This most often occurs between the ages of 40 and 60, and is usually more sudden than an ischemic stroke. The preponderance of women is evident from age 50 on. There is evidence that family history plays a role in this type of stroke; that is, the weakened blood vessel walls can be from congenital aneurysms. It follows logically, however, that even if the condition is inherited, smoking and uncontrolled hypertension will add to the problem. Sudden severe headache with or without a stiff neck and an alteration of consciousness might precede a cerebral hemorrhage. Having headaches for several weeks might possibly represent "warning leaks" from the tiny aneurysms.

When hypertension is not present—in an elderly person, for example—a stroke might be caused by amyloid angiopathy, a waxy protein that forms on the blood vessel wall.

Symptoms of Stroke

Depending on the size and location of the blood clot or hemorrhage, a stroke can begin with sudden stuttering, severe headache, varying degrees of loss of language, loss of motor or sensory function, or a disturbance in the consciousness. Dizziness, numbness of the limbs, nausea, and difficulty with the eyes can also be signs. Loss of consciousness is usually sudden.

The symptoms of a stroke depend upon what area of the brain is affected. The attack can start with dizziness and a sudden severe blinding headache, perhaps on one side. It can cause blindness in one eye if it is in the forward part of the brain, which involves the retinal artery, or loss of various fields of vision if it affects the posterior (occipital) cortex. If it affects the temporal area of the dominant hemisphere, problems develop with speech. Blockage of the middle cerebral artery will cause a weakness of an arm or leg; blockage of one of the posterior cerebral arteries will cause loss of balance, a feeling of unsteadiness when walking, and double vision.

However, many symptoms can be confused with other conditions such as a vitamin deficiency or an overreaction to a drug, such as a tranquilizer. Symptoms such as memory loss, numbness or tremor, difficulty with speech, or partial paralysis should be thoroughly evaluated by a doctor. In fact, if a stroke is diagnosed early enough, much of the later suffering can be avoided.

If you are an elderly person experiencing a sudden loss of strength in the arm or leg, loss of balance, or loss of vision, see a physician or go to an emergency room immediately. Bring all your medications so that the physician can assess what you are taking. He or she can assess whether those medications are responsible for your symptoms or if they are simply insufficient to prevent stroke.

Diagnosis of Stroke

It is important to evaluate a stroke patient with a CT scan or an MRI of the head in order to locate the area of the brain that is affected, and to determine if a hemorrhage has occurred (these tests can differentiate between an ischemic stroke and a cerebral hemorrhage). Certain other tests analyze the electrical impulses of the brain, test nerve and muscle function, and assess how nerves respond to stimuli. Echocardiogram of the heart, and ultrasound of the large blood vessels in the neck, can locate blockage. Spinal fluid can also be tested, and brain, nerve, and muscle tissue can be biopsied. Blood tests detect inflammatory problems.

Angiography. Dye is injected into a catheter that is placed into an artery. By taking X-ray pictures from many angles, doctors can locate a clot in a vessel or detect a narrowing vessel. Carotid angiography will visualize the arterial branches that feed various parts of the brain. This X ray is performed by a neuroradiologist, a physician who treats and diagnoses conditions of the nervous system, including the spine and brain, with radiant energy.

Electrocardiography (EKG). An EKG can detect a pattern of strain on the heart, left ventricular (from hypertension) or right ventricular (from massive pulmonary embolus); a block, partial or complete; arrhythmia; and heart attack.

Electroencephalography (EEG). When the brain is not functioning normally, abnormal patterns can be detected with electroencephalography, which records the brain's electrical activity. Electrodes with suction cups are placed on your scalp and the reading is shown on the screen.

RECOVERING FROM A STROKE

Preventing further tissue damage is a priority in treating a stroke patient. A team approach is needed, with rehabilitation beginning as soon as possible. In addition to the primary care medical doctor, a neurologist, a speech therapist, an occupational therapist, and a psychiatrist might all work with the patient to rehabilitate her emotionally and physically. It is important that family members get involved in the rehabilitation, so they can be of assistance, and also understand what is needed. The patient's level of determination to overcome the disabilities of the stroke determine her degree of recovery.

When a man has a stroke, there is usually a wife at home to care for him. But it is an unfortunate reality that when a woman has a stroke, she is put into a nursing home—either because she is a widow or because her husband is not willing or able to care for her at home.

How fast you can return home after a stroke depends on how well you are able to perform the activities of everyday living. From 35 to 60 percent of patients go directly home, 5 to 20 percent go to a rehabilitation unit, and 15 to 30 percent are placed in nursing homes. Eventually, 85 percent return home. The quality of family support has a great deal to do with recovery.

It has been observed that women who have suffered a stroke regain speech better than men. This is thought to be due to the relative bilaterality of the female brain. Fortunate for us.

The actress Patricia Neal had a stroke many years ago at a fairly young age. With the support of her family, and in possession of all the resources she needed, she made a complete recovery, regaining her speech and the use of her limbs. With the best rehabilitative care available, she eventually returned to acting. The only difference was that she now had an assistant who stood away from the camera, or behind the curtain if she was onstage, and quickly prompted her if she appeared about to forget her lines.

A University of Richmond (Virginia) study reported in 1977 found that stroke patients in managed health care programs (HMOs) tended to go to nursing homes while those with traditional fee-for-service insurance received more comprehensive—and costly—rehabilitation treatment.

A survey in Finland of stroke survivors revealed that after fourteen years, 80 percent of them still lived at home. Women made a better psychosocial adjustment, participated in entertainment activities, and had a better mood than men. Most of the women perceived their health as good or satisfactory.

Prevention is the beginning of treatment of stroke because hypertension can be controlled by not smoking, by managing diabetes carefully, and by avoiding high levels of cholesterol in your diet. Aspirin therapy might be called for to prevent clots. Other medications that prevent clotting are the anticoagulants, such as warfarin and low-molecular weight heparin. Surgery on the carotid artery can repair bleeding aneurysms or correct severe blockage after a TIA. This Roto-Rooter type of surgery clears the plaque from inside the artery walls. To prevent re-closure they place a stent nowadays similar to the kind, but larger, used for coronary angioplasty. Also anticoagulants are usually employed following the procedure. A recent analysis revealed that estrogen use tends to offer women protection from strokes and stroke mortality.

Is Stroke a Brain Attack?

The treatment of an acute stroke is undergoing intensive re-evaluation these days. Encouraged by the results of pro-active treatment of coronary artery occlusion (the use of clot-dissolving medications), some medical centers manage stroke as a "brain attack" and experiment with using similar substances. This treatment is successful in some cases such as in younger patients, and in the early stages of the stroke (within a few hours after the symptoms start). Clot dissolving medications are not for everyone and not adaptable to every medical center. Experiments with anti-platelet agents (substances that interfere with platelets clumping together, thought to be the first step in ischemic stroke as well as in heart attack) are in progress for stroke as well as for heart attacks.

••29••

Alzheimer's Disease

Sometimes when we cannot recall a name or a place during a conversation, we laugh it off with a quip: "Must be early Alzheimer's!" Though we make jokes about it, the fear of losing our memory and mental capacity is the most feared condition of old age.

Most people, even those past 80, maintain high mental competence and neurological function. There is a significant minority, however, who do suffer from disorders of the central nervous system, such as Alzheimer's and Parkinson's diseases. And women are more vulnerable than men to these diseases.

Because there are so many baby boomers entering their sixties as the millennium turns, the medical establishment is expecting an epidemic of Alzheimer's disease to occur early in the twenty-first century. This chronic, degenerative disease that results in death—usually within eight years of onset—most often strikes people over 65. One in ten persons over 65 and nearly half of those over 85 have Alzheimer's disease. Over 14 million are expected to have it by the middle of the twenty-first century, unless a cure or a prevention can be found.

In a 1993 survey by the Alzheimer's Association, 19 million Americans said they had a family member with Alzheimer's, and 37 million said they knew someone with the disease. Half of all nursing home residents—most of whom are women—suffer from Alzheimer's or a related disorder.

The cost to the health care system is enormous—Alzheimer's is the third most costly disease in the nation. The financial impact on families is devastating because none of the current medical insurance programs cover the cost of the long-term care most patients need. A person with Alzheimer's will eventually require around-the-clock care, including help with routine activities such as getting dressed, eating, and going to the bathroom. Almost 75 percent of care for the seven out of ten patients who live at home is paid by families or friends out of pocket. The average lifetime cost for one patient is $174,000. So, while there are an estimated 5 million Americans with the disease, it affects the lives of tens of millions.

Alzheimer's disease is a progressive, degenerative disease—discovered in 1906 by Dr. Alois Alzheimer, a German neurologist—that attacks the brain. It is the most common form of dementia (the loss of intellectual functioning—thinking, remembering, reasoning). It is the fourth leading cause of death in adults after heart disease, cancer, and stroke.

The two primary characteristics of the disease are nerve fiber tangles (twisted protein fibers called *neurofibrillary tangles* inside the neurons) and neuritic plaques coating the nerve cells. The plaque is formed by amyloid, a waxy protein that interferes with the function of nerve cells.

The only treatment known is to delay the process as long as possible.

THE BRAIN AND NERVOUS SYSTEM

Most beliefs about old age and the brain are myths. If you remain involved in the world and life, and continue to use and develop your body and mind, you will remain fit both mentally and physically for a long time.

The central nervous system, like all body systems, does become slightly less efficient with age. We have billions of nerve cells, called neurons, in our brains and spinal cords, and they communicate with each other in networks of synapses, which function like electrical sparks. While we do lose some of these cells with age, the remaining cells have the capacity to compensate.

The brain receives messages from the spinal cord and sense organs in a continuous generation of impulses that oversee all of our functions and actions. Each neuron consists of a cell body, one long extension called *axon,* and many short extensions called *dendrites.* Messages from other nerve cells are received by the neuron through its dendrites, modified, and relayed to other neurons via its long axon. A rich dendritic network ensures proper functioning of the brain (and the rest of the body). Some of the messages travel from groups of neurons within the brain called *nuclei* to other nuclei via axons and dendrites; other messages travel from the spinal cord to the brain and vice versa. Messages from the brain and spinal cord are transmitted to the muscles and glands of the body through the long axons.

Like telephone cables, axons are covered—but are covered by a sheath of *myelin,* which enhances the speed by which the impulses are conducted. Damage or loss of this sheath can result in slowing of the transmission of the impulses. (This is what happens in multiple sclerosis.) Axons carry impulses from the nerve cells, and *dendrites* are the cell extensions that receive the impulses. This dendritic network is central to the preservation of our skills and knowledge. In Alzheimer's disease, this dendritic network thins out, especially in the part of the brain—the hippocampus—where new knowledge is being laid down.

We also have cells, called *glia*, that provide nutritional support to the nerve cells. In order to keep up this work, the nervous system depends on continuous oxygen and glucose from the blood. The brain cannot store blood or oxygen, so any interruption in the supply, even for a few minutes, can cause permanent neurological damage.

Hormones and other chemicals such as adrenalin, noradrenalin, serotonin, and dopamine play key roles, too. Dopamine, or the lack of it, underlies Parkinson's disease. The lack of serotonin is one of the causes of depression.

Loss of critical vitamins can also lead to cell death. Eating a well-balanced diet that includes adequate amounts of vitamins, especially the B vitamins and vitamin E, is important to the health of the central nervous system and the brain. Some strict vegetarian diets are often deficient in vitamin B_{12}.

The Myths of Dementia and Senility

It is estimated that 4 to 5 percent of Americans over 65 have some degree of intellectual impairment. About half of these cases are caused by Alzheimer's disease. A number of other conditions and stroke each cause about a fourth. And at least 25 percent of all dementialike symptoms in the elderly are caused by something else such as depression, drug reactions, infections, anemia, thyroid disease, and some very curable conditions.

Interestingly, elderly people living in nursing homes for more than three months are more likely to develop mental impairment. So, too, are people with poor diets, and those who don't drink enough fluids. Memory loss, forgetfulness, and dementia can be caused by malnutrition, lack of exercise, dehydration, and medications. Cutting down on stimulating life experiences and on contacts with people predisposes to poverty of thought and loss of mental function. Again, it becomes a matter of "use it or lose it."

Despite the advances in medicine and in public education about health care, many problems of the central nervous system are not well understood and are difficult to manage. We do know that smoking in middle age is related to dementia, so here is yet another great reason to quit. Also, many elderly people are drugged into a stupor by psychoactive substances, especially the antianxiety medications and sedatives. Naturally, they will exhibit signs of dementia. Anyone would! A person who is believed to be "senile" needs a total physical examination and some lab tests to determine what is really the problem.

Parkinson's disease, which is slightly more common in men, can also be associated with dementia. More than 1 million Americans are affected by this progressive disorder of the central nervous system. Patients with Parkinson's disease lack *dopamine*, which is important for the central nervous system's control of muscle activity. Thus, patients experience tremors, stiffness in the limbs and joints, speech impediments, and difficulty in beginning movement. The three common features are bent posture, rigidity, and tremor. Later in the course of the disease, dementia sets in. The degree of symptoms varies from one person to another. About one in forty people are affected after the age of 60. A drug called L-dopa has been used since the 1970s to replace the lost dopamine, but it is not completely effective and can cause side effects.

Scientists have been experimenting with brain tissue transplant as a treatment for Parkinson's disease, but it is not yet widely used in this country. Fetal brain cells are used to replace the dead brain cells that cause the symptoms, but this use of fetal tissue, usually from aborted babies, is extremely controversial.

RISK FACTORS

Age, family history, and being female are the only known risk factors for Alzheimer's disease. It is two to three times more prevalent in women, although the Alzheimer's Association claims the gender distribution is equally divided. It might seem to be more prevalent in women because there are more women over 65. The lifetime risk for women is one in three over the age of 65, and after 65 prevalence doubles every five years, so that 50 to 70 percent of women over 80 will have it.

The disease is also associated with thinness, a history of heart attack, hip fracture, and hysterectomy (especially at an early age). All these conditions have something in common—namely, lack of estrogen, which also seems to play a role in Alzheimer's. However, this "guilt by association" is not definitive proof.

It is believed that a gene that is responsible for regulating the production of apolipoprotein E (ApoE) is involved in the development of Alzheimer's disease. ApoE is a protein that transports cholesterol through the bloodstream. We all have two ApoE genes in a variation as ApoE 2, 3, or 4, one from each parent. People who inherit one or two copies of the number 4 variation of ApoE are at higher risk for Alzheimer's disease. Although the E4 variant proves a greater risk for Alzheimer's, we still don't know for sure why some people who have this variant do not get Alzheimer's and others do.

Because there is no cure for Alzheimer's disease, there is a great deal of controversy about genetic testing. What good would it do for a person to know that he or she would probably get Alzheimer's disease?

SYMPTOMS

Severe difficulty with short-term memory is a common early symptom of Alzheimer's disease, but this should not be confused with the common forgetfulness that many people have, even when younger. Memory loss is gradual, as is disorientation, difficulty in learning, loss of language skills, and personality changes. The rate of progression varies in each individual. From the time it begins until death is usually eight years, but it can take as long as twenty years. Alzheimer's patients eventually become totally incapable of caring for themselves. Thinking becomes difficult, and the personality begins to change. Confusion and eventually helplessness will mean total dependence on the care of others.

I remember one woman, Natasha, who got Alzheimer's at a fairly young age—she was only 48—and her progression was fairly rapid. Fortunately, she had a loving husband and son who continued to keep her at home and care for her. Even though Natasha was unable to remember her husband's or her son's name, she would sometimes come into the room where one of them was and say, "I love you."

DIAGNOSIS

There is no single test to identify Alzheimer's disease, but a comprehensive examination is necessary because its early symptoms can often be confused with dementia caused by other conditions, such as depression, reactions to medications, nutritional deficiencies, and salt inbalance.

Symptoms need to be documented over a period of time, and personal and family heath histories need to be considered by the doctor. Clinical tests include neurological and mental status assessments, blood and urine tests, electrocardiogram and chest X rays. CT scanning and electroencephalography EEG (see chapter 28), and formal psychiatric testing are also needed. All of these tests can tell us that a person *probably* has Alzheimer's, but conclusive evidence can only be gotten after death in an autopsy study of the brain.

TREATMENT

Right now there is no cure for Alzheimer's disease, and the only treatment involves delaying the process for as long as possible. It seems to help if an Alzheimer's patient tries to make the most of remaining abilities, such as using memory aids called mnemonics. Making lists of things to do can also help.

Medical and social management can help the patient and family cope, and decisions can be made about care while the patient is still able to reason. It is important that the patient get good nutrition, exercise, and social contact. A well-structured and calm environment makes the disease less stressful. Sometimes medications can be used for some of the symptoms, such as anxiety or sleeplessness.

Tacrine and donepezil hydrochloride are two approved drugs used in treatment. Research is focusing on delaying the process with estrogen, NSAIDs, and vitamin E.

THE LINK BETWEEN ESTROGEN AND ALZHEIMER'S DISEASE

The decline in cognitive functioning after age 50 is thought to be due to generalized "central nervous system aging." Recent studies suggest, however, that estrogen decline at menopause might have a specific role in this process. Estrogen appears to increase the action of a gene in the brain called CREB that plays a critical role in memory. Ironically, this function is so important that it occurs in men and women alike. In men, testosterone, the male hormone, is converted to estrogen for use in the male brain. Because men do not suffer a precipitous drop in hormone levels at midlife, as women do with estrogen loss, it is theorized that this might be the reason men are less susceptible to Alzheimer's disease.

Studies have shown that women who had their ovaries removed, and who were given estrogen replacement, improved their short- and long-term memory as well as their ability to reason. More recent studies suggest that estrogen influences neurons in the regions of the brain most affected by Alzheimer's disease. Estrogen might sensitize neurons to a growth factor responsible for maintaining axon-dendrite connections. It appears to enhance the functioning of these synaptic connections, as well as help in the formation of new ones.

Some studies indicate that women using estrogen replacement therapy seemed to delay the onset of and lower the risk of Alzheimer's disease. A study by the Society for Neuroscience watched twelve women in their seventies, who had mild to moderate Alzheimer's. They were given estrogen via skin patches. Women on the estrogen had memory test scores as much as two and a half times greater than before taking the drug.

Here is a summary of what has been discovered:

- Hormone replacement therapy is effective in some women with Alzheimer's disease.

- Women with mild to moderate disease respond better.

- Memory, orientation, and calculation tasks improve.

- Adding progesterone might be harmful.

- The effect is lost if treatment is stopped.

The clinical effect of estrogen appears to be enhancement of memory, with better results with short-term memory and verbal skills, as well as keeping the thinking process from deteriorating. We need to do a great deal more research into estrogen's role in these and other neurobiologic functions. While we cannot prevent Alzheimer's with estrogen—at least not yet—there is a strong indication that it might play an important role. So convinced are women that estrogen therapy will prevent Alzheimer's disease that clinical studies are in jeopardy. Women have refused to participate because they do not want to risk being the ones who get the placebos rather than the estrogen.

Researchers are also now studying the use of androgens (male hormones) to treat Alzheimer's in men. So far, this has only proved beneficial in the laboratory with female rats programmed for Alzheimer's disease.

ALZHEIMER'S AND VITAMIN E

Scientists are more aware that immune/inflammatory mechanisms can cause brain dysfunction. For example, a study showed that lupus patients have cognitive dysfunction. And when they are treated with the anti-inflammatory/immunosuppressive prednisone, cognition improves.

A great deal of study has revolved around vitamin E and the immune system, because vitamin E might influence the inflammatory response. Inflamed cells release free radicals capable of damaging invading organisms. In inflammatory diseases, the accumulation of free radicals might overwhelm local defenses and contribute to tissue damage. It has been hypothesized that age-related decline in organ function, including the brain, might be related to an imbalance between free radicals and defense mechanisms. Since vitamin E is a potent antioxidant, capable of neutralizing free radicals, it might be useful in protecting tissues from stress caused by oxidation. This is the thinking behind the research into vitamin E and Alzheimer's.

Other Drugs

Other anti-inflammatory drugs such as nonsteroidal anti-inflammatory drugs (NSAIDs) also seem to have a beneficial effect in preventing

Alzheimer's. Experiments have indicated that drugs used for other things, such as antirejection drugs used with organ transplants, may be useful in treating disorders of the central nervous system such as stroke, spinal cord damage, Parkinson's, and Alzheimer's diseases. Cyclosporin used in monkeys and rats seemed to restore damaged nerve cells. The drug has been studied in how it improves regeneration of nerves that have been crushed. It has stimulated regrowth of these nerves, such as those in the face, and in test tubes it also works on the nerve cells important to Parkinson's and Alzheimer's.

WHERE TO GET INFORMATION

• The National Institute on Aging (NIA), part of the National Institutes of Health, sponsors the Alzheimer's Disease Education and Referral Center (ADEAR), where you can get information. The telephone number is 800-438-4380. The e-mail address is: adear@alzheimers.org. The Web site is at: http://www.alzheimers.org/adear.

• The Alzheimer's Association has a twenty-four-hour information line and links families who need assistance to chapters in their area. Telephone: 800-272-3900; Internet: http://www.alz.org.

·· 30 ··

Preventing
Respiratory Infections

There is considerable evidence that aging is associated with a decline of the immune system and that this decline contributes to the increased incidence of infections, cancers, and other conditions in later years. Diminished immunity means it takes longer to recover after an illness, too.

Two infectious diseases—influenza and pneumonia—are the fifth and sixth, respectively, leading killers of women. The most serious types of infections as we age are the ones we cannot perceive right away and whose symptoms are often hidden. For example, a woman might seem tired or have a back pain, but she has no fever or chest pain, so pneumonia is not suspected. Because the immune system is weaker and the symptoms can confuse, it is important to get flu shots and avoid being exposed to contagious disease.

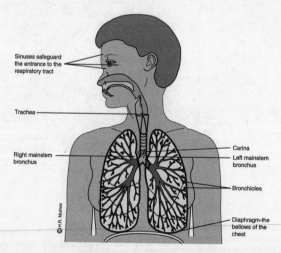

Sinuses safeguard
the entrance to the
respiratory tract

Trachea

Right mainstem
bronchus

Carina

Left mainstem
bronchus

Bronchioles

Diaphragm-the
bellows of the
chest

©H.R. Muños

Figure 32. The respiratory system.

INFLUENZA: A MORE SERIOUS BUSINESS

By striking an aging immune system, the flu can be more serious and can cause pneumonia and other complications, resulting in death. Most flu deaths are among the over-65 population. Elderly residents of nursing homes or chronic care facilities are especially vulnerable, and so are those who already have respiratory conditions such as asthma or chronic bronchitis. People over 65 are at serious risk; 85 percent of those who died from the flu would have survived had they been vaccinated.

Flu has become a catchall word for any malady from a cold to a stomachache that hits us in the fall or winter. But influenza is caused by a very specific virus. The influenza types, A, B, and C, have been known since the 1930s and 1940s. Type A is the worst. This is the influenza that killed 20 million people in a global epidemic in 1918, taking more lives than World War I. This type is also to blame for the 1957 Asian flu epidemic and the 1968 Hong Kong flu epidemic. Type B is also serious but does not cause such widespread epidemics. Type C is the mildest form.

Influenza, or the flu, is highly contagious. You can get it through the air if you happen to be in the same room with an infected person who sneezes or coughs. At the height of flu season, crowded places such as subways, theaters, or parties can put you at risk. Holding hands and kissing are both infectious. It is also contagious indirectly because the virus can live for hours on telephones, faucets, or anything infected people have touched without washing their hands. Once the bug enters a particular community—such as a school or a nursing home—it spreads quickly.

In North America, the flu season is from December to March, with peak season in February. We should be vaccinated in the fall because the vaccine needs some time to take effect. In the tropics the risk is year-round. The virus is not always predictable, however, and has been known to strike before Thanksgiving, the way it did in the southern United States in the early 1990s.

Symptoms
The virus strikes quite suddenly. It causes fatigue, muscle ache, headache, and fever. Also a runny nose, sore throat, and cough. This could be a dry, hacking cough, but could become congested as the other symptoms worsen. Often, people feel weak and tired for weeks after the flu has left them.

Diagnosis
Diagnosis is usually made clinically on the basis of symptoms in the midst of an epidemic. Samples of throat tissue are used by research scientists at the outset of an epidemic to determine the strain of the

virus. This early diagnosis might help at-risk people respond to medication. The flu generally runs its course in three to seven days with care and bed rest.

Complications

There are usually warning signs that you are developing complications—such as pneumonia—from the flu. Call your doctor if you notice pain in your chest, wheezing, difficulty breathing, or green or yellow sputum. These can be signs of pneumonia. This means the virus has infected your lungs or compromised the immune system. This is a secondary infection.

People over 65 are at serious risk for pneumonia, especially if they have other chronic conditions such as diabetes, cancer, chronic heart or lung disease, and if they are in a hospital or nursing home.

Treatment

There is no cure for influenza, but the symptoms can be treated, so that you can feel better while your body fights the infection. The infection must run its course (three to seven days), and your natural defenses will get rid of the virus by developing sufficient antibodies to destroy it. Aspirin or acetaminophen is generally taken to fight the fever and ease the aches and pains.

Sometimes antiviral drugs, such as amantadine hydrochloride and rimantadine hydrochloride, are used for high-risk patients in hospitals or nursing homes. Amantadine is an antiviral drug that is effective against influenza A but not against B or C. Before taking it you must be sure that the flu that "is going around" is of the A variety. It should be taken by vulnerable persons only at the very start of symptoms (it works *only* if you start taking it early; one pill twice a day for three to five days is usually effective in preventing a full-blown case of flu). However, it can have neurological side effects if taken in larger doses and for prolonged periods of time. Ask your physician if amantadine is for you. If it is taken for several days within forty-eight hours of the first symptoms it will shorten the length of the illness and make it milder. Whether or not it reduces the risk of complications is not yet known. It can cause side effects such as anxiety and stomach upset—and, in large doses, seizures.

A newly developed Australian anti-influenza drug, Relenza, is administered by inhalation; it is not available in this country. The best treatment is prevention. Read more about flu vaccines on page 460.

PNEUMONIA

How many times have we shivered in a cold room and said, "Brrrr, I'll catch pneumonia." We do not get pneumonia from being cold unless we are already vulnerable. Just like *flu*, we use the term *pneumonia* to cover a variety of ills. However, pneumonia is much more than a bad cold. It is a severe infection of the air spaces in the lungs. These tissues become inflamed and congested with mucus as the immune system tries to respond to an army of invading bacteria or viruses. As the air spaces become filled with fluid and mucus, the oxygen/carbon dioxide exchange is severely compromised and you feel short of breath. Because of mucus in the airways, you keep coughing instinctively, trying to get rid of the mucus.

Pneumonia can be a primary infection or a complication of another disorder, such as the flu. It can also be caused by fungal infections or by the breathing in of certain dusts, or chemicals, or even food or liquids while unconscious because of anesthesia or intoxication. This last type is called *aspiration pneumonia.*

The bacterial type is the most common, and is responsible for half a million cases of the disease each year. Between 40,000 and 70,000 people in the United States die from this type of pneumonia. It is the sixth leading cause of death. The viral type accounts for half of all cases. When it is caused by the influenza virus, it is extremely serious because the virus multiplies, undermining the integrity of the lung and paving the way to invading bacteria.

Most people recover from pneumonia, but it can also be fatal if it is not diagnosed early and if there are complicating medical conditions, such as emphysema. Other risk factors include alcoholism, smoking, heart and lung disease, a weakened immune system, and respiratory virus infection. Here is a brief description of the different types of pneumonia.

• **Viral pneumonia.** The influenza viruses can cause viral pneumonia. Another microorganism responsible for viral pneumonia is mycoplasma.

• **Hospital-acquired or nosocomial pneumonias** are a recent problem as more and more elderly people are cared for in nursing homes and hospitals. Strains of bacteria have become resistant to many antibiotics. This pneumonia often targets frail elderly people who are in a weakened condition or on ventilators. Treatment usually requires further hospitalization and antibiotics given intravenously.

• **Bacterial pneumonias** can be mild or life-threatening. Normal symptoms are coughing, fever, sputum, and sometimes chest pain.

• **Fungal forms** of the disease occur in damp, moldy climates, and they occur sporadically in people with weakened immune systems. Farmers working in silos are at risk for fungal infections.

- **Parasitic forms** of pneumonia are rare in this country.

- **Lobar pneumonia** is when an entire lobe of the lung is infected (the right lung has three lobes; the left has two lobes).

- **Double pneumonia** is when two lobes—usually one on each side—are involved.

- **Bronchopneumonia** is slower to develop and strikes an area smaller than a lobe in an area surrounding a bronchus or a bronchiole—a subdivision of the airway. The disease remains in a smaller area and is near the bronchial tubes. While this form is not often fatal, it is sometimes more difficult to cure because it can be caused by a mixed group of microorganisms that might resist conventional treatment.

- **Walking pneumonia.** Some people recover without even knowing they had the disease—later called "walking pneumonia." It is the patient who walked through it, not the pneumonia.

Sometimes bronchitis can be confused with pneumonia, but bronchitis cannot be determined with an X ray, as pneumonia can. Bronchitis is an infection of the bronchioles, the small tubes that spread throughout the lung like branches of a tree. Pneumonia is an infection of the alveoli, the tiny balloons at the ends of the bronchioles where oxygen and carbon dioxide are exchanged. The infected alveoli show up on X ray, but the infection inside the alveoli does not show this way.

Symptoms of Pneumonia

Pneumonia might start with a cold and then strike with a sudden shaking chill, pain, cough, shortness of breath, and increased sputum. High fever, rapid pulse, and rapid breathing are also symptoms, as, occasionally, is blood in the sputum. Tiredness, weakness, and muscle aches are also symptoms. Noisy breathing sounds that indicate air is having difficulty getting through the lungs can be heard by the doctor with the stethoscope.

If the lower lobe of the lung is infected, pain might be felt in the upper abdomen.

Diagnosis of Pneumonia

A chest X ray is the most common way to confirm the diagnosis of pneumonia. It is important to check carefully for any signs of pleurisy, abscess, lung cancer, or more serious pulmonary complications.

Adelaide N. was a delightful 85-year-old neighbor I greeted every morning as I rushed off to work and she walked her tiny poodle. Adelaide's daughter was a pediatric colleague of mine and brought her mother to my office one day with symptoms of pneumonia. Adelaide tried hard to be polite and engage in giving me her history but was having obvious difficulty breathing. Her breaths were shallow and rapid; her color—especially her lips—was dusky. She was obviously cyanotic (this happens when there is not enough oxygen and a bluish or cyanotic color tinges the skin and mucous membranes). She looked exhausted by just the effort of breathing, and her pulse was rapid and feeble. Adelaide did not have a fever, and that worried me, because it meant she was bereft of the normal defense mechanisms that her body could muster to withstand the onslaught by an infectious invader. And, indeed, her lungs were full of crackles and rattles. Her white blood cell count was very high, and the blood smear showed a "shift to the left," meaning that immature cells were being summoned from the bone marrow to combat an overwhelming infection. An X ray confirmed the diagnosis of pneumonia. Adelaide had a long-standing heart disease and was on numerous medications for her hypertension, angina, gastroesophageal reflux, and hiatus hernia.

Treatment of Pneumonia

Treatment must begin at once in cases of bacterial pneumonia in older women, and maybe hospitalization. According to the American Lung Association, prompt treatment with antibiotics will usually cure bacterial and mycoplasma pneumonia. Some strains of pneumonia grow resistant. There is no direct cure for viral pneumonia. All that can be done is to provide rest, proper diet, and allow enough time for convalescence and full recovery.

Nursing care includes plenty of fluids, keeping the air humidified, and bringing down the fever. Mucus needs to be drained from the lungs if the patient cannot cough it up. There are many ways to do this. Aerosol medications can be inhaled and thus break up the mucus, making it easier to cough up. If that does not work, the patient can lie on her abdomen with her head lower than her abdomen. This posture, plus another person thumping on the chest, can help dislodge the mucus. If that fails, a tracheotomy tube can be inserted into an opening in the neck. The bronchial tubes and lungs can be cleared with suction. This, naturally, is a hospital procedure.

We put Adelaide into the hospital on a course of antibiotics to cover a number of microorganisms until the culture results were available to target the antibiotics more specifically. We gave her medications to raise her blood pressure from the dangerously low level to which it had fallen. Oxygen was delivered by a nasal tube, and a tracheotomy allowed us to suction the lungs of mucus.

We had a close call with Adelaide, but she survived, and I was eventually able to greet her and her little dog in the mornings again.

PREVENTION WITH IMMUNIZATIONS

Pneumonia and influenza are leading causes of death in people over 65. Maintaining good health and getting your flu shots is important. Currently about half the population gets flu shots every fall, equal among men and women. The percentage is lower for blacks and Hispanics.

Vaccine for Influenza

The flu vaccine is a live viral serum made from purified viruses raised in eggs. The vaccine itself cannot cause the flu. A new vaccine is usually developed each year from the most common strains from the previous winter. The antibodies protect us from that particular strain of the flu.

It takes about two weeks after getting a flu shot before your body produces antibodies to protect you. Months later, the antibodies drop off—and so does protection. This is why we need shots each fall, so by the winter, when the flu season begins, we are protected. Our antibody levels have been marshaled.

The vaccine does not protect an older person as well as it does a younger one, because the immune system does not respond as well. However, you are much less likely to be seriously ill or die from flu complications if you get the vaccination every year.

Some women who are at high risk for the flu might want to get more than one shot per year. For example, a shot in September can wear off by February and afford little protection. Ask your doctor if you should have a booster shot to get you through the remainder of the cold weather.

Side effects are rare, but if you are allergic to eggs, you might not be eligible to use the vaccine. Also, if you have a fever or other condition at the time of your appointment, most doctors will not give you the vaccine.

Amantadine, the antiviral medication mentioned earlier, can be taken daily if there is a particularly serious epidemic of flu present, such as in a nursing home. If given within the context of a vulnerable community such as a nursing home, it must be taken for two weeks to allow for repeated exposure to the virus. Amantadine is also used for those who are allergic to eggs and thus could not be vaccinated.

Vaccine for pneumonia

Pneumococcal vaccine can protect against twenty-three of the most common strains of pneumococcus. Antibodies are produced in about two to three weeks, just like the flu vaccine. Protection lasts, however, for as long as ten years. So you do not need this every year the way you need a flu shot. Anyone over 65; or who lives in a nursing home; or who suffers from chronic diseases of the lungs, kidneys, or heart; or has diabetes or metabolic disorders should get vaccinated.

OTHER PREVENTIVE MEASURES

• Wash your hands frequently after being in public, and always after you touch something that could be infected by flu virus, such as water faucets. You could infect yourself by rubbing your eyes or nose.

• Keep your immune system healthy by getting plenty of antioxidants such as vitamins E, C, and A in your diet from fresh fruit and vegetables. Aging involves oxidative stress, and antioxidative therapy might be suggested. Dietary vitamin E is found in wheat germ, seeds, nuts, fish oils, unsaturated vegetable oils, and green leafy vegetables.

• Wear warm clothing in the cold and protective clothing in wet weather. Although getting cold or wet will not cause the flu, it will make you more susceptible because your body will be more stressed.

• Avoid crowds during flu season, especially if you are not feeling 100 percent healthy. A person across the room can sneeze or cough, and the virus will "work the room" like a good politician.

• Don't share kisses, hugs, cups, or straws of people with the flu.

• Don't smoke. With a damaged respiratory tract, you are more at risk.

A NOTE ABOUT THE RESURGENCE OF TUBERCULOSIS

Although tuberculosis (TB) was almost wiped out in this country years ago, it has lately been making a return, especially in big cities. In 1993, there were 25,000 cases reported in this country, about half in New York, Chicago, Los Angeles, and other cities. This country has witnessed the frightening phenomenon of a multidrug-resistant tubercle bacillus. People with immunodeficiency defects, such as those with AIDS, are especially vulnerable. So are people who use steroids for asthma, rheumatoid arthritis, and other illnesses. Elderly people with weakened immune systems are also vulnerable.

TB strikes men and women equally, but with increasing numbers of women succumbing to AIDS, that ratio is likely to change. TB requires intensive, at least yearlong, treatment and surveillance. Public health measures are planned in most major cities, especially New York.

In the past, TB developed in crowded slums where people were living close together in unsanitary conditions. These conditions can still be conducive to TB, especially for the elderly in crowded nursing homes. Anyone living in such conditions needs to be able to get outside into the fresh air as often as possible.

··31··

Conditions of the Urinary Tract

The most neglected areas of health care for mature women are the urinary and reproductive systems. Women often fail to get regular pelvic exams and Pap smears because they are no longer menstruating, or they are no longer sexually active. If they are, they fail to check for sexually transmitted infection. But it is the lower urinary tract that is most frequently ignored. Many women and some physicians do not realize that estrogen loss causes susceptibility to bladder infections. Women live with urinary incontinence because they don't know—and their doctors rarely tell them—that there is medical treatment for such a condition and that it is not simply a natural consequence of aging.

Women suffer in silence—and ignorance. A 63-year-old woman, Hildy, told me she and her husband plan trips by the number of rest rooms along the highway because both have to urinate so often. Far too many people accept this condition as inevitable, something they can do nothing about. But this does not have to be true, especially for women. Men often urinate more frequently as they age because their prostate gland enlarges naturally and causes pressure on their bladder. In women, frequency of urination or stress incontinence have a host of causes, all of which can be corrected with medical attention. These are explained later in this chapter.

Estrogen deficiency has a profound effect not only on the reproductive organs but also on the lower urinary tract. Without estrogen, the vagina shortens and its lining becomes thin, less acidic, and easily abraded. The pelvic floor muscle becomes flabby without estrogen, and the urinary organs—the bladder and urethra—have a tendency to prolapse, which means they sag into an unnatural position.

With periodic pelvic exams and preventive care these miseries can be avoided.

THE CHANGING ANATOMY

The reproductive and lower urinary tracts are closely associated in the pelvis, and as the pelvic floor, which is usually muscular and taut, loses elasticity with age, they become displaced. The pelvic floor muscle acts like a sling to keep pelvic organs in place. This muscle weakens with childbirth and with decreased estrogen. The pelvic organs such as the bladder, urethra, and uterus shift from their original positions. (The uterus is just above the bladder, and the vagina is just beneath it.) This is *prolapse*. It can cause a feeling of pressure or that something is slipping, and it can cause incontinence.

The brain, spinal cord, and nervous system coordinate the function of the urinary system. The kidneys are suspended above your waist and closer to your back, and are connected to your bladder by two tubes known as ureters. These tubes carry the urine produced by the kidneys to the bladder. The bladder, which is lined with muscles that stretch as the bladder fills up, acts as a reservoir. From the lower portion of the bladder (the neck of the bladder), a short tube (urethra) that leads to the outside of the body emerges through an opening (the urinary meatus) just above the vagina and below the clitoris. The muscle of the body of the bladder (detrusor muscle) and the muscle that closes off the neck of the bladder (sphincter) are coordinated. Once the bladder is filled and you initiate the act of urination, the detrusor muscle contracts and the sphincter of the neck of the bladder relaxes and thus urine is expelled.

The bladder neck joins the urethra, which is the tube that takes urine out of the body. The urethra is surrounded by a muscle—the internal sphincter—that automatically keeps the bladder neck closed or open, depending upon whether or not you want to release urine. The sphincter is actually at the neck of the bladder, not throughout the urethra. The internal sphincter is a smooth—that is, involuntary—muscle that normally keeps the bladder neck closed. It relaxes automatically when the detrusor muscle contracts.

The urethra loses muscle tone with age. The portion of the pelvic floor muscle surrounding the urethra is the external sphincter muscle. This muscle voluntarily contracts to stop and start the flow of urine. This external sphincter can compensate for the internal sphincter.

When you decide you cannot conveniently go to the bathroom, your brain signals your sphincter muscles via the spinal cord. This signals the bladder neck to stay shut. When you are able to go, your signals open the bladder neck.

THE PELVIC EXAM FOR A MATURE WOMAN

The periodic pelvic examination should not be omitted in the mature woman. It should be considered an integral part of a comprehensive annual exam as much as it is in young women. In addition, if a woman suffers from pain, discomfort, change in urinary frequency, incontinence, postmenopausal bleeding, or any other abnormality she should have an additional exam.

Doctors frequently fail to do pelvic exams in mature women, assuming that they are not sexually active. This oversight can have serious repercussions since women in this age group account for almost half the deaths from cervical cancer. These deaths are directly caused by failure to obtain routine annual Pap smears. Another area overlooked in mature women is testing for sexually transmitted infection, especially AIDS, which showed up increasingly in the late 1990s in mature heterosexual women.

Administering estrogen replacement or estrogen/progestin replacement therapy requires careful monitoring, including periodic pelvic examinations.

If you should have a problem with bleeding or pain, and your doctor suggests a hysterectomy, get one or two more opinions. Almost half the hysterectomies done in this country are considered unnecessary. While they are not so often performed at this life phase, it is easy to see that a woman on estrogen replacement therapy who has intermittent bleeding might be, under certain circumstances, a candidate for hysterectomy no matter what her age. In addition, hysterectomy with oophorectomy (removal of the ovaries) would be justified if the patient had an ovarian tumor. Unfortunately, ovarian cancer is seldom caught early enough to be eradicated in time. In a woman who carries the gene for ovarian cancer (with or without the gene for breast cancer), early oophorectomy with hysterectomy might be considered for prevention.

Women often complain of painful pelvic exams because the doctor is insensitive to the changes in the woman's reproductive organs. As we age, we should expect a certain sensitivity from a physician because of the changes in our reproductive anatomy. Your doctor should do a mini exam first to check the pelvic area before inserting any instruments. A "mini pelvic" is a manual exam using one finger only, instead of the customary two. A generous amount of lubricant and a narrower speculum should be used to avoid causing pain. Movements of fingers and instruments should be slow and gentle, and even downward pressure could be uncomfortable because the fourchette can easily be irritated.

Unless a woman is taking estrogen, a physician would expect the uterus to be small and the ovaries to be so tiny they cannot be felt on examination. The presence of an enlarged, or even a medium-sized, uterus is abnormal in an estrogen-deprived woman. This is a call for further investigation. Similarly, if the ovary can be felt at all, an alarm should go off in the physician's mind and further investigation, including a pelvic sonogram, is warranted.

The younger vagina has an S-shaped curve, but with the loss of elasticity the vaginal canal flattens and shrinks, and the walls gape. The vagina narrows, especially at the apex. This makes the visualization of the cervix difficult during an examination. In younger years, the vaginal lining is composed of three layers, the basal, the transitional, and the superficial cell layers. This lining, as we age, thins down and consists primarily of the basal layer. Such thin mucosa is vulnerable to infection and is also more likely to be injured or abraded as a result of unlubricated intercourse or an unlubricated exam. A thin, pale discharge might be present. In an attempt to repair injury, adhesions might form, spanning the walls of the vagina. At first the adhesions are flimsy and crumbly, but eventually they can become firm and fibrous and can narrow the vaginal canal. Such stalactite formations might cause severe discomfort on intercourse or on the insertion of a speculum.

URINARY TRACT INFECTIONS

During most of their lives women have a natural defense mechanism in the walls of the bladder that inhibits bacterial growth. But the bladder walls become less strong with age, and as the sagging urethra and bladder neck expose the urinary bladder to the invading microorganisms, women are more likely to get urinary infections. The vaginal flora change with menopause, too, adding to the problem. High estrogen levels promote an acidic environment that protects the vagina and urethra from bacteria that cause harm.

Postmenopausal women (along with pregnant women) are the population most susceptible to urinary tract or bladder infections. These infections are the most common infections in adult women. Fecal bacteria, *E. coli,* entering the bladder cause most of this. Another bacterium, gardnerella, associated with vaginitis, can cause infection of the urinary tract.

The bacteria from the vagina or rectum travel up to the bladder through the urethra. These infections are fourteen times more common in women because we have a much shorter urethra, the opening to the urethra is continuously contaminated by germs, and bacteria enter the urethra during sexual intercourse.

Cystitis

Cystitis is a bacterial infection of the bladder and is one of the most common ailments of women. As late as the 1970s cystitis was described in medical textbooks as a condition of men, something that so plagued Napoleon that it led to his defeat at Waterloo.

Blood in the urine is often a symptom of cystitis. The bladder can be so inflamed that you might be unable to hold onto urine, even briefly. Symptoms might be acute and sudden or persist in a mild form for some time. With a bladder infection, most women experience burning discomfort when urinating, or feel a frequent need to urinate, or feel as if the bladder is never quite empty.

Cystitis has a tendency to recur. If you experience high fever, shaking chills, and severe pain in your side, with or without occasional nausea and vomiting, that can be a sign that the infection has moved to your kidneys.

Diagnosis must be made by urinalysis; the type of an infecting organism is determined by urine culture.

If left untreated, urinary tract infections can travel to the kidneys and cause serious kidney disease. If the infection involves the kidneys (*pyelonephritis*), you might feel pain in the side and have a fever. It can also cause lower abdominal pain.

Urethritis

Urethritis is an infection of the urethra. A woman might feel constant irritation and go to the bathroom frequently. There is usually no blood in the urine, but there may be occasionally an increase in white cells in the urine.

As described on page 218 both cystitis and urethritis are common in young adult, sexually active women and are particularly troublesome when occuring in pregnancy.

Treatment for Urinary Infections

Antibiotics are needed to treat urinary tract infections for seven days, and you need to drink lots and lots of fluids to flush out your bladder. This dilutes the concentration of the urine as well as the concentration of the infecting agent. Cranberry juice has often been advocated because it increases the acidity of the urine and thus inhibits the growth of bacteria. However, the amount needed is more than most people can drink. Water and all juices are okay.

If the infection reaches your kidneys, stronger antibiotics are needed—and possibly hospitalization so the antibiotics can be delivered intravenously.

Lowering the Risk of Urinary Infection

There is no absolute way to prevent urinary tract infections, but there are ways to lower your risk.

• Keep your vaginal area as clean as possible, and wipe from front to back with a clean moist towelette or moistened cotton balls after a bowel movement (refer to page 27.)

• Empty your bladder soon after you feel urinary urge and make sure it is completely empty. When you hold on to urine, bacteria have a chance to multiply.

• Empty your bladder before and after intercourse.

• Cut down on caffeinated drinks such as colas and coffee, which may irritate the bladder.

• Follow the guidelines for nutrition and exercise to stay healthy.

• Topical estrogen preparations have been shown to prevent recurrent urinary tract infections in postmenopausal women.

INVOLUNTARY URINATION

Weakening of pelvic floor muscle, especially if you have had several children, can result in stress incontinence, or involuntary urination. This is a leakage of urine when you sneeze, cough, laugh, or bend over. When the pelvic floor muscles get weak, the pelvic organs slip out of place and sag (prolapse). This changes the placement of the bladder neck, which is no longer in the correct position. Pressure from sneezing, coughing, or lifting something heavy puts pressure on the abdomen, thus forcing the bladder neck to open. Because it is weak it cannot stay shut, and the external sphincter on the pelvic floor is unable to compensate and keep the urine from leaking out. Stress incontinence can be associated with prolapse of the uterus, nerve damage, infection, medication, reduced mobility, or even drinking too much coffee.

Stress incontinence is common and, given a woman's anatomy, not unexpected. More than a third of the women over 60 in the general population, and half of nursing home residents, have some form of stress incontinence. The decline in estrogen is thought to be a factor, but the cause is not yet known. Needless to say, there has been little research into all of the conditions affecting older women. And most especially conditions that are not fatal.

Despite the fact that urinary incontinence affects about 13 million people in this country—the majority are women—most people do nothing about it. They are not aware that it is a medical condition that can be corrected, or they are too embarrassed to ask their doctors for help. It is hoped that this will change as baby boomers age and demand better health care.

In the twenty-three years between 1969 and 1992, there were twenty-three clinical trials researching the effect of estrogen on incontinence. One genitourinary specialist said results were not objective and that there was no statistical evidence that estrogen replacement therapy helps this condition. We have only anecdotal evidence from what doctors observe with their patients. I have seen in my own practice that if estrogen is started early enough before the deterioration of the tissues sets in, the patient retains a great deal of control over urination. I have always urged my patients to use at least topical estrogen if any urinary symptoms develop after menopause.

While you will not die from incontinence, it certainly impairs the quality of your life. Many women give up their favorite activities and stop socializing because they are afraid they will wet their pants. Part of the problem is that women do not ask for help. One study showed that it took ten years from the time of the first symptom for a woman to ask her doctor about it. This is understandable given the attitudes of most male doctors, and even some women physicians, toward older women. With sexism as well as ageism working, the barriers are tall.

Also, doctors rarely tell women they can treat or prevent incontinence. One unenlightened doctor's response to his patient was, "Well, you had three babies, what do you expect?"

Symptoms of Stress Incontinence
You know you have stress incontinence when you:

- Leak urine when you cough, sneeze, or laugh.

- Go the bathroom more often to avoid accidents.

- Avoid exercise for fear of causing a leak.

- Sleep through the night, but leak when you get up from bed in the morning.

- Sometimes leak urine when you get up from a chair.

Other Types of Incontinence
Overflow incontinence. This is less common than stress incontinence and can result when prolapsed organs or scar tissue narrows the urethra and blocks the flow of urine. The bladder is never emptied completely, so it is always filling. Pressure increases, and the external sphincter cannot prevent leakage. Causes might be childbirth, pelvic surgery, diabetes, constipation, a history of sexually transmitted infection, or medications that hinder contractions of the bladder.

Treatment for this type varies with the cause. You might need medications—or intermittent self-catheterization to drain urine from your bladder. If the urethra is narrowed or the vagina has prolapsed, surgery can often correct the condition.

Symptoms of overflow incontinence include:

- Urine leakage.
- Low back pain.
- Low abdominal pain.
- A feeling of fullness in the vagina.
- A weak urine stream.

Urge Incontinence. Women with stress incontinence might also have urge incontinence. *Urge incontinence* is a result of erroneous signals from the brain. While the bladder might not contain much urine, the brain perceives the need to urinate. The overly sensitive bladder—also called *overactive bladder*—feels full all the time, even with little urine present. It is always contracting and releasing urine. You have urge incontinence if upon receiving a signal from your bladder that it is full, you run to the bathroom at full speed but lose urine just before reaching the toilet. Urge incontinence typically appears in childhood, goes away, and comes back after menopause when hormones change. This is why a doctor will ask you if you ever wet the bed as a child. Your medical history here might include pelvic surgery, back problems, or genitourinary infections.

Overactive bladder—the main cause of frequent urination, urge and urge incontinence—is more common than previously understood. Nearly one in 4 adults, an estimated 17 million Americans have an overactive bladder.

Treatment for urge incontinence varies with the cause. For overactive bladder there is a new medication recently approved by FDA—tolterodine tartrate (Detrol)—that, taken as a tablet twice a day, blocks the receptors on the oversensitive bladder muscles. Side-effects include dry mouth and, less frequently, headache, constipation, indigestion, and dry eyes.

If the cause of urge incontinence is obstruction to the flow, intermittent self-catheterization is sometimes recommended to drain urine from your bladder. If the urethra is narrowed or the vagina has prolapsed, surgery can often correct this.

RISK FACTORS FOR INCONTINENCE

An acute bladder infection can bring on temporary incontinence because of irritation to the bladder or urethra. In older women, however, symptoms are not always present, so any sudden incontinence should be brought to a doctor's attention right away.

The condition can also be caused by:

• Medications, such as diuretics or blood pressure drugs, that weaken the urethra and allow urine leakage.

• Alcohol and caffeine, which also weaken the urethra.

• Medications, such as antihistamines and decongestants, that cause you to retain urine and thus increase chances that overflow incontinence will occur. Some antidepressants and narcotics can also cause this reaction.

• Severe constipation can also cause you to retain urine by compressing the bladder outlet.

• Estrogen depletion.

• Having had several pregnancies.

• Pelvic muscle weakness.

• Stroke.

• Diabetes.

• Delirium, degenerative disease, impaired cognition.

• Obesity.

• Cigarette smoking.

• Low fluid intake.

DIAGNOSIS OF INCONTINENCE

In order to get proper treatment for incontinence, it is important to discuss the condition candidly with your doctor. You should keep a daily record of how often and how many times you leak urine, how often you urinate voluntarily or feel like urinating, and what seems to cause the incontinence. Your doctor should ask you questions like the following:

• How long have you had this problem?

• Do you have any pain when you urinate?

• Do you get up during the night?

• Describe the urine stream. Is it a stream with no force, a dribbling?

• Do liquids such as coffee or colas go right through you?

• Are you taking any medications such as diuretics, high blood pressure medications, sleeping pills, tranquilizers, antihistamines, or decongestants?

• Are you taking hormone replacement therapy?

• Have you had pelvic surgery?

A complete history and physical exam, including a pelvic exam, will enable an initial diagnosis. Certain tests might be done to confirm a diagnosis, such as:

• **Blood test** to look for levels of various medications, chemicals, or bacteria.

• **Urinalysis** to check for signs of infection or blood.

• **Urine flow test** to show how well your bladder is functioning.

• **Cystoscopy,** when a small fiberoptic tube called a cystoscope is inserted through the urethra so that the doctor can see inside the urethra and bladder to look for any abnormalities.

• **Cystometrogram,** when another tube called a catheter is inserted into the urethra and bladder to measure and record bladder pressure.

• **Stress test** to examine urine loss when bladder muscles are stressed by coughing or lifting.

• **Urodynamic testing** to check bladder and urethral sphincter function. The catheter is filled with a special dye so that an X ray can be taken. This makes the bladder visible to the X ray.

• **Postvoid residual (PVR) measurement,** during which the doctor places a tube into the urethra, or uses ultrasound, to measure the amount of urine left in the bladder after urinating.

TREATMENT TECHNIQUES FOR INCONTINENCE

Treatment depends on the degree of incontinence. Sometimes, Kegel exercises alone can strengthen the pelvic floor muscles and stop leakage. Biofeedback or electrical stimulation therapies are also used for mild cases. Estrogen therapy is often used when stress incontinence is caused by hormonal changes. In more severe cases, surgical implants might be needed.

While the problem cannot be entirely eliminated with any one treatment, it can be greatly reduced and managed so it does not interfere with life. There are also many helpful support groups to handle emotional frustration over the condition.

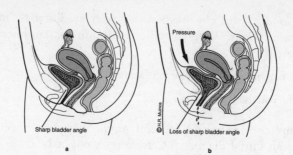

Figure 33. Urinary stress incontinence. See the change in the bladder angle.

Kegel Exercises

When stress incontinence is mild, and your doctor believes it is associated with weakness of the pelvic floor muscles, you might be able to correct it with simple exercises known as Kegels. Because the external sphincter is under your control, you can build up its strength just as you would any other muscle in your body. Regular exercise over a period of a few months will tighten up the pelvic floor muscles and the external sphincter.

First locate the muscle by trying to stop and start the flow of urine while you are on the toilet. Repeat, squeezing shut and opening the muscle several times so you become familiar with where it is located. If you are tightening your abdomen, leg, or buttock muscles, you are not using the right muscles.

You can also insert a small weight, such as a marble, into your vagina and squeeze it shut. Hold the weight for a brief time and then release it. Hold each contraction count to four, release, then repeat. Do a series of at least ten several times a day.

You can do these exercises any time and anywhere. Do them every hour at your desk, or driving, or watching TV. Do them every day for three months.

Kegel exercises can improve bladder control, but they might not always be effective when other bladder problems exist.

Fryda had to take early retirement at 62 because she could not sit at her desk long enough between the trips to the bathroom to get her work done. When I saw her I diagnosed stress incontinence due to a sagging bladder and shrinking pelvic support tissues. With the help of estrogen creams, consistent Kegel exercises, and a newly developed removable plastic urethral cap that snugly covers the opening of the urethra, she improved gradually. Eventually she was able to return to playing tennis without the fear of soiling her underwear.

Bladder Retraining

Try to wait a bit longer before you urinate even when you feel urgency. Try to stop the feeling by contracting the pelvic floor muscles. Each time you do this, you are increasing the time between urinating.

Biofeedback and Electrical Stimulation

More and more physicians are using the simple and painless technique of biofeedback to help patients retrain their bladders. This requires a biofeedback therapist and the equipment, which is usually found in hospitals.

A sensor is placed in your vagina or rectum, and a flat sensor is placed on your stomach. These sensors read the signals given when you contract or relax your pelvic floor muscles. The signals show up on a video screen. By watching the monitor you can learn what the muscles are doing and, thus begin to control them.

Electrical stimulation is like biofeedback. In this therapy, a tiny amount of painless electric current is sent to the pelvic floor muscles and your bladder. This helps the muscles contract so they can get stronger. This works for stress incontinence if you have very weak pelvic floor muscles. If you have urge incontinence, the electric current helps the bladder relax and keeps it from contracting unnecessarily.

Diet

Incontinence can sometimes be managed with changes in the diet. Some foods irritate the bladder, and if you avoid them, you are bothered less. These foods include caffeinated or carbonated drinks, alcohol, citrus fruits and juices, spicy foods, and artificial sweeteners.

Depending upon your particular condition, your doctor might suggest other diet modifications. It is important to always drink enough fluids. People often believe if they drink less, the urge to urinate will be lessened. This is not true. What happens is you dehydrate yourself, which irritates your bladder and makes the condition worse.

Hildy, the woman I mentioned earlier, realized after a thorough physical exam, and a lot of questioning from me, that there were several factors that she could probably control to help eliminate her stress incontinence. Hildy had been taking antihistamines for her allergies, and she loved her coffee, drinking about four cups a day. By controlling these two things—both of which act to produce more urine—and by practicing Kegel exercises to strengthen her pelvic muscles, Hildy was able to reduce her anxiety about needing to always be close to a bathroom.

Temporary Measures

Absorbent Products. Many women seem willing to accept the advice of an aging film actress who hawks disposable adult diapers in a television commercial. They think this is all they can do. Such absorbent products are a stopgap, a temporary measure, not a life sentence—unless a woman is incapable of caring for herself, such as someone with advanced Alzheimer's disease.

Absorbent products come in a variety of sizes and shapes, from thick menstrual pads to diapers to bed pads. When using these it is essential to change them frequently. You can also use special deodorant products to reduce any telltale odors that might exist until you can change the pad.

Self-Catheterization. Another temporary measure is self-catheterization. Your doctor can show you how to drain your urine periodically by inserting a catheter into the urethra and into the bladder. You might need to do this several times a day. This measure is used mainly for women with overflow incontinence.

MEDICAL TREATMENT FOR INCONTINENCE

Estrogen Therapy

Replacing the diminished levels of estrogen might restore urethral function by restoring the muscle tone in the sphincter and vaginal muscles. There are no long-term studies, however, and we still do not know the exact mechanism by which this works. The few clinical studies we do have show that more than a third of the women on estrogen therapy are improved.

Collagen Implants

When other measures are not satisfactory, collagen implants can be injected around the urethra near the bladder neck to bulk up the urethral tissue. This makes the opening narrower so the muscle has a smaller space in which to open and close.

Collagen is a natural protein. With several injections around the urethra near the bladder neck, a seal is created that prevents leaks. It might take more than one treatment to bulk it enough. And you might need to repeat the procedure in a few years.

Surgical Treatment for Stress Incontinence

The goal of surgery is to put the bladder neck back where it belongs and support it properly so it can do its job. Surgery can restore the pelvic floor muscles, connective tissues that support the bladder neck, and the bladder to their correct positions. An artificial urinary sphincter can be inserted to compress the urethra and prevent involuntary urination.

Through an open abdominal incision, the surgeon inserts stitches into the muscle and connective tissue around the bladder neck. This forms a sling that holds the bladder neck in the correct position. If other organs are in the way, some surgeons remove them. For example, the uterus might be removed, or the wall of the vagina repaired, or both. If your uterus is going to be removed, you are getting a hysterectomy, so be sure you and your doctor have discussed all the ramifications of this in advance.

It is very important that you ask about all this *before* surgery. Also be sure to ask about how successful your surgeon has been in relieving incontinence. Ask for statistics. There is wide variation in the skill and actual outcome of these procedures among institutions and among surgeons.

This is inpatient surgery and should be done with general or regional anesthesia. You will need the usual preop testing. The surgery itself typically lasts from one to two hours. The incision will extend from your navel to your pubis. You might go home the next day, but a catheter will remain in your bladder for up to two weeks.

Pain and discomfort could last six to eight weeks. At first you might feel the urge to urinate small amounts. This could take three to four weeks to go away.

You might need to follow up the surgery with Kegel exercises and possibly medication.

WHEN YOU NEED A UROLOGIST

A general internist should be able to treat common urinary tract infections and order and interpret urinalysis, cultures, X rays of the kidneys, and sonograms and CAT scans. The urologist, a surgical specialist for the urinary tract organs in women and the urinary and reproductive organs of men, is called upon when the diagnosis is not clear from the above tests and a surgical procedure is needed to clarify or treat the situation.

WHERE TO GET INFORMATION

There are many organizations and support groups available to provide information on what to do about incontinence.

- Help for Incontinent People (HIP), 800-252-3337.

- Simon Foundation for Continence, 800-237-4666.

- American Foundation for Urologic Disease (AFUD), 800-242-2383.

··32··

Keeping Your Senses and Living Well

Our sensory system probably takes more of the beating of age than any other system. Our senses of taste and smell become less sharp, and we might need corrective eyeglasses or a hearing aid. Very often people do not adapt for these deficiencies, and they miss out on much of life by not being able to see or hear clearly. Very often glasses and hearing devices are not covered by medical insurance, and the expense can be one reason for not getting them. Another reason for diminished senses is being overmedicated, and it is important that if you are taking several different medications you and your doctors monitor their use frequently. There is more about this later in the chapter.

ADAPTING TO CHANGING VISION

Of all the senses, vision is the most complex and most specialized because sensory reception as well as our intellectual judgment account for how and what we see.

The eye works much like a camera. Light passes through the cornea and lens in the front of each eye to converge on the retina in the back of the eyeball and create an upside-down image. Signals from the retina to the brain transport the image and put it right side up. Each eye sees an image slightly differently, and the visual field of one eye overlaps the other field. This adds another dimension, depth, to our vision.

Ciliary muscles automatically respond to the distance of an object by altering the shape of the lens. This changes the angle of the incoming rays and allows for sharper focus on the retina. This is the elasticity that decreases as the body ages.

To focus on objects in the distance, the ciliary muscles relax and the lens flattens and thins. To see things close-up, the muscles contract

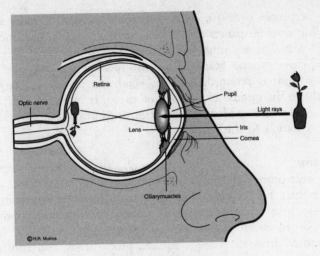

Figure 34. The eye.

and the lens becomes more rounded. The point at which the image of a close object becomes blurred is called the near point of vision. This occurs when the lens reaches its maximum curvature.

The eyeball itself has three layers and is held in place by ligaments.

Even before middle age, our vision changes. The optic lens hardens and loses its ability to change shape to focus on close objects such as the small print on medicine bottles or the classified ads in the newspaper. This can usually be remedied with simple magnifying reading glasses you can buy in the drugstore. If you already have less-than-perfect vision and wear glasses for driving, or the movies, then bifocals become an option. One pair of glasses, or contact lenses, can help you see close and far. Trifocals also adjust to each field of vision but might be difficult to adapt to.

Most of us can see perfectly well if we use the proper corrective lenses and get regular checkups with an ophthalmologist. If you are diabetic, you must be particularly diligent about eye exams to prevent diabetic retinopathy. Any sudden change in vision should be reported right away. (Optic nerves are also an indicator of certain neurological problems such as multiple sclerosis.)

MACULAR DEGENERATION

A condition that affects twice as many women as men is senile macular degeneration. While we do not understand this condition very well, it seems to cause deterioration of the part of the retina that is responsible for sharp, clear, color vision. Macular degeneration affects about 10 percent of people over 70, most commonly women. Whites are more susceptible than Hispanics and blacks. Smokers and former smokers are two and a half times more vulnerable than nonsmokers. High blood pressure, diabetes, and heart disease also increase the risk.

Some sight is retained, but this condition produces a large blind spot right in the middle of the field of vision. It interferes with driving, watching television, and other activities. It is associated with abnormal blood circulation to the retina.

Prevention

Always wear protective sunglasses (see chapter 6), and eat lots of fruits and vegetables, rich sources of antioxidants. Vegetables containing carotenoids—such as carrots—are clearly associated with protection against macular degeneration. Kale, spinach, parsley, greens, celery, broccoli, leeks, lettuce, Brussels sprouts, squash, green beans, and corn are also good.

Treatment

Macular degeneration has been treated with laser therapy in early cases. There are also special vision aids, including magnifiers, telescopic lenses, and closed circuit TV that projects printed matter onto a screen to allow people to continue normal activities.

CATARACTS

The lens of the eye is normally transparent; a cataract causes it to cloud. The lens is the part of the eye that focuses light on the retina so that you see a clear image. A cataract blocks light from passing through the lens, thus vision is blurred or there is double vision or a halo around the image.

More women get cataracts than do men, but we are not sure why. Most cataracts are caused by aging, but some are caused by diabetes, too much exposure to the sun, and certain medications. Nearly everybody over 65 has some degree of cataracts, but only a small portion have cataracts serious enough to require treatment and interfere significantly with vision.

We know now that long-term exposure to ultraviolet rays of the sun can cause cataracts to develop prematurely. Sunglasses are essential.

Treatment

The only way to remove a cataract is with surgery, which is nearly always successful. Special glasses or contact lenses are then needed to replace the function of your own optic lens. An alternative is to replace the natural lens with a plastic lens during surgery, a procedure that has become standard with most eye surgeons.

GLAUCOMA

About 80,000 people in the nation are blinded by glaucoma each year, and glaucoma threatens the sight of nearly a million others. Glaucoma is the leading cause of blindness in the elderly. It occurs when aqueous fluid buildup increases the pressure on the optic nerve, gradually damaging it. When eyes are healthy, the normal drainage system prevents this pressure buildup.

If it is detected early enough, the most common type of glaucoma can be treated with medication to control the pressure and prevent loss of vision. Surgery might be needed in some cases. An annual checkup for this condition beginning at age 40 is essential.

FLOATERS

Seeing spots before your eyes—or squiggles or floating strands—can happen to anyone, but it is more likely to happen with age. These are bits of floating debris behind the eyeball that usually go away by themselves. When they are accompanied by flashes of light, or if they do not go away, see an ophthalmologist right away. These symptoms could be signs that the retina is detaching, which could lead to permanent damage to vision if it is not repaired with laser surgery.

PRESBYCUSIS: HEARING LOSS

Nearly everyone over 80 has some degree of hearing loss. Generally, the loss is so slight as not to interfere with normal activities. Hearing loss is more common in men. Hearing loss associated with aging is called *presbycusis*. About 25 percent of adults in their sixties and seventies are affected by presbycusis, although the exact cause is unknown. Perhaps it is associated with long-term exposure to noise, or circulatory problems common to the elderly, or changes associated with aging. Nerves that control speech and hearing can also be affected by advancing age.

When hearing loss occurs in the elderly it is often the high tones that become difficult to hear. This is why you might think you can hear somebody talking, but you cannot understand what he or she is saying. You might be able to distinguish the vowels but cannot hear the consonants, and you might be losing the last few words of the sentence because many people finish sentences more softly. This can be

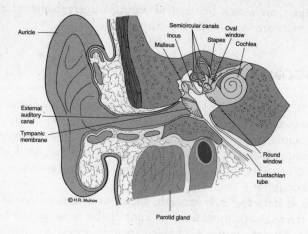

Figure 35. The ear.

very irritating in a social situation when everybody laughs at a joke and you have missed the punch line. Or you might be a fan of "Masterpiece Theater" but no longer can decipher the British English dialogue. While hearing loss cannot be reversed, you can be helped with hearing aids, lip reading, and subtitles on the television screen.

When hearing loss occurs early it is generally caused by trauma to the head, a disease of the middle ear, or constant exposure to loud noise. Rock musicians often become deaf. Heart disease, diabetes, and thyroid disease can also damage hearing, as can some common drugs such as aspirin and antibiotics.

How the Ear Works

There is an external, middle, and inner ear. Each begins where the other ends in the canal. The canal carries sound from your external ear, where it gathers, into the middle ear. In this external canal there are glands that produce wax and hairs that protect you from germs and foreign objects. The external canal ends at the eardrum, which is the outside wall of the middle ear, a chamber containing tiny bones that amplify sound and carry it to the inner ear. The middle ear chamber is connected to the throat through the Eustachian tube. When you go up fast in an elevator or in an unpressurized airplane, the outside air pressure falls slightly, but enough to be recognized by your middle ear. With a higher pressure inside the middle ear there is stress on the walls of that chamber and you might feel discomfort. The best remedy is to swallow. When you swallow, the air pressure in your middle ear equalizes with the pressure outside, you might feel your ears pop, and the discomfort goes away.

When we go down in an elevator, or are in a plane that's going to land, we again experience an imbalance between the pressure of the middle ear and the air pressure. As we automatically swallow, we might hear a popping sound in our ears again. This discomfort normally goes away, but if you have an ear infection, or nasal problems like a stuffy nose or sinus, try a nasal spray in each nostril at the beginning of the descent. Yawning helps; so does chewing gum or drinking fluids. This opens the Eustachian tubes so the pressure will be equalized in your ears.

The inner ear is composed of the *cochlea* (so-called because it resembles the shell of a snail), and the *labyrinth*. It is in the labyrinth that sensory cells are found, and these are responsible for balance. The cochlea is where sound vibrations are transformed into nerve impulses. These impulses are carried to the cortex of the brain through the auditory nerve. This nerve is a bundle of fibers that connects the inner ear with the brain.

TESTING YOUR HEARING

Your primary care physician can examine your ears, give you basic hearing tests, and even manage some hearing disorders. But for more sophisticated evaluation and treatment you might need to visit an otorhinolaryngologist (ear, nose, and throat specialist), an otologist (ear specialist), or an audiologist (technician trained to diagnose and manage hearing problems).

If your doctor cannot prescribe medical treatment to restore hearing loss, then a licensed audiologist can give you a hearing evaluation and prescribe hearing aids. Using a headphone audiometer, he or she measures at different levels how loud the sounds are that you are hearing or not hearing. This is much like getting your eyes examined, when you try different lenses until the right one is found.

If the test indicates you need a hearing aid, the audiologist can help. Be sure the audiologist is a licensed professional who has a variety of hearing devices to show you. Otherwise, you might be in the thrall of a manufacturer's representative who gets a commission on a particular brand or type.

You need to consider many things. The aids have tiny controls that might not be easy to handle if you have arthritic hands. Some can adapt to telephones, but then you might need a special phone, adding another expense.

HELP FROM HEARING AIDS

When people complain about their hearing aids, they are usually not using the proper device and have not been trained well in how to use it. Hearing aids amplify sound, but they do not correct hearing, so their use takes a period of adjustment.

Of the 28 million people with hearing loss in this country, only 6 million wear hearing aids. Profound hearing loss means no device will help, but mild to severe loss can be helped with hearing aids. Modern technology has made vast improvements, and digital hearing aids have been available since 1996. These are available today:

• **Behind the ear (BTE).** These kinds are rarely used today.

• **In the ear (ITE).** These have a shorter life and less power than BTEs. They cost from $700 to $1,000.

• **In the canal (ITC).** These are custom-made to fit inside the ear canal and are almost completely undetectable. Same drawbacks as ITE. Cost: $900 to $3,000.

• **Digital circuitry.** These have microchips in the device so you can program it for different acoustical environments. You can use a remote control, just like with the TV, to get just the right amplification. Some users find programming inconvenient.

Audiologists claim the digital aids have the best potential for the future because they can be programmed to meet individual needs. These mini computers can automatically adjust for levels of sound. They convert sound to an electrical signal, then to a digital signal. A numerical code is activated to adjust the frequency. Manipulating small parts of the hearing device might be difficult for women with arthritis. There are special devices to compensate for this.

There are many types of digital aids being developed, so shop around. Many of these devices, costing thousands of dollars, might be beyond your reach. Health insurance, including Medicare (as of this writing), will not cover the cost of hearing aids. Medicaid programs will, however. Unfortunately, this seems to mean the young have precedence, even when poor.

Staying Tuned In

With a proper hearing device and some training, a woman who is hearing impaired can compensate for the loss. There is individual instruction, and classes are available everywhere for you, family members, employers, and friends.

• Keep background noise to a minimum.

• Ask people to face you when speaking to you so you can learn to read lips and watch facial gestures.

• Remind them not to shout, just to speak clearly. One of my older professors refused to acknowledge that he was hard of hearing; instead, he would admonish the student in a booming voice: "Don't mumble! Speak out!" Leaning toward the speaker and cupping your good ear can accomplish the same thing.

• If you do not understand what people are saying, ask them to rephrase it using different words. The range of sound may be more clear.

• Always repeat important instructions back to the person who told them, to be sure you got it right.

• Ask people to tap your arm or shoulder when they wish to speak to you. Someone calling you from behind might not be heard.

Help and Information

Self Help for Hard of Hearing People is a consumer group in Bethesda, Maryland. It can be reached over the Internet at web site www.shhh.org. It also receives E-mail at national@shhh.org.

MONITORING MULTIPLE MEDICATIONS

If you have several chronic conditions, you might be taking a battery of medications every day. The average older person gets thirteen prescriptions filled each year, and drugs are their biggest out-of-pocket expense. About 11 percent of the population over 65 uses 25 percent of all prescription medication dispensed in this country.

Many people, both men and women, have been taking drugs for chronic conditions for decades—for hypertension, diabetes, heart disease, or arthritis. Yet studies of drugs before they get FDA approval rarely consider the reactions to drugs based on sex differences or on age differences. For example, women have a higher fat-to-muscle ratio than men. So it would seem that fat-soluble drugs, including tranquilizers, would have a longer half-life in women. Yet this difference is rarely considered in prescribing dosages.

As our bodies age, naturally, the way we tolerate medications changes as well. The rate at which our bodies absorb drugs, or eliminate them, can change. This means the doses might change, and it is imperative that you and your doctor monitor periodically the medications you use. This surveillance should include over-the-counter remedies, alcohol, or changes in your diet—and most important, dietary supplements.

Some foods often interact negatively with medications. For example, an antibiotic like tetracycline is not absorbed well if it is taken with milk. Taking mineral oil as a laxative can get in the way of vitamin D absorption. Diuretics can cause loss of potassium.

The Total Drug Profile

It is important to talk with your doctor about everything you are taking, your diet and your medications, when drugs are prescribed. Write down the names and dosages of your medications and periodically go over this list with your doctor. Keep a diary of any reactions you notice.

You need a total drug profile, because some drugs cancel out the effect of others. Most pharmacists keep a computerized prescription record for their customers, and this will often be the first line of discovery that one medication has a contraindication with another. This is especially true if you are getting your medications from several different doctors who do not communicate with one another and you are not telling the other doctors which drugs you are taking.

As was mentioned at other places in this book, many older women live in a drug-induced stupor, especially those who are living in nursing homes. It is likely that the generation of women maturing now will not put up with this kind of treatment. Women have traditionally been given drugs, especially psychotropic drugs, as they age. One of the most dangerous consequences is the occurrence of hip fractures because of falls while on mood-altering drugs. The sad fact that their bodies cannot get around is aggravated by the even sadder fact that their minds can't either!

DO YOU NEED VITAMIN SUPPLEMENTS?

Often, when we get older, we eat less. This is good if we are overweight, but it can also lead to malnutrition, because we are eating less, and therefore not enough, of the vital nutrients we need to protect our immune systems. Many older women are underweight because of poor nutrition or a chronic medical problem. This depresses the immune system, which is already less effective than it was in younger years. As a result older women are more vulnerable to infection.

The National Eldercare Institute on Nutrition believes a quarter of older Americans have such poor diets they are at risk for malnutrition. Even if they are getting a substantial and well-balanced diet, certain medications can cancel out the effects of some nutrients. Some medications can depress appetite as well. Metabolism changes, dental problems, depression, and diminished senses of taste and smell can all play a significant role in what and how much we eat. If we are eating less, then supplements should be taken, especially vitamin E, which helps the immune system.

The U.S. Recommended Daily Allowances (RDAs) developed by the National Research Council to prevent diseases such as scurvy (which no longer is a threat in this country) are much lower than those recommended by the Alliance for Aging Research (AAR), a nonprofit advocacy group in Washington, D.C.

VITAMIN	AAR RECOMMENDATION	RDA RECOMMENDATION
Vitamin C	250–1,000 mg.	60 mg.
Vitamin E	100–400 IU	30 IU
Beta-carotene	17,000–50,000 IU (10–30 mg.)	none established

STAYING HEALTHY WHILE YOU TRAVEL

Many women have reached a point in their lives—that zestful postmenopause—when they finally have the time and the resources to travel. If you are healthy and able, plan ahead so you stay that way on your trip.

There is no reason to stop driving a car if you are correcting your vision and hearing, but keep in mind that you might be more sensitive to glare and have less night vision and a slower reaction time. Most older drivers tend to compensate, and avoid risky driving conditions such as torrential rain storms, ice, and snow.

If you believe you must stop driving, then don't hole up in your house. There are plenty of ways of getting around, even in the suburbs. If you have been used to the independence of a car, this can require a period of adjustment. Make use of public transportation, home pickup services for health care reasons, car services, or cabs. Go out!

Be a cautious pedestrian. The most common cause of accidental death in people 65 to 74 is motor vehicle accidents, either as a driver or a pedestrian. Nearly a quarter of pedestrians killed are those over 65. Carry a flashlight at night. Wear clothing that is visible, such as light or iridescent colors. Give yourself plenty of time to cross the street. Always cross at a designated location, never between cars. Be especially careful walking to or from your car in large parking lots, such as those found at shopping malls.

Immunizations When Traveling

Because your immune system is more vulnerable, consider the appropriate immunizations that are needed before you travel. You might need shots for yellow fever, meningitis, typhoid, encephalitis, rabies, or hepatitis A and B (refer to page 196 for specifics on these immunizations).

If you are planning to travel south of the equator between May and October, keep in mind that it is winter there, and the risk of flu complications are high. Even if you had a flu shot last winter, get a booster shot before you travel. Be sure you have had your pneumococcal vaccine. There is no known risk of getting two shots in one year. Plan ahead, because it takes time for the doctor to get flu vaccine off season, and it takes time to work, too.

High Altitudes

Rapid changes in the atmospheric pressure can cause respiratory problems. If you are planning to do any scuba diving, or if you will be in high-altitude locations on a trek or hike, learn about what to do with pulmonary edema and lung problems during a rapid ascent and improper acclimatization. A medication called acetazolamide might be required—and also a very gradual ascent. It's a good idea to check with your doctor before you go.

Gastrointestinal Infections

If you travel be extra careful about possible gastrointestinal infections from bacteria in food or drinking water. Drink bottled liquids without ice. Salmonella, commonly caused by food contaminated with bacteria, can also be caught through contact with the skin of some lizards, turtles, and snakes. A weakened immune system can make you vulnerable.

Age might be encroaching on your body, but with an efficient hearing aid, proper glasses, even a cane if you need it, you can live well. If your memory needs a jog, then write things down so you don't forget. Many people do this at any age. While we do not know if diet and exercise extend life, we know they improve life, so that, whatever is left, you will feel better.

Above all, don't let others—including your doctors—treat you as if you were old and infirm. Remain an active and informed participant in your health care. And in your life!

Afterword:
A Plea for the Future

My aim in writing this book is not only to educate you but also to make you angry. There should not be such big gaps, so many unknowns, in the care of women's health. I have seen many omissions in women's health, and many tragedies in my fifty years of practice.

Peggy would not have died if she had been informed by her doctor, the media, or the educational system about her high level of vulnerability to heart attack after menopause.

Sarah would have been a happy grandmother now if she had realized that all that sun exposure she got as a young woman would kill her.

Elizabeth did not have to have broken her hip and spent the rest of her life in a nursing home if she had known earlier in her life how to prevent osteoporosis.

Jane would be alive today if her parents had understood how adolescence affects their daughters' self-esteem, and how it can lead to depression, eating disorders, and in Jane's case, suicide.

My mother would not have died at a youthful 54 of widespread endometrial cancer if in the 1950s medicine had not been several decades behind in the realization that unopposed estrogen was dangerous and that progesterone supplementation would have made it safer.

In order to insure good health care for our daughters and our granddaughters, we must organize and become vocal. Look at what the Breast Cancer Coalition accomplished in the 1990s in bringing the attention of legislators and medical researchers to this malignancy. But we need to do much, much more. We need research to answer these questions:

- Why are more women than men suffering from autoimmune diseases and osteoarthritis? We need research into the hormone-related aspects of autoimmune disease, diabetes, multiple sclerosis, rheumatoid arthritis, lupus, and scleroderma.

• Why are women less well equipped to deal with coronary heart disease? We need to know the best way to test for and diagnose heart disease in women. We need to know what changes in technique, equipment, and procedure are necessary to reduce complications and fatalities in women after angioplasty and bypass surgery. We need to know the best regimen and dose of hormone replacement to prevent heart disease.

• Why are the cancer surveillance guidelines of the American Gastroenterological Society the same for men and women when women more often get colon cancer on the right side, which is not detected with a sigmoidoscopy? Sigmoidoscopy visualizes only the left side, or sigmoid colon, which is where men usually get colon cancer.

These questions are only the tip of the iceberg. In every chapter of this book you have become aware of disease and chronic conditions more common to women that are diagnosed and treated without taking the difference into consideration. I would like to see many things get better for women's health—in every phase of life—in the twenty-first century. The task is so daunting, I hardly know where to begin.

I would like to see more sex education in our schools, clinics, and doctors' offices so young women learn how to protect themselves from sexually transmitted infection and unwanted pregnancy. Perhaps we could use Sweden as an example of how prevention has been entrained into teenagers and reduced the number of cases of STIs. What a challenge to multicultural America!

I would like to see this country win the war against cigarettes and other drugs that are setting our young people on the path to death at an early age.

I would like to see an end to violence against women.

I would like to see genetic information used to prevent illness, and not as a basis for denial of work opportunity or insurance.

I would like to see more respect in the medical community and society at large for older women. I would certainly like to see more research dollars going into helping older women live lives free of mobility disorders and hip fractures, so they do not have to spend their lives in a nursing home, lulled into a stupor with sedatives and antianxiety drugs to keep from thinking about everything they are missing.

I would like to see an end to fragmented care for women. Under one roof, women should receive comprehensive routine exams including a breast and painless pelvic exam, Pap smears, and life-phase-specific tests.

I would like to see medical students and residents choose to train in women's health, a discipline separate from gynecology, which is only about women's reproductive health.

As this book has amply demonstrated, women are different from men. Our anatomy, physiology, hormones, psychological and social characteristics, risk factors for disease, and treatment outcomes are all different from those of men.

I hope this book will encourage you to stand up for yourself and demand what is your right—to receive an equitable share of this country's health resources and be a full partner in your health care.

Appendix I:
Health Resources
for Women

If you wish to receive more information on women's health issues, problems, and conditions, here are some sources of reliable information:

- **National Council on Women's Health**
  445 East 69th Street
  Olin Hall, Room 320
  New York, NY 10021
  212-746-6967
  Women's health handbooks, periodical newsletters, health days, conferences, and other programs.

- **Women's Health Observer**
  981 First Avenue, Box 154
  New York, NY 10022
  212-980-8147
  A newsletter.

- **The National Network of Libraries of Medicine**
  800-338-7657
  This network can help you find a nearby medical library that is open to the public.

- **Harvard Women's Health Watch**
  164 Longwood Avenue
  Boston, MA 02115
  617-432-1485

- **National Health Information Center**
  P.O. Box 1133
  Washington, DC 20013-1133
  Maintains a list of 100 toll-free numbers of nonprofit organizations that dispense information by phone. Send $1 for the list.

- **American Medical Women's Association (AMWA)**
  801 North Fairfax Street, Suite 400
  Alexandria, VA 22314
  703-838-0500

DATABASES

- **Infotrac** indexes popular newspapers and magazines as well as the *New England Journal of Medicine* and the *Journal of the American Medical Association.* You can find this at good libraries. Using key words or subjects, you can search out information on the computer.

- **Medline.** Your library might also have Medline, the database of articles from the National Library of Medicine. This includes articles from thousands of medical journals beginning with 1966.

- All major medical associations and institutes, such as the American Cancer Society and the American Diabetes Association, can be found on the **World Wide Web.**

Appendix II:
The Woman's
Health Record[*]

A Woman's Health Record—as opposed to doctor's Medical Record—represents a serious effort on the part of the woman to keep a careful account of her health. Just as your bank record or family stock portfolio, or a car-repair record, your Health Record represents a house-keeping device to keep track of your health, your family's medical history, your own conditions and symptoms, the course of treatment and results.

We do not expect you to use it as a diagnostic tool but as a source of information for yourself and the doctor.

This QUESTIONNAIRE is an integral part of the Woman's Health record. It is to be filled out by the woman in the privacy of her own home any time before the first comprehensive visit with a new doctor (the woman's principal doctor). You should share a copy of your WOMAN'S HEALTH RECORD with your physician while the original stays at home. In your health record folder you should also file any communications to you from doctors, copies of consultation notes if any, copies of laboratory, Pap smear, and mammogram results as well as a list of medications taken with results and side-effects. Update your Health Record after each comprehensive visit.

I. PERSONAL DATA

Date_____

Your name _____ Age _____

Marital Status: S M D___Home Address _____ Phone _____

(include zip code)

_____
* © Lila A. Wallis, M.D.

Business Address _____ Phone _____

Nearest relative or friend _____ Address _____ Phone _____

Referred by _____ Address _____ Phone _____

Other physicians attending you at this time:

Name _____ Address _____ Phone _____

Name _____ Address _____ Phone _____

Name _____ Address _____ Phone _____

Name _____ Address _____ Phone _____

Medical Insurance (if any) _____

II. THE CHIEF COMPLAINT

It asks you "What ails you? What are the most important symptoms or reasons for seeking medical attention?" If you have **symptoms** that concern you, write down on the questionnaire the symptom and how long you have had it. This constitutes your CHIEF COMPLAINT. If you have no symptoms and no particular reasons for the visit but are seeking a "physical" or a "check-up" say so and mark the year and month you had your last checkup.

CHIEF COMPLAINT_____ Duration_____

CHIEF COMPLAINT_____ Duration_____

CHIEF COMPLAINT_____ Duration_____

III. HISTORY OF PRESENT ILLNESS

Take out another sheet of paper and write out a total description of what concerns you. History of Present Illness is the most important part of the information that you can bring to your physician. It is important that you describe your symptoms and events in **chronological** order. What happened first?, When? etc.

If it is **pain** that you suffer from, describe first the **quality** of the pain: is it piercing, stabbing, dull, wrenching, crushing, spasmodic, throbbing, gnawing, needlelike, knifelike, crampy, constricting? Consider its **degree**: mild, moderate, severe. Consider its **duration**; does it last a second, a minute, 5 minutes, half an hour, several hours? Does it recur so many times in a day? Is it pulsatile?

Then consider the precise **location** of the pain in the body. Where exactly is it? In the head, forehead, cheeks, or the back of the head, one side of the head or both?

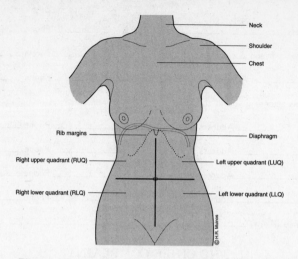

Figure 36. Use this diagram to indicate the location of pain or discomfort.

Is it in the fingers, palms, forearms, arms, shoulders? Is it in the neck, midline front or back or one side? Is it in the front part of the chest, midline, right side or left, or in the back, under the shoulder blade or in the midline? Is the pain in the abdomen? if so, is it in the midline, upper or lower abdomen, is it in the right upper quadrant, left upper quadrant, right lower quadrant, left lower quadrant? Is the pain in the back? lower back, waist, or upper back?

Does the pain go (**radiate**) from one site to another? For instance, does the left shoulder pain radiate into your left hand? or is your right-sided back pain radiating into your right groin?

What has been the **progression** of the pain? How does the pain change with time? does it continue, get worse or is getting better? is it intermittent with long or short pauses in between, lasting a second or a few minutes?

What seems to relieve the pain? what makes it worse (position of the body or the head, sitting, lying down, breathing in, breathing out, food, medication, sleep, bowel movement, urination)? How does the pain affect your sleep, work, working, psychological and mental state?

If your major symptom is a **bowel** disturbance, describe the number of bowel movements in a day, a week. What is the consistency of the stool (hard, small pieces, soft but formed, soft/and forming a pancake, liquid)? What is the color of the stool (black like tar, normal brown, as white as chalk)? Is there blood with the stools and is the blood bright red or dark?

Your observations, perhaps written out on a separate sheet of paper, will help the doctor enormously to arrive at a correct diagnosis. Here is a form that you may want to use:

If your CHIEF COMPLAINT is pain, describe:

quality _____

pain _____

degree _____

duration _____

location _____

radiation _____

progression _____

what relieves it? _____

what makes it worse? _____

If your CHIEF COMPLAINT is bowel disturbance, describe:

\# of bowel movements a day or per week _____

consistency of stool _____

color _____

any blood? _____

color of blood _____

IV. FAMILY HISTORY

Are your parents alive, how old are they? do they suffer from any illnesses? your siblings? If your parent or sibling died, how old were they at the time of death and what did they die from? Use the Table below:

Relative	Age	Is (s)he well? ill? deceased?	Cause of death	Age at death
Father				
Mother				
Brothers				
Sisters				

In your Family History belongs any information about your relatives having the following diseases:

Disease	Which relative	Details
heart disease		
high blood pressure		
stroke		
blood vessel disease		
"cholesterol problem"		
Alzheimer's disease		
osteoporosis (soft bones & fractures)		
diabetes		
obesity		

Ethnic Background: _____ Countries of origin of ancestors: _____
Caucasian _____ Black _____ Hispanic _____ Asian _____
Native American _____

Illness	Which relative	Details
any malignancy		
breast cancer		
ovarian cancer		
cancer of cervix of uterus		
cancer of body of uterus		
cancer of bowel (colon, rectum)		
cancer of lung		
cancer of pancreas		
skin cancer		
birth defects		
Other physical problems		

Illness	Which relative	Details
Other psychological problems		

V. PAST MEDICAL HISTORY

A. Check off your **illnesses** and note your age at which you had it (If you don't know what they are, the chances are you have not had them.):

Illness	Age	Details
measles (rubeola)		
German measles (rubella)		
chicken pox		
whooping cough		
mumps		
scarlet fever, rheumatic fever		
diphtheria		
polio		
hepatitis or other liver ailment		
pneumonia		
lung abscess, emphysema		
typhoid fever		

Illness	Age	Details
malaria		
tuberculosis		
asthma		
hayfever		
AIDS, HIV positivity		
thyroid disease		
ulcer		
irritable bowel		
giardiasis		

B. List injuries, accidents, and surgeries in chronological order by kind, when, where, and the consequences. What were the surgeries for? what were the findings and outcome, success or failure? Dates are always important, at least the year should be noted; all should be presented in a chronological order. Use the Table below:

Event (accident or surgery)	When (year)	Where treated	Consequences

C. List harmful exposures

	Yes	No	Details
Did your mother take DES during pregnancy?			
Did you have radiation to your body (to tonsils, neck, fluoroscopy)?			

	Yes	No	Details
Were you exposed to violence, battering?			
Were you exposed to sexual harrassment, abuse?			
Have you experienced rape?			
Have you been exposed at home or work to Radon?			
. . . to tobacco?			
. . . to lead?			
. . . to radiation?			

VI. PERSONAL HISTORY

A. Marital History:

State age at which you were married (if you were married) _____
Husband's age and state of health or illness _____
If dead, state cause of death and age @ death _____

Husband	Age	Health
1.		
2.		
3.		

List children with their ages and state their health or cause of death

Child	Age	State of health

Have you had any miscarriages, abortions, or stillbirths? _____
What contraceptives have you used and what are you using now? ____

B. Occupational History:

What kind of work do you do at home? _____
(describe own duties, and shared duties, number of hours, intensity)

What kind of work do you do outside your home? _____
(describe your duties, intensity, title, employer, job environment; job satisfaction; aspirations) _____
_____
_____
_____
_____

How many hours a day do you work? _____
    outside the home? _____
    inside the home? _____
    on childcare? _____
    on parent(s)' care? _____
    on care of partner? _____

C. Personal Habits:

This information can help the doctor to evaluate your health risks and plan preventive strategies.
How many hours of sleep do you get? _____
How often do you have sex? _____
    how many times/ day _____ a week _____ a month _____
    a year? _____
    any problems? _____
How safe is your sex life (regarding sexually transmitted infection; and contraception)? _____
How many days a week do you exercise? _____ for how long? _____
    Doing what? _____
Do you smoke? _____ how many packs a day? _____ over how many years? _____
How much alcohol do you drink? _____ a day? _____ a week? _____ a month? _____ what kind? _____
What medicines do you take?(including contraceptives & nutritional supplements):

Name of medication	Dose	How often do you take it?	How long have you taken it?

Name of medication	Dose	How often do you take it?	How long have you taken it?

What "recreational" drugs do you use? (marijuana, cocaine, etc.) _____
Are you taking vitamins? _____ What kind? _____
What is your estimate of your body weight? _____ Approximately how
    much did you weigh last year? _____
When was your last Pap smear taken? _____ result? _____
When was your last mammogram taken? _____ result? _____
Do you use seat-belts when driving or riding? _____
Do you get exposed to sun? _____ when? _____ how
    much? _____
Do you own a gun? _____

D. Nutritional History:
What do you usually have for breakfast? _____ what time? _____
What do you usually have for lunch? _____ what time? _____
What do you usually have for supper? _____ what time? _____
What snacks do you have during the day or night? _____ what time? _____
How many cups of coffee or tea do you drink a day? _____
How many cups of milk or yogurt a day? _____ whole or low fat? _____
How many ounces of cheese do you eat a week? _____
Do you include fruits, vegetables, fiber in your diet? _____
What kind? _____
How many bowel movements do you have a day? _____

E. Menstrual Health:
At what age did the first menstrual period (**menarche**) come? _____
When did the last menstrual period start? _____
(this question requires the **date** of the first day of the last menstrual
period (**LMP**) if the woman is in the young adult phase. If the woman
is postmenopausal the answer to this question is either the age at the last
menstrual period or the year of the last menstrual period (**menopause**).

    The next 5 questions should be answered even if you have not had
a period for a while; the questions pertain to the past or to the present:

Interval _____ (average number of days between first day of one period and first day of the next) **Irregular?** Yes __ No __ Details

Duration _____ (average number of days of flow and/or staining)

Severity of flow _____ (answer either light, moderate, or heavy; or note the average number of napkins or tampons used up for each menstrual period)

Do pains with your period make you lie down? Yes _____ No _____
Details _____
Any kind of pain medicine you use during the menses? _____
Have you been tense and jumpy with your periods? Yes __ No __
Details _____

Inter menstrual bleeding _____ Yes or No _____ Details _____
(refers to bleeding between periods)

F. Genital Health:
Vaginal discharge   Yes _____ No _____
If yes, circle the amount: slight, moderate, or heavy
      color   clear, white, yellow, green
      consistency   thin, mucous, thick, cheese-like
      smell   no-odor, cheesy, fishlike

Circle YES or NO if you have ever been diagnosed with
   vaginitis   Yes __ No __ Details __
   cervicitis   Yes __ No __ Details __
   moniliasis (yeast infection, candidiasis)   Yes __ No __ Details __
   trichomonas infection   Yes __ No __ Details __
   endometriosis   Yes __ No __ Details __
   myomas (fibroids)   Yes __ No __ Details __
   ovarian cyst   Yes __ No __ Details __
   cancer   Yes __ No __ Details __
   pelvic pain   Yes __ No __ Details __
   PMS   Yes __ No __ Details __
   gonorrhea (GC)   Yes __ No __ Details __
   chlamydia   Yes __ No __ Details __
   syphilis   Yes __ No __ Details __
   bacterial vaginosis (BV)   Yes __ No __ Details __
   herpes   Yes __ No __ Details __
   genital warts (HPV, human   Yes __ No __ Details __
   papilloma virus)

(If you don't know what they are, the chances are you have not had them.)

G. History of Pregnancies:

List for each pregnancy: age at which you became pregnant; was it a normal pregnancy?

Full-term pregnancy? Age and health of offspring:

Number	Your age	Compli-cations	Full term	Offspring age now	Offspring health
1.					
2.					
3.					
4.					
5.					

List **miscarriages** and **abortions**: your age; duration of pregnancy before the miscarriage: _____

_____

What contraceptives are you using? _____

H. Menopausal History:

If you are approaching menopause circle presence or absence of the following **Symptoms:**

Have you any hot flushes?	Yes No
sweats (especially nocturnal sweats)?	Yes No
palpitations?	Yes No
mood changes?	Yes No

How bad are the above symptoms? _____

how long did they last? _____

how long have you been free of them? _____

Have you had any back pain? Yes No

Have you had fractures? Yes No

(if yes, where in the body) _____

Have you had any heart problems or blood vessel problems? Yes No

H. Allergies:
List history of reaction to substances and medications.

Substance you had a reaction to	When	What was the reaction?	How was it treated?

I. Immunization Record:
Obtain from your previous internist or pediatrician.

Type   Date
DPT
Tetanus
Rubella
Chicken pox
Mumps
Hepatitis B
Hepatitis A
Polio
BCG
Pneumonia
Other

VII. REVIEW OF SYSTEMS
System Review is a recital of presence or absence of any symptoms belonging to the following organ systems: Head and Neck, Eyes, Ears, Nose and Throat, Pulmonary system, Cardiovascular, Gastrointestinal tract, Urinary, Reproductive, Musculoskeletal, Immune, Thyroid and other Endocrine gland system, the Neurologic system, Psychiatric entities, and General state of Health. The following questions test each of the systems.
Circle Yes or No after each question: If yes, give details.

1. SKIN AND APPENDAGES
Have you had any significant infections or diseases of
   the skin?   Yes No
Has your skin changed in character or texture recently?   Yes No
Are you bothered with severe itching?   Yes No
Do you bruise easily?   Yes No
Has your hair changed in amount or texture?   Yes No
Does your hair fall out easily?   Yes No
Do you use hair dyes?   Yes No
Do you perspire excessively?   Yes No
Details: _____

2. HEAD

Do you suffer frequent headaches? Yes No
Do you have sick headaches (migraine)? Yes No
Do you faint easily? Yes No
Have you ever been knocked unconscious? Yes No
Do you have light-headedness or giddiness? Yes No
Did you ever have severe dizziness? Yes No
Details: _____

_____

3. EYES

Do you wear glasses? Yes No
Did you ever see double? Yes No
Have you had any loss of vision? Yes No
Have you had inflammation of the eyes? Yes No
Do you have difficulty distinguishing colors? Yes No
Do you have spots before your eyes? Yes No
Details: _____

_____

4. EARS

Have you had any loss of hearing? Yes No
Have you ever had earaches or discharge from your ears? Yes No
Do you have buzzing or ringing in your ears? Yes No
Details: _____

_____

5. NOSE

Do you have frequent colds? Yes No
Do you have excessive nasal discharge? Yes No
Did you ever have frequent or severe nosebleeds? Yes No
Have you had sinus trouble? Yes No
Details: _____

_____

6. MOUTH

Have you had excessive trouble with your teeth? Yes No
Do your gums bleed frequently? Yes No
Do you where false dentures? Yes No
Is your tongue frequently sore or sensitive? Yes No
Details: _____

_____

7. THROAT

Have you had frequent or severe sore throats? Yes No
Have you had tonsillitis? Yes No

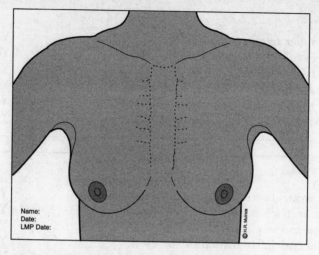

Name:
Date:
LMP Date:

©H.R. Muinos

Figure 37. Use this diagram for recording and comparing
changes in your breasts.

Do you have difficulty in swallowing?   Yes   No
Are you subject to hoarseness?   Yes   No
Details: _____

8. NECK

Have you had swollen or discharging glands in your neck?   Yes   No
Have you had a goiter or thyroid trouble?   Yes   No
Have you had a basal metabolism test or another thyroid test?
                                                             Yes   No
Does cold or hot weather bother you excessively?   Yes   No
Details: _____

9. BREASTS

Have you noticed any strange lumps in your breast?   Yes   No
Have you noticed a bloody discharge from your breasts?   Yes   No
Have you had an operation on your breast?   Yes   No
Details: _____

10. LUNGS

Do you have a chronic cough?   Yes   No
Do you raise more than one tablespoon of sputum daily?   Yes   No
Have you ever coughed up blood?   Yes   No
Do you have night sweats?   Yes   No
Have you been told that you have any lung or
    bronchial trouble?   Yes   No

Have you had pleurisy?	Yes	No
Have you noticed a wheeze or whistle in your chest on breathing?	Yes	No
Have you had close contact with a person who had tuberculosis?	Yes	No
Have you had an x-ray of your chest?	Yes	No

Details: _____

11. HEART

Have you been told you have heart disease or heart murmurs?	Yes	No
Have you been told you have high blood pressure?	Yes	No
Do you become winded on climbing two flights of stairs?	Yes	No
Do you have pain or a tight feeling in your chest on exertion?	Yes	No
Do you have to sleep propped up in bed?	Yes	No
Do your ankles swell?	Yes	No
Do you have palpitation (heart beating rapidly)?	Yes	No
Have you been refused life insurance?	Yes	No

Details: _____

12. GASTROINTESTINAL (STOMACH, INTESTINE, LIVER)

Have you noticed any loss of appetite?	Yes	No
Do you like only a few foods?	Yes	No
Do you eat at irregular hours?	Yes	No
Do you have indigestion or excessive gas?	Yes	No
Do you have pain in your stomach?	Yes	No
Do you have nausea and vomiting?	Yes	No
Have you vomited blood?	Yes	No
Are you constipated?	Yes	No
Have your bowel habits changed in the past 6 months?	Yes	No
Do you have attacks of diarrhea (frequent loose stools)?	Yes	No
Have you passed blood in your stools?	Yes	No
Have you had **black** or **tarry** stools?	Yes	No
Do you pass mucus in your stools?	Yes	No
Do you have hemorrhoids (piles)?	Yes	No
Have you been jaundiced (yellow eyes and skin)?	Yes	No
Have you had intestinal worms?	Yes	No
Have you lost weight?	Yes	No

Details: _____

13. URINARY

Do you get up every night to urinate?	Yes	No
Do you have burning pain when you urinate?	Yes	No

Have you had pus in the kidneys or urine?   Yes   No
Do you have trouble starting your stream when you urinate? Yes   No
Have you passed stones or gravel in your urine?   Yes   No
Have you passed blood in the urine?   Yes   No
Have you had albumin in the urine?   Yes   No
Do you ever lose control over your bladder?   Yes   No
Has a doctor ever said you had kidney or bladder disease? Yes   No
Have you had sugar in the urine?   Yes   No
Have you had or suspected you had venereal disease?   Yes   No
Details: _____

14. MISCELLANEOUS
Did you ever have painful, swollen joints or rheumatism?   Yes   No
Have you ever been told you have anemia?   Yes   No
Do you have varicose veins?   Yes   No
Are you subject to dizziness, fainting, twitching,
    spells, or fits?   Yes   No
Was any part of your body every paralyzed?   Yes   No
Do you have neuralgia or neuritis?   Yes   No
Have you ever had bursitis or back pain?   Yes   No
Do you have numbness or tingling   Yes   No
    (pins and needles) in your fingers or toes?   Yes   No
Details: _____

15. MENTAL AND PSYCHOLOGICAL
Have you ever had a nervous breakdown?   Yes   No
Do you cry easily?   Yes   No
Do you worry very much?   Yes   No
Do you regard yourself as being nervous?   Yes   No
Do you tire easily?   Yes   No
Are you depressed and blue much of the time?   Yes   No
Is it difficult for you to make up your mind?   Yes   No
Are your feelings easily hurt?   Yes   No
Are you easily irritated and upset?   Yes   No
Does every little thing get on your nerves?   Yes   No
Are you extremely shy or sensitive?   Yes   No
Do people often annoy or irritate you?   Yes   No
Are you constantly keyed up and jittery?   Yes   No
Is your home life unpleasant?   Yes   No
Is your work unpleasant?   Yes   No
Do you bite your fingernails?   Yes   No
Details: _____

Appendix III:
Books on
Women's Health

There are now scores of books about women's health in most large bookstores. These books are usually devoted to a particular aspect of women's health such as pregnancy and childbirth, or breast cancer, and so on. Finding good information will take some research on your part, but here are a few books we know that offer reliable information for women.

Chronic Illness and the Family: A Guide for Living Every Day, by Dr. Linda Welsh and Marian Betancourt, 1996, Adams Media, Boston.

The Complete Book of Menopause: Every Woman's Guide to Good Health, by Carol Landau, Ph.D.; Michele G. Cyr, M.D.; and Anne W. Moulton, M.D., 1994, Putnam, New York.

The Doctor's Book of Home Remedies for Women, by the editors of Prevention Magazine Health Books, 1997, Rodale Press, Emmaus, Pa.

The Doctor's Case Against the Pill, by Barbara Seaman, 25th anniversary edition, 1995, Hunter House.

Dr. Susan Love's Breast Book, by Susan Love, M.D., and Karen Lindsey, 1990, Addison-Wesley, Reading, Mass.

Dr. Susan Love's Hormone Book: Making Informed Choices About Menopause, by Susan Love, M.D., and Karen Lindsey, Random House, 1997.

Estrogen: Revised and Expanded, by Lila Nachtigall, M.D., and Joan Rattner Heilman, 1991, Harper Perennial, New York.

The Evaluation of Sexual Disorders: Psychological and Medical Aspects, by Helen Singer Kaplan, M.D., 1993, Brunner/Mazel, New York.

The Female Body: An Owner's Manual, by the editors of Prevention Magazine Health Books, 1996, Rodale Press, Emmaus, Pa.

The Female Heart: The Truth About Women and Coronary Heart Disease, by M. J. Legato and C. Colman, 1991, Simon and Schuster, New York.

The Hormone of Desire: The Truth About Sexuality, Menopause, and Testosterone, by Susan Rako, M.D., 1996, Harmony Books, New York.

The Menopause Book: A Guide to Health and Well-Being for Women After Forty, by Sheldon H. Cherry, M.D., and Carolyn Runowicz, M.D., 1994, Macmillan, New York.

New Choices in Natural Healing for Women: Drug-Free Remedies from the World of Alternative Medicine, by Barbara Loecher, Sara Altshul O'Donnell, and the Editors of Prevention Magazine Health Books; Medical Adviser, Adriane Fugh-Berman, M.D. 1997, Rodale Press, Emmaus, Pa.

The Osteoporosis Handbook: Every Woman's Guide to Prevention and Treatment, by Sydney Lou Bonnick, M.D., 1994, Taylor Publishing, Dallas.

Our Bodies, Ourselves, self-published by the Boston Women's Health Book Collective, 1969, reissued by Simon and Schuster, New York, in 1972, 1984, 1992.

Our Health, Our Lives: A Revolutionary Approach to Total Health Care for Women, by Eileen Hoffman, M.D., 1995, Pocket Books, New York.

Outrageous Practices: The Alarming Truth About How Medicine Mistreats Women, by Leslie Laurence and Beth Weinhouse, 1994, Fawcett, New York.

Outsmarting the Female Fat Cell: The First Weight-Control Program Designed Specifically for Women, by Debra Waterhouse, M.P.H., R.D., 1993, Hyperion, New York.

The Real Truth About Women and AIDS: How to Eliminate the Risks Without Giving Up Love and Sex, by Helen Singer Kaplan, M.D., 1987, Fireside Books, Simon and Schuster, New York.

Relative Risk: Living with a Family History of Breast Cancer, by Nancy C. Baker, 1991, Viking, New York.

The Sexual Desire Disorders: Dysfunctional Regulation of Sexual Motivation, by Helen Singer Kaplan, M.D., 1995, Brunner/Mazel, New York.

Textbook of Women's Health, editor-in-chief, Lila A. Wallis, M.D., 1998, Lippincott-Raven.

Total Health for Women, by Ellen Michaud; Elisabaeth Torg; and the editors of Prevention Magazine Health Books, 1995, Rodale Press, Emmaus, Pa.

Unequal Treatment: What You Don't Know About How Women Are Mistreated by the Medical Community, by Eileen Nechas and Denise Foley, 1994, Simon and Schuster, New York.

What to Do If You Get Breast Cancer, by Lydia Komarnicky, M.D.; Anne Rosenberg, M.D.; and Marian Betancourt, 1995, Little, Brown, and Co., New York.

What to Do If You Get Colon Cancer, by Paul Miskovitz, M.D., and Marian Betancourt, 1997, John Wiley and Sons, New York.

What to Do When Love Turns Violent: A Practical Resource for Women in

Abusive Relationships, by Marian Betancourt, 1997, HarperCollins, New York.

Woman to Woman: A Leading Gynecologist Tells You All You Need to Know About Your Body and Your Health, by Yvonne S. Thornton with J. Coudert, 1997, Dutton Penguin Books, New York.

A Woman's Book of Choices: Abortion, Menstrual Extraction, RU-486, by Rebecca Chalker, Carol Downer, Suzann Gage (illustrator), 1996 Seven Stones Press, New York.

A Woman's Guide to Osteoporosis, by Yvonne R. Sherrer, M.D., and Robin K. Levinson, 1995, Hyperion, New York.

The Woman's Heart Book: The Complete Guide to Keeping Your Heart and What to Do if Things Go Wrong, by J. Fredrick Pashkow, M.D., and Charlotte Libov, 1993, Penguin Books, New York.

The Woman in the Body: A Cultural Analysis of Reproduction, by Emily Martin, 1992, Beacon Press, Boston.

Women and Doctors: A Physician's Explosive Account of Women's Medical Treatment and Mistreatment in America, by John M. Smith, M.D., 1992, Atlantic Monthly Press, New York.

Women's Encyclopedia of Health and Emotional Healing, by D. Foley, E. Nechas, and the editors of *Prevention Magazine*; medical adviser, Lila A. Wallis, M.D.; 1993, Rodale Press, Emmaus, Pa.

Index